RECENT DEVELOPMENTS IN
ALCOHOLISM

VOLUME 12
ALCOHOLISM AND WOMEN

RECENT DEVELOPMENTS IN

Edited by

MARC GALANTER

New York University School of Medicine
New York, New York

Associate Editors

HENRI BEGLEITER, RICHARD DEITRICH,
DONALD GALLANT, DONALD GOODWIN,
EDWARD GOTTHEIL, ALFONSO PAREDES,
MARCUS ROTHSCHILD, and DAVID VAN THIEL

Assistant Editor
HELEN EDWARDS

An Official Publication of the American Society of Addiction Medicine
and the Research Society on Alcoholism.
This series was founded by the National Council on Alcoholism.

ALCOHOLISM

VOLUME 12
ALCOHOLISM AND WOMEN

PLENUM PRESS • NEW YORK AND LONDON

The Library of Congress has catalogued this work as follows:

Recent developments in alcoholism: an official publication of the American Medical Society on Alcoholism, and the Research Society on Alcoholism, and the National Council on Alcoholism—Vol. 1— —New York: Plenum Press, c1983–
  v.:ill.; 25 cm.
  Cataloging in publication.
  Editor: Marc Galanter.
  ISSN 0738-422X = Recent developments in alcoholism.

  1. Alcoholism—Periodicals. I. Galanter, Marc. II. American Medical Society on Alcoholism. III. Research Society on Alcohol (U.S.) IV. National Council on Alcoholism. [DNLM: 1. Alcoholism—periodicals. W1 RE106AH(P)]

| HV5001.R4 | 616.86'1'05—dc19 | 83-643791 |
| Library of Congress | [8311] | AACR 2 MARC-S |

ISBN 0-306-44921-8

© 1995 Plenum Press, New York
A Division of Plenum Publishing Corporation
233 Spring Street, New York, N. Y. 10013

10 9 8 7 6 5 4 3 2 1

Printed in the United States of America

Contributors

Kimberly T. Ackerman, California School of Professional Psychology, Los Angeles Campus, Alhambra, California 91803-1360

Catherine R. Ager, Institute of Health and Aging, Department of Social and Behavioral Sciences, University of California, San Francisco, California 94143

Andrea G. Barthwell, Interventions, Chicago, Illinois 60605

Fred Beauvais, Tri-Ethnic Center for Prevention Research, Department of Psychology, Colorado State University, Fort Collins, Colorado 80523

Linda J. Beckman, California School of Professional Psychology, Los Angeles Campus, Alhambra, California 91803-1360

Betty A. Blanchard, Department of Pathology and Anatomical Studies, School of Medicine, University of Missouri, Columbia, Missouri 65212

Frederic C. Blow, University of Michigan Alcohol Research Center, Ann Arbor, Michigan 48108-3318

Terry C. Blum, School of Management, Georgia Institute of Technology, Atlanta, Georgia 30332-0520

Karen T. Britton, Department of Psychiatry, VA Medical Center and University of California, San Diego, California 92161

Michelle D. Brot, Department of Neuropharmacology, Scripps Research Institute, La Jolla, California 92037

James H. Carter, Department of Psychiatry, Duke University Medical Center, Durham, North Carolina 27710

Richard A. Deitrich, Department of Pharmacology, Alcohol Research Center, University of Colorado Health Sciences Center, Denver, Colorado 80262

William R. Downs, Center for the Study of Adolescence, University of Northern Iowa, Cedar Falls, Iowa 50614

Mary C. Dufour, Division of Biometry and Epidemiology, National Institute on Alcohol Abuse and Alcoholism, National Institutes of Health, Rockville, Maryland 20892

Ruth W. Edwards, Tri-Ethnic Center for Prevention Research, Department of Psychology, Colorado State University, Fort Collins, Colorado 80523

Heidi P. Ferrer, Institute of Health and Aging, Department of Social and Behavioral Sciences, University of California, San Francisco, California 94143

Kaye Middleton Fillmore, Institute of Health and Aging, Department of Social and Behavioral Sciences, University of California, San Francisco, California 94143

Richard K. Fuller, Division of Clinical and Prevention Research, National institute on Alcohol Abuse and Alcoholism, National Institutes of Health, Rockville, Maryland 20892

Judith S. Gavaler, Oklahoma Medical Research Foundation, and Oklahoma Transplantation Institute, Baptist Medical Center, Oklahoma City, Oklahoma 73112

Susan Wagner Glenn, Department of Psychiatry and Behavioral Sciences, University of Oklahoma Health Sciences Center, Oklahoma City, Oklahoma 73104

Stanley D. Glick, Department of Pharmacology and Toxicology, Albany Medical College, Albany, New York 12210

Jacqueline M. Golding, Institute of Health and Aging, Department of Social and Behavioral Sciences, University of California, San Francisco, California 94143

Edith S. Lisansky Gomberg, Department of Psychiatry, Alcohol Research Center, University of Michigan, Ann Arbor, Michigan 48104

Edward Gottheil, Department of Psychiatry and Human Behavior, Thomas Jefferson University, Philadelphia, Pennsylvania 19107

Ellen F. Gottheil, Department of Psychiatry and Behavioral Sciences, University of Washington Medical School, Seattle, Washington 98195

Eileen M. Harwood, Institute for Behavioral Research, University of Georgia, Athens, Georgia 30602-2401

Shirley Y. Hill, Alcohol and Genetics Research Program, Department of Psychiatry, University of Pittsburgh School of Medicine, Pittsburgh, Pennsylvania 15213

Byron C. Jones, Program in Biobehavioral Health, Pennsylvania State University, University Park, Pennsylvania 16802-6508

Steven Kneip, Institute of Health and Aging, Department of Social and Behavioral Sciences, University of California, San Francisco, California 94143

George F. Koob, Department of Neuropharmacology, Scripps Research Institute, La Jolla, California 92037

Francine E. Lancaster, Department of Biology, Texas Woman's University, Denton, Texas 76204

E. Victor Leino, Institute of Health and Aging, Department of Social and Behavioral Sciences, University of California, San Francisco, California 94143

Gerald E. McClearn, Department of Biobehavioral Health and Center for Developmental and Health Genetics, Pennsylvania State University, University Park, Pennsylvania 16802

Brenda A. Miller, Research Institute on Addictions, Buffalo, New York 14203

Sara Jo Nixon, Department of Psychiatry and Behavioral Sciences, University of Oklahoma Health Sciences Center, Oklahoma City, Oklahoma 73104

Alfonso Paredes, Residential Treatment Center, West Los Angeles Veterans Administration Medical Center, University of California School of Medicine, Los Angeles, California 90024

Sylvia Rodriquez-Andrew, College of Social Work, San Jose State University, San Jose, California 95192

Paul M. Roman, Institute for Behavioral Research, University of Georgia, Athens, Georgia 30602-2401

Beatrice A. Rouse, Office of Applied Studies, Substance Abuse and Mental Health Services Administration, Rockville, Maryland 20857

Laura Schmidt, Alcohol Research Group and Department of Sociology, University of California, Berkeley, California 94709

Carlisle Shoemaker, Institute of Health and Aging, Department of Social and Behavioral Sciences, University California, San Francisco, California 94143

Holly S. Thomasson, Eli Lilly and Company, Lilly Laboratory for Clinical Research, Wishard Memorial Hospital, Indianapolis, Indiana 46202

Pamela Jumper Thurman, Tri-Ethnic Center for Prevention Research, Department of Psychology, Colorado State University, Fort Collins, Colorado 80523

Patricia F. Waller, University of Michigan Transportation Research Institute, Ann Arbor, Michigan 48109-2150

Constance Weisner, Alcohol Research Group and School of Public Health, University of California, Berkeley, California 94709

Keith E. Whitfield, Program in Biobehavioral Health, Pennsylvania State University, University Park, Pennsylvania 16802-6508

Sharon C. Wilsnack, Department of Neuroscience, University of North Dakota School of Medicine, Grand Forks, North Dakota 58202

Richard W. Wilsnack, Department of Neuroscience, University of North Dakota School of Medicine, Grand Forks, North Dakota 58202

Preface

From the President of the Research Society on Alcoholism

This twelfth volume of the *Recent Developments in Alcoholism* series highlights the remarkable evolution of alcoholism research during the past few years. The importance of gender in alcohol actions and consequences is finally receiving the attention it deserves. Furthermore, epidemiological, clinical, and psychosocial approaches are assuming increasing importance in alcohol research and investigators on the leading edge are beginning to integrate these formerly segregated approaches. I am impressed at how the content of these volumes reflects the changes in the Research Society on Alcoholism: our membership is increasingly female and the diversity of research interests has grown even more rapidly than our Society.

From the viewpoint of a basic scientist, gender differences are critically important because they provide clues to the biological and thus genetic basis of alcohol actions. The remarkably consistent observations that women drink less than men but are more sensitive to harmful actions of alcohol should provide a powerful approach to dissecting out the factors that contribute to both consumption and organ damage. Section II presents the physiological data on gender differences in alcohol action as well as the genetic underpinning of these differences. The application of animal genetic and neurochemical approaches shows that the strong foundation established by so many alcohol researchers during the past decade will be fruitfully applied to analysis of gender differences. Section II, on epidemiology, raises the important, and doubly neglected, area of alcoholism in older women. Many of the issues presented in the epidemiological and sociocultural sections will have important consequences for treatment and are discussed in Section III.

The editor and associate editors deserve thanks and congratulations from our field for providing excellent coverage of such timely topics.

R. Adorn Harris, Ph.D.
President, Research Society on Alcoholism

From the President of the American Society of Addiction Medicine

The American Society of Addiction Medicine is honored to be cosponsoring with the Research Society on Alcoholism the current issue of *Recent Development in Alcoholism*, Volume 12, *Alcoholism and Women*. It is only in the last decade that a substantial effort has been dedicated to examining the spectrum of alcohol effects. Even now a literature search with women as the topic in substance use disorders will consist preponderantly of articles relating to pregnancy.

It is to the credit of the excellent editor of this series that the current volume covers a broad range of topics relating to women and alcohol, including animal studies as well as sociocultural issues. It is also heartening to note that women have contributed most of the chapters. With an increasing number of women who are heavy drinkers there has been a rising interest among physicians to learn more about the specific ways in which women are affected by alcohol. This volume will contribute toward their education. As a woman I am consistently amazed that half of the world is treated as women so often were in alcohol studies as "special populations."

It is to be hoped that in future volumes of *Recent Developments in Alcoholism,* gender effects will be automatically included where they could be relevant.

Anne Geller, M.D.
President, American Society of Addiction Medicine

Contents

Chapter 3

Older Women and Alcohol: Use and Abuse
   Edith S. Lisansky Gomberg

Chapter 4

Violent Victimization among Women with Alcohol Problems
Brenda A. Miller and William R. Downs

Chapter 5

Women, Alcohol, and Driving
Patricia F. Waller and Frederic C. Blow

Chapter 6

**Employed Women with Alcohol Problems Who Seek Help from
Employee Assistance Programs: Description and Comparisons**
  Terry C. Blum, Paul M. Roman, and Eileen M. Harwood

II. Physiology

Mary C. Dufour and Richard K. Fuller, Section Editors

Overview
Mary C. Dufour and Richard K. Fuller

Chapter 7

**Gender Differences in Alcohol Metabolism: Physiological Responses
to Ethanol**
  Holly S. Thomasson

III. Behavior and Treatment Issues

Alfonso Paredes, Section Editor

Overview
Alfonso Paredes

Chapter 15

Women, Alcohol, and Sexuality
Linda J. Beckman and Kimberly T. Ackerman

Chapter 16

Cognitive Psychosocial Performance and Recovery in Female Alcoholics
Sara Jo Nixon and Susan Wagner Glenn

Chapter 17

The Emergence of Problem-Drinking Women as a Special Population
in Need of Treatment
Laura Schmidt and Constance Weisner

IV. Social and Cultural Issues

Edward Gottheil and Ellen F. Gottheil, Section Editors

Overview
Edward Gottheil and Ellen F. Gottheil

Chapter 18

Race/Ethnicity and Other Sociocultural Influences on Alcoholism
Treatment for Women
Beatrice A. Rouse, James H. Carter, and Sylvia Rodriguez-Andrew

Chapter 19

Patterns of Alcohol Use among Ethnic Minority Adolescent Women
Ruth W. Edwards, Pamela Jumper Thurman, and Fred Beauvais

Chapter 20

Alcoholism in the Family: A Multicultural Exploration
Andrea G. Barthwell

Chapter 21

Gender Differences for the Risk of Alcohol-Related Problems in Mulitple National Contexts: A Research Synthesis from the Collaborative Alcohol-Related Longitudinal Project
Kaye Middleton Fillmore, Jacqueline M. Golding, Steven Kniep, E. Victor Leino, Carlisle Shoemaker, Catherine R. Ager, and Heidi P. Ferrer

I

Epidemiology

Mary C. Dufour and Richard K. Fuller, Section Editors

Overview

Mary C. Dufour and Richard K. Fuller

The final years of the twentieth century are a fitting time to examine recent developments in the epidemiology of alcohol use, abuse, dependence, and other consequences among women and to highlight gender differences. The past century has witnessed spectacular advances in science and medicine. While infectious disease epidemiology has long been an established discipline, chronic disease epidemiology is of more recent origin, coming to the fore in the last 50 years. Alcohol epidemiology is among the youngest of the epidemiology disciplines. Methods of survey research were first applied to a detailed study of drinking practices in a survey of college students in 1949. Since the 1960s, nationwide surveys of drinking practices have applied the requisite statistical sampling methodology for making national estimates of the patterns and levels of alcohol consumption.[1] Initial studies of the epidemiology of alcohol use disorders were conducted in populations of individuals in alcohol treatment facilities.[2] In the last 20 years, development of standard definitions and structured interviewing techniques for identifying and assessing psychiatric disorders has enabled researchers to begin to establish the prevalence of alcohol abuse and dependence in the general population as well as in specific subgroups.[2] The early studies of Wilsnack and colleagues[3] on the drinking behavior of a national sample of women were landmarks in bringing women's drinking behavior to the attention of the scientific community and were pivotal in legitimizing further research in the field.

Finally, advances in mathematical statistics and computer science have enabled researchers to move from simple descriptive epidemiology of inci-

Mary C. Dufour • Division of Biometry and Epidemiology, National Institute on Alcohol Abuse and Alcoholism, National Institutes of Health, Rockville, Maryland 20892.   Richard K. Fuller • Division of Clinical and Prevention Research, National Institute on Alcohol Abuse and Alcoholism, National Institutes of Health, Rockville, Maryland 20892.

Recent Developments in Alcoholism, Volume 12: Women and Alcoholism, edited by Marc Galanter. Plenum Press, New York, 1995

dence and prevalence of particular patterns and conditions to analytic epidemiology with a focus on elucidation of etiologic, contributing, and protective
factors. Ultimately, application of analytic epidemiology to gender differences
in alcohol use, abuse, and consequences will facilitate the development of
prevention, intervention, and treatment strategies uniquely tailored for opti-
mal outcome. The authors in this section rank among the leading researchers
in this field of endeavor.

As advances in epidemiology have occurred, the decade of the nineties
marks the flowering of research on women's health. In 1991, the Office of
Research on Women's Health was created in the National Institutes of Health
(NIH). The following year the *Journal of Women's Health* began publication.
The NIH has mounted the Women's Health Initiative, the largest study of its
type in history, to investigate major causes of death and disability among
older women, including heart disease and stroke, breast and colorectal cancer, and osteoporosis.[4]

Much time and effort has been invested in striving for equality for
women—equality in education, in the workplace, in partnerships, and society as a whole. In the heat of battle, it has sometimes been forgotten that
equality is not synonymous with sameness. Different does not imply unequal
—merely different. The next logical step toward conquering the important
women's health issue of alcohol abuse and dependence is research into gender differences. Knowledge is empowering. The more women know about
gender differences related to alcohol, particularly differential strengths and
susceptibilities, the more control they will have over their own health and
well-being.

The roles of women in American society have evolved dramatically in the
last half century. Women are entering the labor force in record numbers,
comprising 45.3% of the civilian labor force in 1990.[5] In the past 30 years, the
proportion of married women in the labor force has nearly doubled, while the
proportion of married women in the labor force with children under the age
of 6 has more than tripled.[5] With 60% of these mothers working, alternative
child care arrangements are now the rule rather than the exception. With
employment has come unprecedented economic independence. Since 1970,
the average age of first marriage has increased by nearly 3 years for both men
and women.[5] Divorce rates have doubled.[5] In 1990, 55% of households consisted of married couples compared with 70% 20 years ago.[5] Single-parent
households and blended families are becoming more common. How have all
these factors impacted on alcohol consumption and problems in both men
and women? The time is right to survey the state of our knowledge of the
epidemiology of gender differences in alcohol use, abuse, and consequences.
What are some of the research questions that can be answered?

Examinations of the patterns and trends in drinking and drinking problems in the general population provide a background and framework for
ascertainment of gender differences. As a whole, American women remain
less likely to drink, to drink frequently or heavily, and to report alcohol-

related problems than their male counterparts. Levels and patterns of women's drinking, however, have fluctuated over time as well as from group to group. Women are far from a homogeneous group, differing widely in age, employment, marital status, and ethnicity, to name a few key factors. What are the patterns of women's drinking and drinking problems and how have these varied over time and among groups? Multiple cross-sectional studies provide a general sense of differences in drinking patterns by variables such as age. Prospective longitudinal studies provide the opportunity to follow individual women over time to find out how drinking changes with age as well as what factors predict the development of alcohol problems and what factors predict recovery.

Further complicating the picture are rapidly changing societal expectations and cultural milieu. Has this societal upheaval influenced women's drinking, and if so, how? Do role overload and role conflict represent stressors that encourage drinking? How does the stress of struggling to be a wife, mother, and professional coupled with differing drinking norms of co-workers impact on drinking? How do patterns of consumption and problems of women in the work force compare with those of their male co-workers? Is there a differential impact by gender of alcohol problems on performance and attendance? Who are the women who use employee assistance programs (EAPs) for alcohol problems. How do they compare with men using similar services? How do these women vary by occupational category? Are there differences in patterns of alcoholism treatment services offered by gender and what are the mediating factors? What are the characteristics of women employees with probable alcohol problems who are not assessed as such by EAP personnel and what are the implications for improving detection and intervention? Critical questions in this era of health care reform are how do gender differences in health insurance coverage and benefits drive EAP referral patterns and do women receive less than ideal care as a result?

Age is a critical factor. Both ends of the age spectrum require special attention. Younger women report the highest levels of alcohol consumption and related problems as well as the largest fluctuations in levels of consumption. What factors account for these findings? Do the numerous role transitions required of women in this age group play a role?

The population of the United States aged 65 or older is burgeoning at a rate unprecedented in history. Average life expectancy has risen from 47.3 years at the turn of the century to 75.7 years in 1991.[5] Women have outstripped men in this regard to the point where a present-day middle-aged woman can expect to outlive her male counterpart by nearly 7 years. What are the nature and extent of alcohol problems among older women and what implications do these findings have for future cohorts of older women? In 1989, nearly 70% of men aged 75 and older were married and about 25% were widowed.[5] One fourth of the women in the same age group were married and two thirds widowed.[5] This suggests that when older men lose a spouse they soon remarry. Following the death of her husband, an older woman is much less likely to remarry. What are the implications of these findings for detection and treatment of the woman who drinks heavily with a spouse or companion and following whose death continues to drink abusively? The problem-drinking older woman is saddled with the triple stigmata of being female, elderly, and alcoholic, and so is most likely to underplay her drinking and alcohol problems and may very reluctant to seek treatment. In addition, decreasing body water, osteoporosis, and prescription drug use may cause older women to get into trouble at levels of consumption that are not hazardous to younger women. Two types of alcoholism are distinguished in older individuals—early onset and late or recent onset. Are there gender differences in age at onset and recovery? Are there gender differences in factors that predict late onset alcoholism?

The increasing need for transportation to work coupled with increasing financial freedom has led to dramatic increases in the number of women obtaining drivers licenses and owning cars. How have the increasing numbers of women on the road influenced trends in drinking and driving and alcohol-related traffic crashes? Do recent trends in drinking and driving differ by gender? Are there gender differences in the behavior required of a driver in order for a law enforcement official to suspect the individual of drinking and driving? Are there gender differences in recidivism (repeat offenders)? What gender differences exist in crash risk and performance impairment? What are the differential effects, by gender, of acute as well as chronic, long-term alcohol consumption on injury severity and healing? Although not of the same magnitude, the trends in drinking and driving among women are reminiscent of those seen in relation to smoking and lung cancer. Lung cancer deaths due to smoking have been decreasing among men while at the same time rapidly increasing among women to the point where lung cancer has surpassed breast cancer as the leading cause of cancer death among women.[6] This raises the serious question of why existing prevention efforts targeted at reducing alcohol-related traffic deaths (or smoking) in young people are working for young men but not young women.

It is now quite clear that alcoholism in both men and women is mediated by genetic factors. What is the contribution of genetics to alcoholism in women? How is this genetic vulnerability moderated by factors such as age, ethnicity, and psychiatric comorbidity? Are there gender differences in the cultural and familial environmental factors that serve as predictors? What have twin and adoption studies contributed to clarification of gender differences in the genetic epidemiology of alcoholism?

Recent research has disclosed that one familial environmental factor that contributes significantly to the development of alcohol problems in adult women is violent victimization in childhood. How do childhood sexual abuse and father-to-daughter violence predict the later onset of alcohol abuse? What key variables link experience of childhood victimization and development of alcohol problems later in life? This is a new and challenging field of scientific endeavor. What are the possible explanations for how and why childhood violence predicts adult alcohol abuse? What are the strengths and weaknesses of research to date and what direction should future research take? Research also suggests that alcohol-dependent women have an increased risk of becoming victims of violence as a direct consequence of their abusive drinking. In using alcohol to cope with childhood trauma, these women are unwittingly opening themselves to further violence, which in turn may escalate drinking problems. Clearly, recognizing the existence of and understanding the nature and dynamics of this vicious cycle are critical for intervention and recovery.

Integrating the information in this section into one coherent explanatory model is not possible at this time. This is not surprising since scientists examining biological and environmental factors have not yet developed a good model for biology–environment interaction in men either. The epidemiology of alcohol use, abuse, dependence, and consequences in women is a rapidly evolving field. The chapters in this section provide an excellent account of the state of the art.

References

1. Midanik LT, Room R: The epidemiology of alcohol consumption. *Alcohol Health Res World* 16:183–190, 1992.
2. Bucholz, KK: Alcohol abuse and dependence from a psychiatric epidemiologic perspective. *Alcohol Health Res World* 16:197–208, 1992.
3. Wilsnack, RW, Wilsnack SC, Klassen AD: Women's drinking and drinking problems: Patterns from a 1981 national survey. *Am J Public Health* 74:1231–1238, 1984.
4. Healy B: A celebration and new resolve. *J Women's Health* 1:xvii, 1992.
5. U.S. Bureau of the Census: Statistical abstract of the United States: 1991, ed 111. Washington, DC, Government Printing Office, 1991.
6. National Center for Health Statistics: Health United States, 1992. DHHS Pub. No. (PHS)93–1232. Hyattsville, MD, Government Printing Office, 1993, p 46.

Vulnerability to Alcoholism in Women

Genetic and Cultural Factors

Shirley Y. Hill

Abstract. The etiology of alcoholism in women is no longer a question of nature or nurture. Most observers would agree that alcoholism, both male and female, is mediated by genetic factors. The question is how much of the variance is explained by genetic factors and to what degree is this genetically mediated disorder moderated by personal characteristics of the woman. Among the most salient personal characteristics moderating the genetic vulnerability may be factors such as age, ethnicity, and presence of psychiatric comorbidity. Cultural factors and familial environmental factors are most likely predictors as well. Therefore, the chapter will discuss the genetic epidemiology of alcoholism in women.

Genetic heterogeneity will be discussed and evidence presented that suggests the existence of two forms of alcoholism in women: one more environmentally determined and one more influenced by genetic mediation. Evidence for the existence of a genetic diathesis in women will be presented, noting extant literature involving twin and adoption designs. Suggestions for what might be transmitted from generation to generation (e.g., neurobiological factors, temperament) with special reference to preadolescent and adolescent girls will also be discussed.

1. Introduction

Significant progress has been made in understanding at least some of the factors promoting alcoholism.[1] However, if the development of alcoholism in women varies significantly from that of men, a separate review of the existing literature concerning the etiology of alcoholism in women appears to be war-

Shirley Y. Hill • Alcoholism and Genetics Research Program, Department of Psychiatry, University of Pittsburgh School of Medicine, Pittsburgh, PA 15213.

Recent Developments in Alcoholism, Volume 12: Women and Alcoholism, edited by Marc Galanter. Plenum Press, New York, 1995.

ranted. What evidence may be offered for there being separate etiological pathways to alcoholism by gender? First, alcoholism occurs less frequently among women than men. A recent survey places the ratio of male to female alcoholism at 2:1 in the general population,[2] differences that could reflect either cultural or genetically mediated factors. Second, while having another coexistent psychiatric disorder is associated with poorer treatment outcome for alcoholics, the presence of comorbidity, particularly the presence of depression, is associated with poorer outcome for men but more favorable outcome for women with respect to drinking-related measures.[3] Schuckit and Winokur[4] found that alcoholic women who had a primary diagnosis of affective disorder did comparatively better than alcoholic women whose primary diagnosis was alcoholism.

One speculation might be that the clinical heterogeneity one sees among alcoholics by gender may represent two separate genetic diatheses, or alternatively there may be a single genetic diathesis with variable expression by gender. The difficulty lies in untangling which of these alternatives represents the true state of affairs. The existence of a genetic vulnerability to alcoholism continues to be debated by some workers in the alcoholism research field.[5,6] Most observers, however, would support the notion that some genetic mediation occurs. The real question is how much of the variance is explained by genetic factors and to what degree are they moderated by personal factors (gender, age, and psychiatric comorbidity) and environmental ones (cultural milieu, shared familial environment).

2. Epidemiology of Alcohol Abuse and Alcoholism in Women

Wilsnack et al.[7] determined the rates of abstention and light, moderate, and heavy drinking among women in the general population as part of a national household survey (National Survey of Women's Drinking Practices). Although this survey did not attempt to diagnose alcoholism per se, the rates of "heavy drinking" reported by this group probably reflect the majority of women who are at greatest risk for developing alcoholism. Here, the highest levels of heavy drinking reported were for women between the ages of 35 and 49 (9%), with those aged 21 to 34 showing slightly lower rates (6%).

At the same time that the Wilsnack study was being conducted with the aid of the National Opinion Research Center (NORC), the Epidemiological Catchment Area (ECA) program was conducting a national survey of specific psychiatric disorders in the community. The ECA project used trained interviewers to assess the number and variety of symptoms reported by the respondents and compared these with established DSM-III criteria. This study[8] reported rates of Alcohol Abuse and/or Dependence by sex and age, allowing comparison with the Wilsnack data gathered at approximately the same time (1980–1982). While more recent household survey data are available,[2] rates by sex and age are not available. Thus, for the present discussion rates of alcoholism taken from the ECA survey and heavy drinking rates from the NORC survey for women by age are considered together.

Combining information from these two sources, what is striking is that while the peak for heavy drinking appears to be between the ages of 35 and 49 (NORC survey), the peak for Alcohol Abuse and/or Dependence reported is between the ages of 18 and 24 (ECA data). Moreover, the ECA data shows a dramatic drop in problems suggestive of abuse after age 24 to only 1.8% in the 25–44 age group and 0.9% among 45 to 64-year-olds. Because every alcoholic woman must first pass through a heavy drinking stage (be it brief or prolonged), these results suggest that those young women who become alcoholic early (between 18 and 24) are probably not typical of the female drinking population as a whole. Could it be that the majority of women who develop alcoholism after the age of 35 are the same women who, having experienced the lifetime peak for heavy drinking, later succumb to dependence on alcohol? If so, women who develop alcoholism between the ages of 18 and 24, the peak for alcoholism in women found by the ECA survey, may be another subset of alcoholic women. These women develop alcoholism after a much shorter duration of drinking (by definition) because of their young age.

Thus, two types of alcoholism may occur in women.[9-12] The etiology of early-onset alcoholism in women could result from factors other than societal sanctions or lack of such sanctions, whereas the later-onset may arise in response to changes in the woman's milieu. Thus, early-onset female alcoholism, though much less common in the population, may well be a more severe form with greater genetic mediation. As will be explored further in later portions of this chapter, we suggest that the familial form of alcoholism seen in women may resemble that seen in men, (e.g., early onset, multiple affected relatives, relative independence from environmental antecedents).

3. Evidence for Genetic Mediation

3.1. Family Data

The first attempt to model alcoholism transmission using empirical data that included rates by gender was completed by Cloninger and co-workers.[13] Using a multifactorial model of disease transmission in which the collective influence of all genetic and environmental factors that influence an individual's risk for developing a disorder are subsumed under a single variable termed *liability*, Cloninger and colleagues considered the relative contribution of these factors by gender. In considering both environmental and genetic influences, further delineation of the environmental influences were made: those arising from cultural or ecological variables and those originating within the family.

Using predictions from the more general multifactorial model, three specific models were tested: (1) the independent model, (2) the isocorrelational, and (3) the environmental. Testing of these models requires the availability of nuclear families.

Utilizing information from 365 first-degree relatives of 259 alcoholics who were consecutive admissions to a psychiatric hospital in St. Louis, Cloninger and colleagues[13] concluded that the environmental model provided the best fit to the observed family data. This model assumes that differences in prevalence of alcoholism in men and women are due entirely to nonfamilial environmental influences. In this model it is assumed that one gender is exposed to greater pressure to drink (or not drink) as a function of their gender. Even though alcoholism among women is less common than it is among men in the general population, the fact that there were equal numbers of affected relatives among both male and female probands suggested that differences in prevalence were due to nonfamilial environmental factors. In other words, both genders have *equal* likelihood that their disorder is genetically mediated. The difference in prevalence (rates for men exceed those for women) is due entirely to cultural differences.

Although the conclusions of this study have been modified by more recent analyses of family data[14] emanating from the St. Louis group, the results of this early study have implications for current theoretical approaches to the etiology of alcoholism. If the differences in prevalence are due entirely to variations in societal sanctions for drinking (based on the best-fit model being the environmental model), then one can assume that genetic factors may be as relevant to the etiology of alcoholism in women as they are in men. Unfortunately, the salience of the conclusions of the early study appear to have been overlooked in more recent discussions.

For example, it is noteworthy that Cloninger and colleagues use the term *femalelike* to describe a less severe and less genetically mediated form of alcoholism in men (type I alcoholism), presumably on the assumption that alcoholism in women less often requires involvement of genetic factors in its etiology.[14] This conclusion was based on separate analyses of family data acquired for male proband alcoholics and a similarly selected group of female alcoholic probands and their family members.[14] Analysis of alcoholism in relatives from the families of the 55 female probands best fit a multifactorial model. A similar analysis of a group of 140 families of male probands was found to best fit a mixed model with a recessive major locus. Because the latter model more strictly implies a genetic factor operating than does the multifactorial model, it may be concluded that the Gilligan study[14] implies greater genetic involvement in male alcoholism than female alcoholism.

The conclusions of this study have been questioned, however.[15] Particular methodological limitations of the Gilligan and colleagues' analysis may have led to premature conclusions. The three limitations previously noted[15] include the following: (1) nuclear families rather than extended families were classified as *malelike* and *femalelike*; (2) testing for heterogeneity within the sample was not performed; and (3) in the absence of testing, there was an assumption of no heterogeneity among these 55 families of female probands (heterogeneity was not directly tested). With respect to the first issue, a nuclear family consists of a proband, siblings, and parents, whereas an extended family includes multigenerational information. Nuclear families were classified as "malelike" if their likelihood under the recessive mixed model (seen in male proband families) exceeded their likelihood under the multifactorial model (seen in female probands). All others were classified as "femalelike." When a segregation analysis was applied to the data to determine the best fit for each subset of families ("malelike" or "femalelike"), a different mode of transmission was found for each; the "malelike" demonstrated a dominant gene mode of inheritance while the "femalelike" followed a multifactorial mode of transmission.

With respect to the question of genetic heterogeneity, Gilligan and colleagues[14] contrasted the male and female families for the presence or absence of heterogeneity. Genetic heterogeneity may be defined as quantitative evidence that more than one type of inheritance explains the transmission of a disease within families. Geneticists commonly use statistical tests to evaluate the likelihood of homogeneity relative to heterogeneity by evaluating the observed sample relative to a theoretical one using a χ^2 distribution. Gilligan and colleagues[14] may have incorrectly concluded that heterogeneity existed for the male families because of improper nesting of alternative hypotheses (see Aston and Hill[15] for details). Furthermore, no formal tests of heterogeneity were applied to the female families, though the authors state that they were not heterogeneous.

The alcoholism field appears to have bought the notion of two types of male alcoholism (one more severe and derived more clearly from a genetic predisposition and the other more environmentally based), while assuming that only one type of alcoholism exists in females. Moreover, it has been assumed without scientific evidence that this single form does not have a genetic etiology. Because the assumption is based on incomplete information, it may not be correct. Thus, based on currently available family history data, we conclude that there is every reason to believe that the etiology of female alcoholism (at least one form of it) has as much likelihood of being mediated through genetic factors as it does in men.

3.2. Adoption Data

Transmission of alcoholism within families appears to occur at higher probability than most psychiatric disorders, including the affective disorders.[16] The now classic adoption study which concerned etiology in males[17] suggested that such transmission can occur even in the absence of exposure to the alcoholic parent. Fewer adoption data are available for women, so that the conclusions that can be reached are somewhat tentative.[18,19] To summarize, three adoption studies have been conducted in Sweden,[20] Denmark,[21] and the United States.[22] The Swedish and Danish studies had too few alcoholic women to draw firm conclusions. However, Cadoret and colleagues employed a reasonable sample size and sophisticated data analytic techniques, and concluded that genetic factors operate in the etiology of alcoholism in both men and women.

3.3. Twin Studies

Further evidence for genetic mediation of alcoholism in women can be gained from studies that have utilized adult twin pairs. Both concordance for drinking[23] and alcohol dependence[24-28] have been studied. While some studies[24,25,27] did not find monozygotic (MZ)/dizygotic (DZ) rates suggestive of genetic mediation in female twin pairs, recent publications[26,28] are quite convincing. Pickens and colleagues[26] studied 114 male and 55 female twin pairs and concluded that a genetic component was operating in female alcoholism as well. Finally, Kendler et al.[28] studied 1030 MZ and DZ twin pairs and found substantially higher correlations in MZ than DZ twins, with over 50% of the variance in alcoholism risk explained by genetic factors.

In summary, we have previously noted that the etiology of female alcoholism has as much likelihood of being mediated through genetic factors as it does in men.[19] The evidence includes two persuasive twin studies of female alcoholism[26,28] and the adoption study of Cadoret et al.[22] Moreover, alcoholism appears to be heterogeneous in women, with one form more clearly mediated by genetic factors. Studies by Glenn and Nixon[11] and Lex et al.[12] give evidence for greater severity of symptoms in the early-onset groups of women, along with greater familial density of alcoholism in the severe form. Preliminary results from our own laboratory suggest a very early onset of alcoholism for female alcoholics who had multigenerational alcoholism running in their families. The median age of onset for alcoholic women ascertained by familial alcoholism density was 16 years.[29]

4. Premise: Two Types of Alcoholism in Women

Cloninger et al.[9] have described the characteristics of male type I alcoholics in contrast to type II alcoholics as those whose likelihood of drinking depends much more heavily on the environmental milieu in which the individual resides. The latter, or type II, males tend to be of the familial form and display earlier onset. Quite possibly two forms of alcoholism may exist in women: one that is largely the result of environmental pressures and grows out of late-onset heavy drinking (peak ages 35–49) and another early-onset form that occurs between the ages of 18 and 24 and is much more likely to be genetically mediated.

Thus, at least two types of alcoholism have been identified in men[9,10] based largely on the severity that is exhibited, as well as on the proportion of genetic variance explaining the emergent behavior. It is very likely that there are two types of alcohol abuse/dependence in women. One type would appear to be part of a youthful rebellion that "matures out" as the individual is acquiring new responsibilities of young adulthood (career, marriage, child rearing). This form may be most responsive to environmental pressures. In contrast, it is proposed that familial alcoholism appears to be of greater severity, being part of an intergenerational pattern of substance abuse that reappears in multiple generations and is present even in families where the environment is relatively propitious (the family has a higher socioeconomic status, is intact, and subscribes the traditional values) as we have seen in our ongoing family study of male alcoholic probands.[10]

Further evidence for two types of alcoholism comes from studies by Glenn and Nixon[11] and Lex *et al.*[12] Glenn and Nixon showed that when women are classified by age of onset, a number of significant differences emerged with respect to severity of alcoholism exhibited. In general, the early-onset alcoholism group displayed greater severity of symptoms and more affected relatives. Lex *et al.* studied women with more severe alcohol problems who come to the attention of the courts as a result of their drinking (DWI offenses) and found that these women exhibited a greater density of familial alcoholism than those who did not.

4.1. Evidence for Genetic Mediation of the Early-Onset Form

Thus, early-onset female alcoholism, though much less common in the population, may well be a more severe form with greater genetic mediation. It is suggested that the familial form of alcoholism seen in women may resemble that seen in men (e.g., early onset, multiple affected relatives, relative independence from environmental antecedents). If there are two forms, with the early-onset, severe type being characterized by multiple affected relatives, evidence for familial transmission should be apparent. The question arises, however, as to whether or not the familial transmission could be genetically mediated. Although the available data necessary to draw firm conclusions are missing with respect to female alcoholism, a brief review of the extant literature is provided in support of the position that alcoholism in women is as likely to be found to be genetically mediated in women as it is men.

5. The Need to Integrate Neurobiological and Sociocultural Perspectives

Any model of alcoholism vulnerability that supports a purely neurobiological–genetic perspective without taking into account the sociocultural factors that mitigate against drinking, and heavy drinking in particular, is incomplete. Moreover, a "process" model may be a more accurate representation of the waxing and waning, episodic nature of alcoholism through the life course than a "static" one.[30,31] In this view, the alcoholic is thought to have certain neurobiological characteristics at birth that may predispose her to becoming alcoholic. The likelihood of that happening will be determined by the consequences of drinking (both biological and psychosocial), which in turn become antecedent conditions for maintenance of abusive drinking (see Fig. 1). Thus, the following sections will first discuss possible neurobiological factors transmitted from generation to generation in families of alcoholics, and second will discuss the sociocultural factors relevant to initiation and maintenance of drinking in women, along with those rendering some women more vulnerable to becoming alcoholic.

5.1. Characterizing the Neurobiological Factors That May be Transmitted

A large number of research efforts have been initiated in the past 20 years in an attempt to identify reliable and valid markers for alcoholism risk. Broadly defined, these appear to belong within the domains of personality or temperament, on the one hand, and neurocognitive on the other. The notion of an "alcoholic personality" has been a common theme in discussions both by clinicians and researchers. However, whether or not temperament/personality factors have etiologic significance is dependent on the research designs used to test these personality theories. Studying alcoholics does not allow one to separate cause from consequence. Neurocognitive and neurobehavioral theories have also been plentiful among the etiologic models proposed for alcoholism.

These capacities for processing information may prove to be relevant to why one individual is more suited or motivated to pursue intellectual pursuits, endeavors that may be incompatible with long-term abusive drinking. The neurobehavioral characteristics deserve mention because they reflect both the "neurological health" of the brain and the "final common pathway" for the behavioral expression of this capacity. For example, it has long been known that children with "minimal brain dysfunction" have problems inhibiting the motor system and have variously been described as hyperactive or attentionally deficient. If high-risk individuals are born with a subtle neurological wiring handicap, this may be expressed as motoric hyperactivity and impulsivity and may additionally be reflected in higher levels of tonic autonomic arousal or increased response to environmental stressors than do individuals who are at low-risk for developing alcoholism.

Alcohol metabolism may play a role in the development of alcoholism. Theoretically, any living organism can be addicted to alcohol if sufficient quantities are ingested over a period of time. In fact, passive dependence on alcohol can easily be achieved in laboratory rats by restricting their fluid to alcohol-adulterated water.[32] Whether or not some individuals are born with a greater or lesser capacity to metabolize alcohol, a tendency that might be enhanced by being from a high-risk family, is currently unknown. Although it may be the case that some groups of individuals who are low consumers of alcohol (e.g., those with Asian background) appear to have altered metabolism, it is necessary to show that high-risk groups from the same ethnic

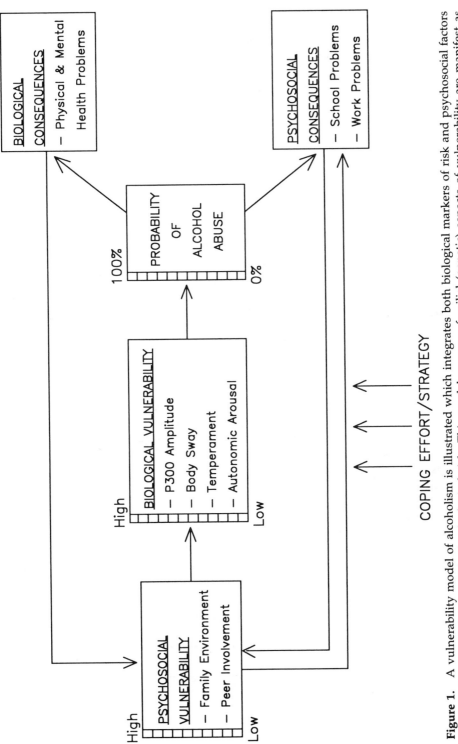

Figure 1. A vulnerability model of alcoholism is illustrated which integrates both biological markers of risk and psychosocial factors that may be expected to modify this biological risk. This model assumes familial (genetic) aspects of vulnerability are manifest as biological markers.

background have elevated rates of metabolism in order for the observed difference to be of major etiologic significance. Also, it is possible that high- and low-risk groups have similar rates of metabolism but differ in their innate tissue tolerance for alcohol or differ in the rate at which they develop acute tolerance. Women may be at greater risk for developing alcohol dependence than men because at the same level of consumption (corrected for body weight, e.g., grams per kilogram) they exhibit reduced levels of alcohol dehydrogenase (ADH) in the gastrointestinal tract relative to men.[33]

Of course, within the neurocognitive–neurobehavioral domain one must include possible differences in subjective, behavioral, and motoric response to alcohol as a function of the individual's familial risk for alcoholism and information-processing capacities. However, the individual's response to alcohol will also be conditioned by the person's unique metabolism of alcohol, state of alcohol tolerance, and beliefs about alcohol effects. These beliefs are derived from the culture he or she lives in and are also dependent on whether or not the individual grew up in a family in which an alcoholic(s) resided. Additionally, the individual's personality/temperament will determine his or her response to alcohol (e.g., is the subject in the test environment cooperative and compliant or disbelieving and difficult?). For these reasons, it may be very difficult to learn about the unique characteristics of high-risk individuals that predispose them to becoming alcoholic by utilizing only those tests that involve alcohol administration.

As part of a program designed to uncover neurobiological factors contributing to alcoholism vulnerability in alcoholic women, we have uncovered a number of differences between alcoholic women and their children compared to control women and children with respect to the neurocognitive–neurobehavioral domains. We speculate that at least some of these differences may contribute to higher risk for alcoholism and specifically early-onset female alcoholism.

5.2. Neurobiological Characteristics

The primary areas of inquiry have been with respect to event-related potential characteristics of adults[34,35] and children,[36–38] cardiovascular responding,[39] and body sway (static ataxia) in children.[40,41] Event-related potential (ERP) characteristics including particular components of the waveform (e.g., P300, N250) are of interest for a number of reasons. The N250 component is a negative wave occurring approximately 250 msec after the onset of a stimulus and is thought to become less negative during a child's development. P300 is a scalp-positive wave that occurs after an informative event occurs. These components are of particular interest because (1) long-latency components of ERPs, including P300, are associated with particular sensory and cognitive aspects of information processing,[42,43] (2) the ERP waveform appears to be under genetic control,[44–49] and (3) the P300 component of the event-related potential has received considerable attention as a possible neurophysiological risk marker for the development of alcoholism, both in our own laboratory and in others.

5.2.1. Event-Related Potentials and Alcoholism Risk.

Although there has been some controversy surrounding whether or not P300 is a risk marker for alcoholism, it should be noted that there are now a number of laboratories showing consistent results[50–52] besides our own.[36–38] Decrements in P300 are usually seen when high-risk minor children are tested with sufficiently difficult paradigms and when the density of the alcoholism in the high-risk group is sufficient to allow the variation between high-risk (HR) and low-risk (LR) groups to be explored (see Hill and Steinhauer[37] and Steinhauer and Hill,[38] for discussion). We have reserved the use of the term "high-risk" to denote cases where the familial constellation is of sufficient density to produce lifetime risk of 50% or greater for young males, a more stringent requirement than the family history positive (FHP) designation used by many.[53] For an individual to have a predicted recurrence risk of this magnitude, multiple relatives must be alcoholic.[54]

5.2.2. Children of Female Alcoholics and Children of Male Alcoholics.

We are in a unique position to compare children of alcoholics from male alcoholism families with children from female alcoholism families. As part of a large-scale family study of alcoholism in which families are identified through multigenerational alcoholism and the presence of at least two alcoholic brothers per family, we are studying children prospectively. We have observed remarkable consistency in our findings of reduced P300 in HR children utilizing an auditory oddball paradigm. Two studies have been published utilizing two *different* samples of children ascertained through male alcoholic probands that found P300 amplitude reduction.[36,38] P300 amplitude reduction in HR children is also seen utilizing a visual task.[37]

In a separate study, using a similar ascertainment scheme requiring multiple alcoholic family members, we have been studying families of alcoholic women. We have chosen this design because we believe that in those families where female alcoholism is multigenerational, with multiple affected relatives, one might expect an early onset of the problem. These families are much more likely to transmit alcoholism to the next generation, thereby increasing risk to offspring. Also, because this subtype is more severe, a minority of affected individuals will achieve remission simply as part of a maturing-out process.

Analysis of data obtained from offspring of female proband alcoholism families indicates, once again, that the amplitude of the P300 component is smaller in HR children ($p = 0.016$) compared with control children (see Fig. 2). Nonparametric analysis of data supports this result; 9 of 28 HR children were one or more standard deviations below the mean of age- and gender-matched controls, while only 3 of 28 controls were found to be this deviant. Because of the importance of these findings, we looked for other explanations for why children from female alcoholism families (CFA) would show reduced P300. The

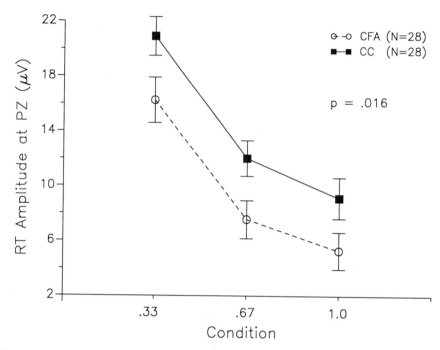

Figure 2. Using the auditory RT task, amplitude reduction is seen among high-risk children in comparison to low-risk ones, illustrating that biological differences may precede the development of alcoholism in women.

variables we considered were: (1) drinking during pregnancy; (2) presence of "other psychopathology" in mothers, especially antisocial personality disorder which has been linked to P300 reduction by some, though not all, laboratories; and (3) lower socioeconomic status. None of these explanations could explain our data, leading us to conclude that a diathesis for alcoholism was a strong predictor of P300 reduction in children from these female alcoholism families.

Even in families with an extremely high density of alcoholism, the recurrence risk for alcoholism in offspring will be less than 1.0; that is, only a proportion of offspring will become alcoholic. Therefore, one would *not* expect every child from a HR family to carry the marker (reduced P300 amplitude) even if the marker were perfectly correlated with affection status. Therefore, it is not surprising that one third of HR boys and one fifth of HR girls show P300 reductions that place them one or more standard deviations below the mean of an age- and gender-matched control group (these proportions based on visual data for children from the male alcoholism families[37]).

Although only a preliminary analysis, we were recently excited by the fact that a greater proportion of girls from HR female alcoholism families (30%) than girls from the HR male alcoholism families (20%) showed P300 reduction (1 or more SDs below mean). In view of the more frequent female-to-female transmission reported than cross-gender transmission seen in the Swedish adoption study,[20] we are speculating that more girls from these HR for female alcoholism families may carry a neurobiological diathesis for alcoholism than do girls from similarly matched HR for male alcoholism families.

Establishing that P300 deficits occur in female alcoholics is another important step. Our laboratory has an extensive database on adult relatives of male proband alcoholics (both alcoholic and nonalcoholic) and low-risk subjects.[34,35,55] A now more modest data set of HR women has enabled us to determine that those who develop alcoholism exhibit a 50% reduction in the amplitude of P300 in comparison to their nonalcoholic sisters and to controls in response to information processing demands.[35] Recent history of drinking (past 7 and past 30 days) was entered into these analyses as covariates without significant effect. Thus, we ask, is the absence of a P300 decrement protective for the HR nonalcoholic sister?

5.3. Sociocultural Aspects of Alcoholism Vulnerability

In order for women to become alcoholic they must make a decision to drink alcohol, a decision to continue using alcohol, and to either moderate their ongoing use of alcohol or drink as often or as much as they wish. As seemingly simplistic as this statement may seem, it summarizes the enormous variability between drinking patterns between men and women, particularly in some cultures. Sociocultural factors determine the likelihood that women will drink and the manner in which they drink. The following review will highlight some of the sociocultural aspects of women's drinking that alter their vulnerability to becoming alcoholic. These include familial–environmental factors, the cultural tradition with which they identify, and secular trends in alcohol use.

5.3.1. Familial–Environmental Factors. Although environmental effects are usually not thought of as "markers" for alcoholism risk, nevertheless, the effects of environment, if they are nonrandom and occur at a developmentally critical stage, may endure beyond childhood. Therefore, certain kinds of environmental exposures may be thought of as markers of risk. For example, suppose that the same behavioral characteristic shows up in all children whose alcoholic mothers failed to achieve remission during their preschool years. This behavioral trait might be thought of as etiologic if these children have higher rates of alcoholism as adults than they would by virtue of having a family history without environmental exposure. Currently, we know very little about the effects of early experience on later development of alcoholism or substance abuse. However, it is interesting to note that even laboratory rats, when differentially reared (impoverished vs. enriched), show differences in drug preference as adults.[56] Specifically, rats reared in enriched environments display a greater preference for cocaine solutions, when offered a choice between plain water and cocaine-adulterated water, than do rats reared in impoverished environments. These results are intriguing in view of reported differences in brain development in rats differentially reared in similar environments.[57] Extrapolating to the human condition one could argue that the immature brain may be open to "tuning" by environmental stimuli such that those reared in highly stimulating environments (good or bad) may seek similar levels of stimulation. The change of state that alcohol or drug intoxication provides may satisfy this craving for excessive stimulation. This need for excessive stimulation is embodied in the concept of "sensation seeking" frequently described for substance-dependent individuals.[58]

In addition to possible environmental effects on neurobiological "fine tuning," there is also the clear possibility that expectations concerning the effects of alcohol may be transmitted within families. There is a growing body of evidence that suggests that expectancies are learned early in life and are predictive of later development of alcohol use patterns.[59,60] Johnson et al.[61] studied members of families of college students living in Hawaii, finding moderate to high correlations between parents and their offspring with respect to expected physiological and subjective effects of alcohol. Whether or not these expectancy effects are as salient for girls and young women is unclear. Beliefs about the substantive effects of alcohol were correlated for pairs of family members to reflect resemblance in beliefs. Data presented indicate that the father–son and mother–son correlations were higher than the father–daughter or mother–daughter correlations. Thus, expectancy effects may be transmitted within families but to a lesser degree among females.

5.3.2. Cross-Cultural Variation in Drinking Practices Among Women.

Examining cross-cultural variation in rates of drinking, abuse of alcohol, and alcohol dependence is instructive not only with respect to understanding how cultural variation influences the likelihood that individuals will develop alcoholism, but also elucidates those factors influencing vulnerability to alcoholism in women relative to those found in men.

The fact that more men than women become alcoholic in most cultures has led to a number of misconceptions about women's drinking. One of these has to do with the notion that women traditionally have not had as much freedom with regard to access to alcohol. Child et al.[62] examined records concerning drinking in 139 societies, finding adequate data for analysis from 113, only 4 of which did not allow women to drink. Only in one society was drunkenness forbidden in women. Moreover, in some cultures women actually have greater access to alcohol than do men. As noted by Heath,[63] in Latin America and parts of Africa women are the primary producers and distributors of grain or vegetable-based homebrews that are used both as foods and intoxicants. In some of these societies women own and operate public drinking establishments where they market the alcohol they produce. In some tribal societies the homebrew business is the focus of the economy.

Because a greater proportion of men than women become alcoholic in most societies much of the current thinking that presupposes a greater genetic (biological) vulnerability to alcoholism for men than for women[14] may have been influenced by this observation. Yet, formal tests of heterogeneity among women alcoholics have not been performed in any of the family studies of women performed to date[14] so that it is not possible to rule out the possibility of two (perhaps, more) types of alcoholism in women. We suspect that there may be an equal number of more genetically determined cases of male and female alcoholism in the population, but the higher rates overall in men are largely due to the fact that environmental pressures to drink heavily are much greater for males. This conclusion is, in part, based on analysis of our high-density families selected through male alcoholic probands. In these families the age of onset for females who become alcoholic is as early as it is for brothers who become alcoholic.[18] Also, families selected through female probands for their high density of alcoholism and multigenerational affectation show that female alcoholism can be as severe as the most familial form identified in men. We have found the median age of onset for alcoholism in these women to be 16 years.[1]

If the discrepancy between alcoholism rates among men and women is largely due to variations in environmental pressures to not drink heavily in the first place, one should find widely varying ratios between male and female rates from society to society. This is exactly what one sees in reviewing the ratio of male to female alcoholism across those societies that permit women to drink, which as noted previously include the majority of societies. For example, reanalysis of data provided by epidemiological surveys in Israel and the United States[64] reveals a 6-month prevalence for the male : female ratio for alcoholism of approximately 6 : 1 in the United States versus 14 : 1 in Israel. Another cross-national study utilizing the Diagnostic Interview Schedule (DIS), the instrument originally developed for the US Epidemiological Catchment Area study, compared the lifetime prevalence of alcohol abuse and alcohol dependence in the United States, Canada, Puerto Rico, Taiwan, and South Korea.[65] This study found ratios of 5.4 : 1, 4.7 : 1, 9.8 : 1, 29 : 1, and 20 : 1, respectively. Clearly, cultural variation changes the likelihood that individuals will become alcoholic. This variation is not equally effective by gender. This observation is further illustrated in an intriguing study in which the Korean version of the DIS was administered to Korean men and women living in two sites, Kangwha, Korea and Yanbian, China.[66] All were native Koreans but lived in different sociocultural environments, with those living in China subject to more traditional and conservative attitudes toward drinking. A significant difference in lifetime prevalence of alcohol abuse and alcohol dependence was reported by the authors. What is of interest with respect to sociocultural influences on female drinking and alcoholism was the widely varying male-to-female ratios in alcohol abuse. For Kangwha, the ratio was 17.5 : 1, whereas the ratio for Yanbian, China, where traditional societal values are more salient, was 115 : 1!

In contrast, in those societies that are more permissive of drinking, the male : female ratio is much less discrepant. Brown et al.[67] examined alcoholism in Southern Cheyenne Indians and found a ratio of 1.7 : 1. Moreover, the majority of both male and female alcoholics had an early onset (< 25 years) of the disorder. In fact, there are cases where females drink more than males as noted by Weibel-Orlando.[68] She found that Sioux women drank more frequently than Sioux men, and appear to consume more alcohol per occasion than do the men.

Finally, a word is in order regarding possibly different mechanisms involved in alcohol use and alcohol dependence. Societies that have shown rapid changes in attitudes and behaviors related to substance use provide the opportunity to evaluate whether alcohol dependence and alcohol abuse are equally influenced by societal changes. Hwu et al.[69] have reported that prevalence of alcohol abuse is five times more likely than alcohol dependence in current (post-World War II) Taiwanese society, suggesting that alcohol abuse may be more responsive to changes in societal norms than is alcohol dependence.

Because alcohol use is culturally, and in many societies, legally controlled, it is not surprising that women are less likely to drink abusively and to consume less alcohol overall than men. However, if some alcoholism is genetically mediated (perhaps a greater proportion of female than male alcoholics), then one might expect that the manifestations of alcoholism would be equivalent in men and women once they become alcoholic. Several recent studies would appear to support this conclusion. The World Health collaborative project has been collecting data concerning the prevalence of harmful levels of alcohol consumption in six countries: Australia, Bulgaria, Kenya, Mexico, Norway, and the United States. For all national groups the level of consumption for men is significantly higher than for women. However, among alcoholics the average daily intake for women was 74% of the intake for men (176 g for women and 200 g for men). Correcting for body weight differences would indicate that women alcoholics may be drinking more in terms of gram per kilogram intake than are alcoholic men.

Further, Kawakami et al.[70] found that among a sample of over 2500 employees of a computer factory in Tokyo, 15% of the men and 6% of the women could be classified as having alcohol problems using an alcoholism screening test (Kurihama Alcoholism Screening Test) designed for use among Japanese, and embodied similar concepts to those utilized in DSM-III definitions of alcoholism. Importantly, there was no significant gender difference in the prevalence of alcohol-related problems for a given amount of alcohol consumption. These results support the conclusions reached by Edwards et al.[71] that women have the same susceptibility for alcohol-related problems when they drink the same amount as males.

6. Conclusions

In summary, there is as much evidence that at least one form of alcoholism in women is genetically mediated as it is in men. For women with the more severe form of alcoholism, onset of the disorder is as early as it is in men. Gender differences in rates of alcoholism probably have more to do with cultural variations that have greater impact on women than men, preventing them from becoming heavy drinkers. Once they become heavy drinkers, their chances of developing alcohol problems are equivalent to that of men. Neurobiological risk factors identified in very-high-risk men appear to apply equally well to women and girls who are at very high risk for becoming alcoholic by virtue of the high density, multigenerational nature of the alcoholism running in their families.

ACKNOWLEDGMENTS. Preparation of this manuscript was supported in part by awards from the National Institute on Alcohol Abuse and Alcoholism AA005909 and AA05808.

References

1. Hill SY: Etiology, in McCrady B and Frankenstein W (eds.): *Annual Review of Addiction Research and Treatment*, vol. 3. New York, Pergamon Press, 1994, pp 127–148.
2. Kessler RC, McGonagle KA, Zhao S, *et al*: Lifetime and 12-month prevalence of DSM-III-R psychiatric disorders in the United States. *Arch Gen Psychiatry* 51:8–19, 1994.
3. Rounsaville BJ, Dolinsky ZS, Babor TF, *et al*: Psychopathology as a predictor of treatment outcome in alcoholics. *Arch Gen Psychiatry* 44:505–513, 1987.
4. Schuckit MA, Winokur G: A short-term follow-up of women alcoholics. *Dis Nerv Syst* 33:572–578, 1972.
5. Murray RM, Clifford CA, Gurling HMD: Twin and adoption studies: How good is the evidence for a genetic role? in Galanter M (ed): *Recent Developments in Alcoholism*, vol. 1. New York, Plenum Press, 1983, pp 25–48.
6. Peele S: Implications and limitations of genetic models of alcoholism and other addictions. *Gen Stud Alcohol* 47:63–73, 1986.
7. Wilsnack RW, Wilsnack SC, Klassen AD: Women's drinking and drinking problems: Patterns from a 1981 national survey. *Am J Public Health* 74:1231–1238, 1984.
8. Robins LN, Helzer J, Weissman MN, *et al*: Lifetime prevalence of specific psychiatric disorders in three sites. *Arch Gen Psychiatry* 41:949–958, 1984.
9. Cloninger CR, Bohman M, Sigvardsson S: Inheritance of alcohol abuse: Cross-fostering analysis of adopted men. *Arch Gen Psychiatry* 38:861–868, 1981.
10. Hill SY: Absence of paternal sociopathy in the etiology of severe alcoholism: Is there a type III alcoholism? *J Stud Alcohol* 53:161–169, 1992.
11. Glenn SW, Nixon SJ: Applications of Cloninger's subtypes in a female alcoholic sample. *Alcohol Clin Exp Res* 15:851–857, 1991.
12. Lex BW, Sholar JW, Bower T, *et al*: Putative type II alcoholism characteristics in female third DUI offenders in Massachusetts: A pilot study. *Alcohol* 8:283–287, 1991.
13. Cloninger CR, Christiansen KO, Reich T, *et al*: Implications of sex differences in the prevalences of antisocial personality, alcoholism, and criminality for familial transmission. *Arch Gen Psychiatry* 35:941–951, 1978.
14. Gilligan SB, Reich T, Cloninger CR: Etiologic heterogeneity in alcoholism. *Genet Epidemiol* 4:395–414, 1987.
15. Aston CE, Hill SY: Segregation analysis of alcoholism in families ascertained through a pair of male alcoholics. *Am J Hum Genet* 46:879–887, 1990.
16. Merikangas KR, Leckman JF, Prusoff BA, *et al*: Familial transmission of depression and alcoholism. *Arch Gen Psychiatry* 42:367–372, 1985.

17. Goodwin DW, Schulsinger F, Hermansen L, et al: Alcohol problems in adoptees raised apart from alcoholic biological parents. Arch Gen Psychiatry 28:238–243, 1973.
18. Hill SY, Smith TR: Evidence for genetic mediation of alcoholism in women. J Subst Abuse 3:159–174, 1991.
19. Hill SY: Genetic vulnerability to alcoholism in women, in Gomberg E, Nirenberg TD (eds): Women and Substance Abuse. Norwood, NJ, Ablex Publishing, 1993, pp 42–61.
20. Bohman M, Sigvardsson S, Cloninger CR: Maternal inheritance of alcohol abuse: Cross-fostering analysis of adopted women. Arch Gen Psychiatry 38:965–969, 1981.
21. Goodwin DW, Schulsinger F, Knop J, et al: Alcoholism and depression in adopted-out daughters of alcoholics. Arch Gen Psychiatry 34:751–755, 1977.
22. Cadoret RJ, O'Gorman TW, Troughton E, et al: Alcoholism and antisocial personality: Inter-relationships, genetic and environmental factors. Arch Gen Psychiatry 42:161–167, 1985.
23. Heath AC, Jardine R, Martin NG: Interactive effects of genotype and social environment on alcohol consumption in female twins. J Stud Alcohol 50:38–48, 1989.
24. Gurling HMD, Murray RM, Clifford CA: Investigations into the genetics of alcohol dependence and into its effects on brain function, in Gedda L, Parisi P, Nance, WE (eds): Twin Research 3: Epidemiological and Clinical Studies. New York, Alan R. Liss, 1981, pp 77–87.
25. McGue M, Pickens RW, Svikis DS: Sex and age effects on the inheritance of alcohol problems: A twin study. J Abnorm Psychol 101:3–17, 1992.
26. Pickens RW, Svikis DS, McGue M, et al: Heterogeneity in the inheritance of alcoholism: A study of male and female twins. Arch Gen Psychiatry 48:19–28, 1991.
27. Pickens RW, Svikis DS: The twin method in the study of vulnerability to drug abuse, in Biological Vulnerability to Drug Abuse, Research Monograph vol. 89, 1988, pp 41–51.
28. Kendler KS, Heath AC, Neale MC, et al: A population-based twin study of alcoholism in women. JAMA 268:1877–1882, 1992.
29. Hill SY: Familial risk for alcoholism in women: Is P300 a marker? Proc Am College Neuropharmacol 39, 1993.
30. Hill SY: A vulnerability model for alcoholism in women. Focus on Women: J Addict Health 2:68–91, 1981.
31. Hill SY: Biological consequences of alcoholism and alcohol-related problems among women, in Alcohol and Health Monograph No. 4, Special Population Issues. (DHHS Pub. No. [ADM] 82-1193), Rockville, Maryland, US Department of Health and Human Services, National Institute on Alcohol Abuse and Alcoholism, 1982.
32. Hill SY: Addiction liability of Tryon rats: Independent transmission of morphine and alcohol consumption. Pharmacol Biochem Behav 9:107–110, 1978.
33. Frezza M, di Padova C, Pozzato G, et al: High blood alcohol levels in women. The role of decreased gastric alcohol dehydrogenase activity and first-pass metabolism. N Engl J Med 322:95–99, 1990.
34. Hill SY, Steinhauer SR, Zubin J, et al: Event-related potentials as markers for alcoholism risk in high density families. Alcohol Clin Exp Res 12:545–554, 1988.
35. Hill SY, Steinhauer SR: Event-related potentials in women at risk for alcoholism. Alcohol 10:349–354, 1993.
36. Hill SY, Steinhauer SR, Park J, et al: Event-related potential characteristics in children of alcoholics from high density families. Alcohol Clin Exp Res 14:6–16, 1990. (Reprinted in Annu Rev Addict Res Treat 1:177–192, 1992.)
37. Hill SY, Steinhauer SR: Assessment of prepubertal and postpubertal boys and girls at risk for developing alcoholism with P300 from a visual discrimination task. J Stud Alcohol 54:350–358, 1993.
38. Steinhauer SR, Hill SY: Auditory event-related potentials in children at high risk for alcoholism. J Stud Alcohol 54:408–421, 1993.
39. Hill SY, Steinhauer SR, Zubin J: Cardiac responsivity in individuals at high risk for alcoholism. J Stud Alcohol 53:378–388, 1992.
40. Hill SY, Armstrong J, Steinhauer SR, et al: Static ataxia as a psychobiological marker for alcoholism. Alcohol Clin Exp Res 4:345–348, 1987.

41. Hill SY, Steinhauer SR: Postural sway in children from pedigrees exhibiting a high density of alcoholism. *Biol Psychiatry* 33:313–325, 1993.

42. Sutton S, Braren M, John ER, *et al*: Evoked potential correlates of stimulus uncertainty. *Science* 150:1187–1188, 1965.

43. Donchin E: Event-related potentials: A tool in the study of human in formation processing, in Begleiter H (ed): *Evoked Brain Potentials and Behavior*. New York, Plenum Press, 1979, pp 13–88.

44. Bock F: Pupillary dilation and vertex evoked potential similarity in monozygotic and dizygotic twins and siblings. Unpublished doctoral dissertation, City University of New York, 1976.

45. Surwillo WW: Cortical evoked potentials in monozygotic twins and unrelated subjects: Comparisons of exogenous and endogenous components. *Behav Genet* 10:201–209, 1980.

46. Polich J, Burns T: P300 from identical twins. *Neuropsychologia* 25:299–304, 1987.

47. Aston CE, Hill SY: A segregation analysis of the P300 component of the event-related potential. *Am J Hum Genet* 47(Suppl):A127, 1990.

48. Rogers TD, Deary I: The P300 component of the auditory event-related potential in monozygotic and dizygotic twins. *Acta Psychiatr Scand* 83:412–416, 1991.

49. Aston C, Hill SY: Segregation analysis of alcoholism in families ascertained through a pair of male alcoholics. *Am J Hum Genet* 47:A127, 1990.

50. Begleiter H, Porjesz B, Bihari B, *et al*: Event-related brain potentials in boys at risk for alcoholism. *Science* 225:1493–1496, 1984.

51. Whipple S, Parker ES, Noble EP: An atypical neurocognitive profile in alcoholic fathers and their sons. *J Stud Alcohol* 49:240–244, 1988.

52. Berman SM, Whipple SC, Fitch RJ, *et al*: P300 in young boys as a predictor of adolescent substance use. *Alcohol* 10:69–76, 1993.

53. Polich J, Bloom FE: Event-related brain potentials in individuals at high and low risk for developing alcoholism: Failure to replicate. *Alcohol Clin Exp Res* 12:368–373, 1988.

54. Aston CE, Hill SY: Segregation analysis of alcoholism in families ascertained through a pair of male alcoholics. *Am J Hum Genet* 46:879–887, 1990.

55. Steinhauer SR, Hill SY, Zubin J: Event-related potentials in alcoholics and their first-degree relatives. *Alcohol* 4:307–314, 1987.

56. Hill SY, Powell BJ: Cocaine and morphine self-administration: Effects of differential reading. *Pharmacol Biochem Behav* 5:701–704, 1976.

57. Krech D, Rosenzweig MR, Bennett EL: Effects of environmental complexity and training on brain chemistry. *J Comp Physiol Psychol* 53:509–519, 1960.

58. Zuckerman M: Sensation seeking and the endogenous deficit theory of drug abuse. National Institute on Drug Abuse, Research Monograph Series No. 74, 1986, pp 59–70.

59. Christiansen BA, Smith GT, Roehling PV, *et al*: Using alcohol expectancies to predict adolescent drinking behavior after one year. *J Consult Clin Psychol* 57:93–99, 1989.

60. Miller PM, Smith GT, Goldman MS: Emergence of alcohol expectancies in childhood: A possible critical period. *J Stud Alcohol* 51:343–349, 1990.

61. Johnson RC, Nagoshi CT, Danko GP, *et al*: Familial transmission of alcohol use norms and expectancies and reported alcohol use. *Alcohol Clin Exp Res* 14:216–220, 1990.

62. Child IL, Barry H, Bacon MK: A cross-cultural study of drinking: III. Sex differences. *Q J Stud Alcohol* 3:49–61, 1965.

63. Heath DB: Women and alcohol: Cross-cultural perspectives. *J Subst Abuse* 3:175–185, 1991.

64. Levav I, Kohn R, Dohrenwend BP, *et al*: An epidemiological study of mental disorders in a 10-year cohort of young adults in Israel. *Psychol Med* 23:691–707, 1993.

65. Helzer JE, Canino GJ, Yeh EK, *et al*: Alcoholism—North America and Asia: A comparison of population surveys with the diagnostic interview schedule. *Arch Gen Psychiatry* 47:313–319, 1990.

66. Namkoong K, Lee HY, Lee MH, *et al*: Cross-cultural study of alcoholism: Comparison between Kangwha, Korea and Yanbian, China. *Yonsei Med J* 32:319–325, 1991.

67. Brown GL, Albaugh BJ, Robin RW, *et al*: Alcoholism and substance abuse among selected Southern Cheyenne Indians. *Cult Med Psychiatry* 16:531–542, 1993.

68. Weibel-Orlando J: Women and alcohol: Special populations and cross-cultural variations, in *Women and Alcohol: Health Related Issues*. Rockville, MD, National Institute on Alcohol Abuse and Alcoholism, 1986, pp 161–187.
69. Hwu HG, Yeh EK, Yeh YL: Risk factors of alcoholism in Taiwan Chinese: An epidemiological approach. *Acta Psychiatr Scand* 82:295–298, 1990.
70. Kawakami N, Haratani T, Hemmi T, *et al*: Prevalence and demographic correlates of alcohol-related problems in Japanese employees. *Soc Psychiatry Psychiatr Epidemiol* 27:198–202, 1992.
71. Edwards G, Chandler J, Hensman C, *et al*: Drinking in a London suburb: II. Correlates of trouble with drinking among men. *Q J Stud Alcohol* [Suppl] 6:94–119, 1972.

2

Drinking and Problem Drinking in US Women

Patterns and Recent Trends

Sharon C. Wilsnack and Richard W. Wilsnack

Abstract. General population surveys suggest that the percentage of US women who drink declined slightly during the 1980s. Comparisons of 1981 and 1991 national surveys using the same drinking measures show that fewer women drank heavily in 1991, and women drinkers drank less frequently and had fewer episodes of heavy drinking, although younger drinkers reported more frequent intoxication. Longitudinal analyses of 5-year changes in drinking behavior indicate that movement both into and out of problem drinking is greatest among women aged 21 to 34.

Subgroups of women with elevated rates of heavy drinking and/or adverse drinking consequences include younger women; women lacking social roles or occupying unwanted social statuses; women in nontraditional jobs; cohabiting women; and ethnic minority women experiencing rapid acculturation. Risks of heavy and/or problem drinking are also greater among women with a heavy-drinking husband or partner; depression; sexual dysfunction; or violent victimization in childhood or adulthood.

Future research should focus on (1) the causes and consequences of recent declines in women's drinking; (2) antecedents and consequences of specific patterns of multiple substance use in women; (3) social and relational contexts of women's drinking, including occupational influences, drinking behavior of significant others, sexual dysfunction, and relationship violence; (4) longitudinal predictors of both problem drinking onset and "spontaneous" remission of women's alcohol problems; and (5) childhood sexual abuse as a potentially powerful risk factor for later alcohol abuse in women.

This chapter describes patterns and recent trends in the drinking behavior and drinking-related problems of women in the United States. The chapter

Sharon C. Wilsnack and Richard W. Wilsnack • Department of Neuroscience, University of North Dakota School of Medicine, Grand Forks, North Dakota 58202.

Recent Developments in Alcoholism, Volume 12: Women and Alcoholism, edited by Marc Galanter. Plenum Press, New York, 1995.

makes use of general population surveys reported during the last 10 years, with an emphasis on longitudinal survey data where available. These surveys are used to describe general trends in women's drinking and heavy drinking between 1971 and 1991, and to show more detailed 10-year and 5-year comparisons of our own 1981, 1986, and 1991 national surveys. Subsequent sections discuss variations in women's drinking across demographic subgroups, describe personal and social factors that are possible risk factors for problem drinking in women, and suggest directions for further epidemiological research on women.

1. Trends in Women's Drinking and Drinking Problems

1.1. Historical and Cross-National Perspectives

In all countries and historical periods for which there are general population survey data, the two strongest predictors of drinking behavior are gender and age. Men consistently drink more than women, and the young drink more than the old. Meta-analyses of data from 39 longitudinal general population surveys in 15 countries show that in every country and age group represented, women were less likely than men to drink, to drink frequently or heavily, and to report drinking-related problems.[1,2] Although gender differences are robust, levels and patterns of women's drinking vary greatly between nations and within nations over time. Societies also show different levels of concern about women's drinking behavior at different periods in their history. Some scholars suggest that concerns about women's use of alcoholic beverages tend to increase during periods of gender-role change, perhaps reflecting more general social discomfort with changing gender relationships and the expanding roles of women.[3,4]

1.2. Drinking and Heavy Drinking in US Women, 1971–1991

One period of heightened concern about women's drinking began in North America in the early 1970s. Despite public perceptions and media reports of an "epidemic" increase in women's drinking, analyses of trends in nine US surveys between 1971 and 1981[5] showed that women's drinking was relatively stable during this period, except for a modest increase in any alcohol use (nonabstention) among women aged 35 to 64. In all nine surveys, men were more likely than women to drink and to drink heavily, with no evidence of "convergence" in rates of either drinking or heavier drinking. Hilton[6] extended the analyses from 1964 to 1984. Although abstention was significantly rarer among women in 1984 (36%) than in previous surveys (39–47%), men in all age groups still had much higher rates of drinking and heavy drinking than women. Age group analyses found that women by 1984 were more likely to drink lightly (less than 0.22 ounces ethanol/day) at ages 18 to 20, to drink heavily (60 or more drinks per month) at ages 21 to 34, and to drink at all (nonabstention) at ages 50 to 64.

Consistent with declining per capita alcohol sales in the United States in the 1980s,[7] Williams and DeBakey[8] found signs of a shift toward reduced alcohol consumption in the later 1980s. Using data from the 1983 and 1988 National Health Interview Surveys (with measures differing slightly from Hilton's), Williams and DeBakey found significant increases in abstention and/or decreases in heavy drinking among both women and men in a number of demographic subgroups.

We have recently evaluated changes in women's drinking between 1971 and 1991, using data from 15 US national surveys, including the 1983, 1988, and 1990 National Health Interview Surveys, the Alcohol Research Group's 1990 national survey, and our own 1991 national survey.[9] Data for four different age groups (Table I) did not reveal any sudden or dramatic changes in the percentages of women drinking or drinking heavily, although the 1983 NHIS had the highest percentage of women drinkers in each age group.

We used segmented regression analysis[12] to learn whether women's drinking and heavy drinking from 1971 to 1991 showed two trends rather than one, with a more recent downward trend. Results showed that a model in which rates of drinking increased through the 1970s but declined modestly in the 1980s fit the data better than a model that assumed that drinking rates had followed a simple linear trend since 1971. A two-slope model of *heavy* drinking rates fit the data better only for women under age 50; heavy drinking rates in women over 50 did not vary enough to show clear trends.

1.3. Ten-Year Changes in Women's Drinking and Drinking Problems, 1981–1991

The trend analyses from multiple surveys have several limitations. It is unclear when a downturn in women's drinking may have begun; turning points at 1981 and 1983 produced equally good fits with the data. Irregular intervals between the surveys prevented us from testing statistically the superiority of the two-slope models. And variations in how surveys measured drinking and heavy drinking may have obscured or distorted trends.[13] For example, women's drinking was most prevalent in the 1983 and 1990 NHIS surveys, perhaps because these surveys had questions that could detect very infrequent drinking. To get beyond some of these limitations, we compared data from our 1981 and 1991 national surveys, which used exactly the same questions about drinking behavior and drinking consequences.

1.3.1. Methods. In 1981, 1986, and 1991, the National Opinion Research Center (NORC) gathered national data on women's drinking through personal interviews. The stratified 1981 sample of 911 women included 498 moderate-to-heavy drinkers (who consumed four or more drinks per week) and 413 lighter drinkers and abstainers; NORC also interviewed a comparison sample

Table I. Percentages of Women Who Are Drinkers and Heavy Drinkers, by Age Group, 1971–1991

	Investigator									
Age group	Harris 1971	Harris 1972	Harris 1973	Harris 1973	Harris 1974	ORC 1975	RAC 1976	SRG 1979	UND 1981	NHIS 1983
				1971–1983						
21–34										
Drinkers	71	67	72	65	71	68	71	77	71	79
Heavy drinkers	6	4	5	3	6	5	4	5	6	4
35–49										
Drinkers	64	56	63	55	65	57	73	65	73	74
Heavy drinkers	5	4	8	5	6	3	3	8	8	5
50–64										
Drinkers	47	44	43	50	49	48	50	49	53	67
Heavy drinkers	5	4	5	4	4	1	3	3	5	4
65 and over										
Drinkers	26	42	29	28	36	32	37	40	33	53
Heavy drinkers	0	5	2	2	2	1	0	2	2	3

	Investigator				
	1984–1991				
Age Group	ARG 1984	NHIS 1988	ARG 1990	NHIS 1990	UND 1991
21–34					
Drinkers	73	71	73	76	74
Heavy drinkers	7	3	3	2	4
35–49					
Drinkers	64	68	64	74	65
Heavy drinkers	6	4	2	2	3
50–64					
Drinkers	62	59	57	66	52
Heavy drinkers	4	4	2	2	2
65 and over					
Drinkers	44	45	32	52	29
Heavy drinkers	2	2	1	2	1

Sources: R. Wilsnack et al. (1984),[5] Williams & DeBakey (1992)[8] (reanalyzed by SF DeBakey), Hilton (1986),[6] Midanik & Room (1992)[10] (reanalyzed by LT Midanik), Williams et al. (1993)[11] (reanalyzed by SF DeBakey).

of 396 men. In 1986, NORC reinterviewed two subsamples of women: 143 women who in 1981 reported at least two of three indicators of potential problem drinking (one or more drinking-related problems in the past 12 months, one or more alcohol-dependence symptoms in the past 12 months, average daily consumption of one ounce or more of ethanol) and 157 women who drank more than once a month but reported none of the three problem-drinking indicators. In 1991, NORC reinterviewed 696 women from the 1981 sample (85% completion among women not deceased and not incapacitated), plus a new sample of 403 women aged 21 to 30 (91% of those eligible), again stratified to oversample moderate-to-heavy drinkers. Weighting of responses compensated for oversampling moderate-to-heavy drinkers and for variations in nonresponse rates. The analyses reported below are based on sample sizes reduced to correct for design effects of sampling.

The 1981 and 1991 surveys asked identical questions about (1) typical frequency and quantity of beer, wine, and liquor consumption in the past 30 days; (2) frequency in the past 12 months of (a) having six or more drinks in a day, and (b) drinking enough to feel drunk; and (3) lifetime and 12-month experience of drinking-related problems and symptoms of alcohol dependence. Other questions asked about drinking attitudes, contexts, and companions, and about many possible antecedents and consequences of drinking behavior. More information about the 1981, 1986, and 1991 surveys is provided elsewhere.[5,9,14]

1.3.2. 1981–1991 Comparisons. Comparisons between the 1981 and 1991 national samples used 10-year age groups instead of the 15-year age groups in the 1971–1991 trend analyses, to avoid overlaps of comparison groups. The 1981–1991 comparisons in Table II show declines in some but not all aspects of women's drinking. In five age groups, the percentages of women who abstained from alcohol did not change significantly between 1981 and 1991. The apparent increase in abstention suggested by the trend analyses might be an artifact of measurement differences across surveys, or the result of a peak in women's drinking after 1981, or a change as yet too small and too unstable to be statistically significant. A clearer pattern was that the percentages of all women who were heavy drinkers (averaging one or more ounces of ethanol per day) were consistently lower in 1991 than in 1981 in all age groups, although the decline was statistically significant only for women in their 40s.

Among women *drinkers* in five age groups (Table III), some drinking patterns declined between 1981 and 1991 while others did not. There were no consistent changes in the rates of reporting drinking-related problems or alcohol-dependence symptoms, although women aged 21 to 30 were significantly less likely to report drinking-related problems in 1991. Women drinkers did drink less frequently in 1991 in all five age groups, with significant declines among women in their 30s, 40s, and 60s. Women drinkers also typically had fewer drinks per drinking day in 1991, a decline significant for women in their 20s and 40s. Four of five age groups reported fewer occasions of having six or more drinks in 1991, a decline significant in all age groups

Table II. 1981 and 1991 Drinking Patterns among Women of the Same Age

Age range	Percent of all women abstaining	Percent of all women who are heavy drinkers[a]	(N)
21–30			
1981	24.3	6.8	(275)
1991	27.1	4.4	(405)
31–40			
1981	29.8	4.2	(194)
1991	31.1	3.5	(235)
41–50			
1981	32.8	9.9	(147)
1991	33.6	2.3[b]	(162)
51–60			
1981	44.5	5.2	(132)
1991	49.1	1.4	(122)
61–70			
1981	64.0	4.1	(104)
1991	60.1	1.1	(99)

NOTE: Percentages are based on weighted responses. Ns are actual numbers of respondents in each age group. Numbers of respondents in their 70s and 80s were too small for reliable comparisons.
[a]Average consumption of one ounce ethanol (2 standard drinks) or more per day.
[b]$p < .05$, one-tailed t-test.

under 50. In contrast, feeling drunk became *more* prevalent in four of five age groups, particularly among women under 40. Reporting fewer heavy drinking episodes but more occasions of feeling drunk may not be paradoxical, if public education campaigns and cultural changes have made women more aware of the intoxicating effects of alcohol, and if this awareness may be curtailing heavier consumption.

Comparisons of the 1981 and 1991 surveys lead to four general conclusions: (1) Women's drinking declined during the 1980s in ways that are not simply artifacts of measurement. (2) Some drinking patterns declined more than others; changes in women's drinking cannot be detected solely from rates of abstinence or volumes of alcohol consumed. (3) Contrasting changes in rates of intoxication and episodes of heavy drinking among younger women suggest important cultural (and perhaps cohort) changes in how US women perceive drinking and the effects of alcohol. (4) Any declines in women's drinking during the 1980s have been neither as sharp nor as consistent as reported downturns in alcohol sales during the same period.[7] The possibility that declines in women's drinking may be later or slower than declines in men's drinking is discussed further at the end of this chapter.

1.4. Five-Year Stability and Change in Women's Drinking: A Longitudinal Analysis

Longitudinal analyses of drinking by individual women in the 1981 and 1986 surveys show considerable change in drinking behavior over 5 years.[14]

Table III. 1981 and 1991 Drinking Patterns among Women Drinkers of the Same Age

Age	Year	Frequency >1/Mo.[a]	Quantity >1 Drink[a]	Days of ≥6 Drinks ≥1[a]	Days Felt Drunk >1[a]	Problem Consequences ≥1[a]	Dependence Symptoms ≥1[a]	(N)
21–30	1981	52.7	74.2	51.7	48.1	42.7	30.2	(238)
	1991	50.0[b]	67.4[c]	37.5[d]	55.8[f]	35.0[c]	29.7	(305)
31–40	1981	49.5	58.7	30.5	24.3	19.7	13.3	(162)
	1991	38.0[c]	61.9	24.7[c]	50.0[f]	25.0	14.9	(182)
41–50	1981	57.3	55.2	29.9	21.2	19.5	16.0	(116)
	1991	33.8[e]	38.5[d]	14.2[d]	19.7	13.2[b]	11.4	(124)
51–60	1981	52.3	52.6	16.6	14.2	11.3	7.1	(91)
	1991	44.3	49.1	20.5	24.1	13.4	7.2	(78)
61–70	1981	60.5	47.7	22.6	8.9	9.0	4.7	(58)
	1991	27.5[e]	36.2[b]	14.5[b]	9.1	7.5	2.6	(55)

NOTE: Percentages are based on weighted responses. Ns are actual numbers of respondents in each age group. Numbers of respondents in their 70s and 80s were too small for reliable estimates.

[a] In past 12 months.

[b] $p < 0.10$,   [c] $p < 0.05$,   [d] $p < 0.01$,   [e] $p < 0.001$, one-tailed, Kendall's tau$_c$ for the full ranges of drinking measures.

[f] $p < 0.05$, two-tailed, Kendall's tau$_c$ for the full range of reported days that respondents felt drunk.

Among the 157 women with no indicators of problem drinking in 1981, 11% reported at least one such indicator in 1986; among the 143 women with at least two problem-drinking indicators in 1981, 33% reported no such indicators in 1986. Over the five years, women aged 21 to 34 were most likely to develop some sign of problem drinking (27% of the 1981 nonproblem drinkers) *and* most likely to discontinue problem drinking (38% of the 1981 problem drinkers). Younger women's drinking also fluctuated more than older women's in meta-analyses of 27 surveys from 15 different countries[1] and in a 1984–1992 national longitudinal survey of three US ethnic groups (white, black, and Hispanic).[15] The changeability of young women's drinking may relate to more prevalent and more frequent changes in drinking contexts, drinking partners, and social roles (employment, marriage, and parenthood) during the third decade of life.

2. Subgroup Variations in Women's Drinking and Drinking Problems

Early research that compared drinking of women as a relatively homogeneous group with drinking of equally homogeneous men[16] has evolved into research on important differences among women. The sections that follow describe how women's drinking behavior is differentiated by age, employment, marital status, and ethnicity.

2.1. Age

2.1.1. Young Women. The 1991 survey data confirm that young women have the highest rates of alcohol consumption and alcohol-related problems.[5,6,17] Women aged 21 to 34 in the 1991 sample were considerably more likely (74%) to be drinkers (nonabstainers) than women in any other age group (Table I); rates of heavy drinking were also highest (4%) in this age group. Table II shows similar patterns for 10-year age intervals. Table III shows that women drinkers in their 20s in 1991 had higher rates of heavy episodic drinking, intoxication, and drinking-related problems and symptoms than women at older ages.

As in the 1981 survey,[5] younger women differed more from older women in heavy episodic drinking and intoxication (Table III) than in average consumption levels (Tables I and II). Younger women's greater tendency to have multiple drinks at one time may pose greater risks of adverse effects than older women dispersing the same number of drinks over longer periods of time. One adverse effect is alcohol-impaired driving. A recent rise of alcohol-related crashes among younger women[18] may reflect gender-role changes, with women more likely now to drive themselves to and from social occasions where drinking may occur.

2.1.2. Older Women. Despite low rates of heavy drinking and adverse drinking consequences among women over 60, older women's drinking is receiving increased attention for several reasons: (1) As the US population ages, a projected increase in numbers (if not rates) of older problem drinkers has stimulated general concerns about issues of alcohol and aging. (2) There is speculation that rates of heavier drinking among the elderly may rise as cohorts who grew up during Prohibition are replaced by cohorts who grew up after Prohibition was repealed.[19-21] (3) There is concern that the "triple stigma" of being female, elderly, and alcoholic[22] may make older women particularly likely to underreport their drinking and drinking problems.[23] (4) Alcohol may interact with other characteristics and behaviors of older women (e.g., reduced body fluids, osteoporosis, prescription drug use) to make drinking much more hazardous for these women.[24,25]

Several findings from the trend analyses and 1981–1991 comparisons address concerns about alcohol use among older women who learned to drink after Prohibition. The 20-year trend analysis (Table I) shows no recent increase in the percentage of women aged 65 or older who are heavy drinkers. Table III compares women drinkers in their 60s in 1981 (born in 1911–1920, with childhood/adolescent exposure to Prohibition) with women drinkers in their 60s in 1991 (born in 1921–1930, with much briefer exposure to Prohibition earlier in childhood). The post-repeal cohort (1991) shows *declines* in most categories of alcohol use and adverse consequences, with a sharp drop in the percentage of these women drinkers who drink more than once a month. Although numbers of cases are relatively small, these findings tentatively suggest that any increase in older women's drinking from growing up after repeal of Prohibition has not been large enough to outweigh more recent historical influences, which seem to be leading women to avoid or reduce high-risk patterns of alcohol consumption.

2.2. Employment

2.2.1. Paid Employment and Women's Drinking. Early research often predicted that paid employment would adversely affect women's mental health and increase drinking, particularly if jobs were combined with marriage and family roles.[26] Too many responsibilities (role overload) or conflicting role demands would hypothetically create stress that drinking might seem to soothe. However, research in the 1980s and 1990s has not found that women's employment and multiple roles increase risks of problem drinking. In most studies women employed away from home report higher rates of drinking (nonabstention) and/or more frequent drinking than homemakers, but the two groups generally do not differ in rates of heavy drinking or adverse drinking consequences.[27-29] Recent efforts to learn why employed women drink more frequently than homemakers suggest that differences are based not on stress[30] but on employed women's greater access to alcohol.[31]

2.2.2. Role Deprivation and Women's Drinking. Several recent studies suggest that having too *few* social roles is riskier for women's drinking than having too many roles. In our 1981 survey, women in certain age groups who lacked social roles (e.g., who were unmarried or had no fulltime work role) or who had lost roles (e.g., by separation, divorce, or the "empty nest") were more likely to report problem drinking than women with multiple roles.[32] Women in our 1986 sample were more likely to be problem drinkers if they had never married, had lost a job between 1981 and 1986, or had worked only parttime in 1981 or between 1981 and 1986.[14] Other studies suggest that multiple roles may restrain drinking behavior. Shore[33] found that business and professional women with more children drank less and had fewer alcohol-related problems. Hammer and Vaglum[30] found that women working fulltime consumed less alcohol if they had children. A New Zealand survey found that women were less likely to report alcohol-related problems if they had multiple social roles rather than just one or two.[34] Multiple roles may reduce use of alcohol because employment and family roles increase self-esteem and social support, or because greater responsibilities and performance demands, and increased social monitoring and feedback, may discourage drinking and reduce drinking opportunities.

Evidence to link role deprivation with increased risks of problem drinking is not entirely consistent. Analyses of our 1986 survey data[35] found that 1981 problem drinkers unemployed in 1981 who began working for pay reported more heavy drinking episodes and other problem-drinking indicators by 1986.[29] Clearly, more research is needed to learn which aspects of women's jobs and work environments (e.g., actual and perceived control of job demands, fulltime vs. parttime employment) may accentuate or reduce potential benefits of employment for women's drinking.

2.2.3. Nontraditional Employment. Drinking among employed women may be affected by occupational gender composition. In the United States, Wilsnack and Wright[36] found that women drinkers in male-majority occupations scored higher on a problem-drinking index than women drinkers in female-majority occupations. LaRosa[37] found that women in high-level professional or executive positions were more likely to be at least moderate drinkers than other employed women of comparable age and education. In contrast, Lennon[38] did not find significant differences in drinking among US women in traditional versus nontraditional ($\geq$ 60% male) occupations. Elsewhere, among women in a large national survey in Norway,[30] employment in male-dominated occupations was associated with more frequent drinking. In a Prague community survey,[39] Czech women in traditionally male occupations reported significantly more frequent wine and liquor consumption, and higher daily alcohol consumption, than women in other occupations. Finally, a large survey of women in Helsinki[40] found that women with more male co-workers reported more frequent drinking.

Additional research is needed to specify the drinking patterns most affected by occupational gender composition, and to distinguish effects of occupational gender ratios from effects of gender composition and status in work teams and work sites. Future research could also clarify *how* traditionally male jobs may affect women's drinking, such as through the presence of heavier drinking peers and increased drinking opportunities; stress related to a woman's minority or "token" status; obligations to conform to gendered occupational cultures that include drinking norms; and women's use of drinking to assert or express power in predominantly male occupations or work environments.

2.3. Marital Status

In US drinking surveys, rates of heavy drinking and drinking problems are highest among the never-married and the divorced or separated, lowest among the widowed, and intermediate among the married. However, age differences confound these patterns: the young are more likely to have drinking problems and to be never-married, while the aged are more likely to abstain or drink little and to be widowed.

2.3.1. Cohabitation. Risks of alcohol problems may be particularly high among women who are cohabiting (living with an unmarried partner in a marriage-like relationship). Cohabiting women in our 1981 survey exceeded all other marital categories in rates of drinking and heavy drinking; among drinkers they had the highest rates of intoxication, drinking problems, and alcohol-dependence symptoms.[41] In our 1991 survey, cohabiting women were again the marital category with the highest rates of heavy drinking, drinking problems, and alcohol-dependence symptoms. Longitudinally, 1981 nonproblem drinkers who cohabited were more likely than other nonproblem drinkers to report heavy episodic drinking in 1986, and 1981 nonproblem drinkers who subsequently began cohabiting had higher rates than other 1981 nonproblem drinkers on several 1986 problem drinking indicators.[14] Cohabitation possibly adds to risks of women's problem drinking by (1) creating stress (e.g., related to ambiguity, uncertainty, and lack of institutional support) that drinking may seem to relieve; and by (2) giving women partners who are more likely than husbands to model and encourage heavier drinking. Also, unmarried women living with partners may feel less bound by conventional social rules, including traditional norms restraining women's drinking.

2.3.2. Divorce and Separation. In most US surveys, divorced or separated women have had higher rates of heavy drinking and/or adverse drinking consequences than married women.[5,26,42,43] This pattern must be interpreted with some caution for at least three reasons: (1) Studies of nonwhite women have not consistently replicated these patterns[44–46]; (2) two national surveys in the mid to late 1980s[17,47] found less pronounced differences between divorced/separated and married women than in most earlier surveys, raising the possibility that historical changes have weakened associations between divorce and women's drinking[48,49]; and (3) cross-sectional data in most surveys cannot distinguish to what extent women's drinking is a cause, effect, or accompaniment of marital dissolution.

In three *longitudinal* studies, divorce predicted later increases in drinking: (1) a macroeconomic analysis (not gender-specific) of US divorce rates and alcohol consumption between 1933 and 1984[50]; (2) an analysis of national surveys from 1982 through 1988 that found increased drinking among women aged 24 to 32 who divorced or separated, and decreased drinking among women who married or remarried[51]; and (3) a meta-analysis of 12 longitudinal studies, in which divorce or separation predicted increased alcohol consumption among both women and men.[52] A large British longitudinal study, however, found that heavy drinking predicted partnership dissolution: marriages and cohabiting relationships ended more often among female and male young adults who had been heavier drinkers at age 16.[53] Finally, in 1965 and 1974 surveys from Alameda County, California,[54] divorce was followed by more drinking among some women and less drinking among others.

Our 1981 and 1986 surveys suggest that the dynamics of divorce and drinking may differ for women with different drinking histories.[14] In bivariate analyses of nonproblem and problem drinkers, women drinking more heavily in 1981 were more likely to become divorced or separated between 1981 and 1986. Multiple regression analyses of nonproblem drinkers showed that the few ($n=11$) who divorced or separated during the follow-up interval were more likely to report intoxication and alcohol-dependence symptoms in 1986, but the numbers were too small to be statistically significant. In contrast, among 1981 problem drinkers, divorce or separation predicted *reduced* alcohol-dependence symptoms by 1986 and near-significant reductions in intoxication. Divorce and separation were most strongly associated with remission of problem drinking among women in 1981 marriages characterized by a frequent-drinking partner and/or sexual dysfunction,[55] suggesting that the end of marriage may give some women an escape from stressful relationships that contributed to their alcohol abuse. It appears that marital dissolution can have several different relationships with women's problem drinking, depending on the marital and drinking histories preceding the breakup.

2.3.3. Unwanted Statuses and Women's Drinking. In the 1981 sample, risks of problem drinking were higher among women in "unwanted statuses," social positions they would prefer not to have.[56] An index of unwanted statuses included two employment statuses (involuntary unemployment, and employment the individual would leave if she didn't need the income), two marital statuses (being involuntarily unmarried, and being married with two or more indicators of marital distress), and two parenthood statuses (involuntary childlessness, and having children but feeling there were too many of them or that they were unimportant). Unwanted statuses were related to heavier drinking and adverse drinking consequences specifically among women who drank more than monthly and who had access to alcohol at home, and the relationships persisted after controlling for age, socioeconomic status, and prior anxiety and depression. Unwanted statuses did not predict problem drinking over the 5-year follow-up interval, perhaps because effects of such statuses are more rapid. Cross-sectional relationships between unwanted statuses and drinking behavior were *not* concentrated among the heavier drinkers, casting doubt on any hypothesis that unwanted statuses were more a result than a cause of problem drinking. Relationships between unwanted statuses and drinking were considerably stronger among women than in the smaller 1981 sample of men. Reasons for this gender difference require further research, but may include women's greater distress about the damaged social relationships inherent in many of the unwanted statuses.[57,58]

2.4. Ethnicity*

2.4.1. Ethnic Comparisons in Large Survey Samples. National surveys with large enough numbers of nonwhite respondents for comparisons of major ethnic categories generally find that non-Hispanic whites are most likely to drink, non-Hispanic blacks are least likely to drink, and Hispanics are intermediate.[8,59–61] In these three ethnic categories at all age levels, men exceed women in rates of drinking, heavier drinking, drinking-related problems, and alcohol disorders. With some exceptions, age, employment, and marital status have similar relationships to drinking within gender × ethnicity subgroups, although even large national samples typically have too few black or Hispanic heavy-drinking women for analyses of most demographic correlates of women's heavy or problem drinking. National surveys also typically have too few respondents from other ethnic categories (such as Asian-Americans and American Indians) to allow reliable prevalence estimates or gender comparisons.

2.4.2. Variations within Ethnic Categories. Research on ethnicity and alcohol use has been criticized[62] for using broad ethnic categories that gloss over heterogeneity *within* categories[63] and that overemphasize comparisons between minorities and European-Americans. One recent review[64] deals with these issues by examining differences within and between minority groups, in studies of drinking and alcohol problems of Asians and Asian-Americans, Latinos, African-Americans, and American Indians. In these ethnic categories (and all subcategories studied) men were more likely than women to drink, to drink heavily, and to have drinking-related problems. Drinking decreased with age among women and men in all ethnic groups. However, there was great variation within categories. For example, among Asian-Americans in Los Angeles, Japanese women were much less likely to abstain and more likely to drink heavily than Chinese, Korean, Filipino, and Vietnamese women; and going to bars or restaurants predicted drinking among Japanese women but not among other Asian-American women.[65]

Data on ethnic minorities from the Alcohol Research Group's 1984 nation-

---

* Throughout this chapter, the terms used to denote various ethnic groups are generally those used by the authors of the studies being reported.

al survey showed that men were much more likely than women to drink and to drink heavily in three Latino groups (Mexican-Americans, Cuban-Americans, and Puerto Ricans).[66] However, among the women there was ethnic diversity, with Mexican-American women reporting not only the highest rates of abstention but also the highest rates of heavy drinking and recent drinking-related problems. The 1984 survey showed that among African-Americans also, men were more likely than women to drink, to drink heavily, and to report physical, social, and behavioral problems related to drinking.[67–69] Heavy drinking by African-American women was more common among women who were unmarried and middle-aged (40–59), unmarried and not employed outside the home, or unemployed.

The most heterogeneous ethnic category in the United States may be American Indians, whose numerous tribal groups differ greatly in culture and in experiences with alcohol.[70] American Indian men drink more and report more drinking-related problems than American Indian women, but gender differences may be considerably smaller among younger Indian persons and in Plains Indian tribes such as the Sioux,[71–73] and may be decreasing in some Southwestern tribes where women's roles and drinking behavior are changing.[74]

In many nonindigenous ethnic categories women's drinking is strongly predicted by *acculturation*, the process by which attitudes, values, and behavior of immigrants change to resemble those of the society they have entered.[64] Comparing data from Japan and from Japanese-Americans in California, Kitano *et al.*[75] found that a 45% abstention rate of women in Japan fell to 26% among Japanese-American women, and that 20% of women in Japan but 27% of Japanese-American women were light-to-moderate drinkers. Mexican-American women show particularly clear acculturation effects; rates of heavy drinking in one study[76] were 4% in immigrants, 7% in the first US-born generation, and 32% in later generations. Acculturation may be more closely related to women's heavier drinking than men's.[76,77] The prevailing patterns of female abstention and gender-segregated drinking in most Asian and Latino countries make it likely that women from these countries who begin to adopt US gender roles and drinking norms will make greater changes in their drinking patterns than men will.

2.4.3. Drinking Changes among Whites, Blacks, and Hispanics, 1984–1992.
In 1992 the Alcohol Research Group followed up its 1984 national samples of ethnic minorities, generating the first national longitudinal data on changes in drinking behavior of different ethnic groups. The 1984 survey, which included representative samples of 1947 blacks, 1453 Hispanics, and 1821 non-Hispanic whites, found higher rates of abstention among black and Hispanic women than among white women, and lower rates of frequent heavy drinking among Hispanic women (1%) than among black or white women (both 4%). Rates of drinking problems were generally lower among black and Hispanic women than among white women or black or Hispanic men. Drinking problems were more common among younger or single white and His-

panic women, but age and marital status were not related to drinking problems among black women.[68,69,78,79]

The 1992 survey followed up all respondents who in 1984 reported (1) four or more lifetime drinking-related problems and/or (2) at least one recent occasion of having five or more drinks. A random sample of other respondents were also followed up.[15] Follow-up interviews were completed with 788 whites (75% completion), 723 blacks (68% completion), and 703 Hispanics (63% completion). Like earlier studies,[14,80,81] the 1992 follow-up survey found that drinking patterns fluctuated considerably over 8 years, for both women and men in all three ethnic categories.

Drinking declined and abstention increased from 1984 to 1992 in all ethnic categories, but more among whites than among blacks or Hispanics. Among women abstention increased the least among Hispanics (47% to 48%) compared with whites (31% to 36%) and blacks (46% to 51%); and Hispanic women abstaining in 1984 were more likely to begin drinking by 1992 (29%) than black or white abstainers (19% of both). There were fewer male frequent heavy drinkers among whites in 1992 (from 19% to 12%) but not among blacks (16% to 15%) or Hispanics (21% to 23%). The much rarer female frequent heavy drinkers changed little (4% to 3% for whites, 4% to 5% for blacks, 1% to 3% for Hispanics). These results confirmed earlier evidence of drinking declining more among whites than among blacks or Hispanics, from comparison of the 1984 survey with the Alcohol Research Group's 1990 national survey.[82] However, changes from 1984 to 1992 in drinking within ethnic categories were modified by other demographic factors. Drinking was more likely to increase among younger women and men in all three ethnic categories; among more educated black women (perhaps through association with employment); and among more acculturated Hispanic women.

Apparent ethnic differences in 1984–1992 drinking changes should be interpreted with caution. The 1992 follow-up sample analyzed by Caetano and Kaskutas included no respondents under age 26 (the youngest respondents were 18 in 1984), so results may have differed from national samples that included younger ages. Some of the ethnic differences observed might be due to aging of the sample; in previous cross-sectional analyses drinking decreased with age among white men but increased in middle age among black and Hispanic men. And if more of the whites than blacks or Hispanics were middle-aged or older, this would have made declines in white drinking look greater. Additional cross-sectional surveys with ethnic oversamples could help clarify to what extent minorities may be less affected by a general cultural shift toward decreased drinking.

3. Multiple Substance Use in Women

The focus here on women's *drinking* typifies a tendency of research to focus on women's use of either alcohol *or* one other drug, with only secondary attention to concurrent or alternating use of more than one substance. Separate funding agencies for alcohol research and for drug research, plus different legal issues and treatment traditions, encourage substance-specific studies. One result has been a neglect of research on the prevalence, causes, and consequences of multiple substance abuse in women.

Clinical evidence suggests that alcoholic women in treatment have elevated rates of drug abuse and dependence. In early studies, women alcoholics typically abused prescription drugs such as minor tranquilizers and sedatives.[83–85] More recent evidence suggests that concurrent use of alcohol and illicit drugs may be increasingly common among younger women in treatment for alcohol problems.[86,87]

Measuring combined use of alcohol and other drugs is underdeveloped for women in the general population. Surveys of substance use typically ask enough about both alcohol and other drugs to learn the prevalence of individual substances. However, questions are rarely designed to identify *simultaneous* use of two or more substances (e.g., drinking while smoking marijuana), *concurrent* use of multiple substances (e.g., using tranquilizers and alcohol in the same 24-hr period), or *alternating* use of several substances (e.g., using diet pills, alcohol, and sleeping pills at different points in a 12-month period).

Different combinations of drinking and other drug use may have different probabilities and histories among women in the general population. For example, drinking is positively associated with women's use of tobacco[88,89] and marijuana,[90] but may have minimal or even negative associations with the use of some prescribed psychoactive drugs (e.g., if tranquilizers or sleeping pills "substitute" for alcohol among some women, such as those objecting to alcohol use on religious grounds).[91,92] Certain substance use patterns (e.g., alternating use of a variety of substances at different points in one's life) may be stronger predictors of the *onset* of women's problem drinking, while other patterns (e.g., concurrent use of multiple substances) may be more predictive of continued or *chronic* problem drinking.[14] Closer attention to patterns of multiple substance use may discover whether different combinations and sequences of women's substance abuse have different antecedents or effects, and may require distinctive approaches to treatment and prevention.

4. Other Findings from Recent Epidemiological Research on Women's Drinking

Recent epidemiological studies have identified not only patterns and problems of women's drinking in the general population, but also a number of personal and environmental factors that may increase women's risks of problem drinking. While such variables are discussed in detail in other chapters in this volume, the epidemiology of some major social and psychological risk factors is summarized briefly here.

4.1. Influence of Partner's Drinking

Women's drinking is consistently, positively associated with the drinking behavior of their husbands or partners: in clinical samples of female and male alcoholics[93-95]; in general population surveys in Hawaii[96] and Norway[30]; and among lower-socioeconomic status Mexican-American couples[97] and Asian-American college students and their families.[98] Results of our 1981 national survey[99] found that husbands' problem drinking was not associated with how they perceived their wives' drinking, but wives' frequencies of intoxication, drinking problems, and alcohol-dependence symptoms were associated with their perceptions that their husbands drank frequently. Women may be more influenced by men's drinking than vice versa, if males are culturally given preeminence in defining drinking norms. A stronger effect of men's drinking on women's drinking may help explain, in the NIMH Epidemiological Catchment Area surveys, why older female problem drinkers were more likely to be married than older male problem drinkers,[21] if the women would be more likely to be involved in drinking partnerships.

Risks of problem drinking may be also increased by *discrepancies* between how women and their partners drink. In analyses of 1981 and 1986 survey data for married women, discrepant drinking patterns (e.g., a frequent-drinking wife and an infrequent-drinking husband, or vice versa) were associated with more adverse consequences of the wife's drinking than would otherwise have been expected,[99] and with several indicators of marital distress or dysfunction.[100] Discrepant marital drinking patterns were also linked with serious alcohol problems among *men* respondents in the 1977 wave of the Tecumseh County (Michigan) Community Health Study.[101] Mismatched drinking patterns between spouses may be a source, a sign, or an expression of conflict in the relationship. Therefore, women who drink very differently from their partners, as well as women involved with heavy-drinking partners, may merit special attention in alcohol education campaigns, marital interventions, or other prevention efforts.

4.2. Depression and Women's Drinking

Clinical studies find considerable comorbidity of alcohol abuse or dependence with other psychiatric disorders. Consistent gender differences are that depression is more commonly diagnosed in alcoholic women, while antisocial personality disorder and other substance use disorders are more common in alcoholic men.[102,103]

General population surveys also link women's drinking with depression. In a 1979 national survey,[104] alcohol problems were more strongly associated with depressive symptoms in women than in men, a gender difference more pronounced in those with more severe alcohol problems. Meta-analysis of longitudinal surveys from the United States, Canada, and Scotland[105] found that higher levels of depression predicted higher levels of alcohol consumption later on only among women. The reciprocal pattern also occurred: earlier alcohol consumption predicted later depression, with the relationship stronger among women than among men. Longitudinal analyses of our 1981 and 1986 surveys indicated that depression more consistently predicted chronicity of problem drinking among women who already had alcohol-related problems than it predicted initial onset of problem drinking.[14]

4.3. Sexual Experience and Women's Drinking

The recent growth of research on relationships between sexual experience and drinking behavior has included general population surveys, smaller questionnaire and interview studies, clinical investigations of alcoholics in treatment, psychophysiological and hormonal studies, and behavioral studies in controlled laboratory settings.[106] Detailed descriptions are provided elsewhere in this volume (see Chapters 9 and 15), but several contributions of recent epidemiological research deserve to be highlighted here.

4.3.1. Alcohol Expectancies and Reported Effects of Drinking on Sexual Behavior. There is ample evidence that both women and men *expect* drinking to have beneficial effects on sexual experience, although alcohol *physiologically* tends to reduce sexual arousal.[107–109] In both our 1981 survey[110] and our 1991 survey, approximately 60% of women drinkers reported that drinking reduced their sexual inhibitions. In both surveys, heavier drinkers were even more likely to report these positive effects, suggesting that such beliefs may be one motivation for heavier drinking among women.

Despite women's positive expectancies about drinking and sexuality, drinking may not have strong effects on their sexual *behavior*. For example, only 22% of drinkers in our 1981 survey said that they had ever become "sexually forward" when drinking, and only 8% reported ever becoming "less particular in choice of sexual partners." In an early longitudinal study of college students,[111] while a majority of female and male students said that drinking increased their sexual excitement, only 11% reported that drinking facilitated necking and petting, and only 1% reported that it increased the likelihood of sexual intercourse. Studies using diaries have failed to discover links between drinking and risky sex on specific occasions of sexual activity.[112,113] Such findings underscore the need for research on factors that modify how alcohol expectancies and consumption affect women's sexual behavior in specific situations.[114]

4.3.2. Sexual Orientation. Studies in the 1970s found high rates of alcohol problems—generally around 30%—among both gay men and lesbians.[115,116] However, many of the studies obtained their samples at least in part through gay bars, thereby overrepresenting heavier drinkers. The AIDS epidemic has led to well-designed probability sample surveys of gay communities, producing considerably improved estimates of alcohol use and abuse among gay men. In revised estimates, homosexual men are higher than heterosexual men on some drinking measures, but rates of alcohol abuse are substantially lower than in the earlier studies.[117]

Unfortunately, efforts to study gay men more carefully have for the most part not extended to lesbians. One exception is a large Chicago study[118] that included 748 women among 3400 gay respondents recruited from several community sources. In comparisons with a 1979 national survey, Chicago lesbians were not more likely to be heavy drinkers (9% vs. 7%), but were more likely to report alcohol problems (23% vs. 8%). In a 1984–1985 national study of health concerns among 1917 lesbians,[119] 83% reported drinking at least occasionally, 6% reported daily drinking, and 14% said that they were worried about their alcohol use. These rates are only slightly higher than rates for all women in our 1981 survey, and the small differences may result from higher educational and occupational levels of the lesbian sample. But in both the Chicago and national samples, lesbian drinking did not decline with age as it does among most women. In fact, daily drinking in the national lesbian sample *increased* with age, from 3% of women aged 17 to 24 to 21% of women aged 55 and older.

Isolation and alienation in response to homophobia and discrimination are thought to increase alcohol abuse in both lesbians and gay men.[115,120] However, data about risk factors for lesbian alcohol abuse are scarce. Among Chicago respondents who went to bars and expected drinking to reduce tension, measures of social discrimination and alienation were related to alcohol problems among gay men but not among lesbians.[118,121] Other risk factors for alcohol abuse in lesbians may include underemployment, a heavy-drinking partner, physical or sexual abuse, and relationship violence.[122,123]

4.3.3. Sexual Dysfunction. Problems of sexual adjustment may have a curvilinear relationship to drinking levels among women in the general population. In our 1981 survey, moderate drinkers (consuming 4 to 13 drinks per week) scored lower than lighter or heavier drinkers on an index of female sexual dysfunctions.[110] Social restraints or personal inhibition may affect both sexual functioning and drinking among women who drink little or nothing. Among the heaviest drinkers, drinking may be both an attempt to self-medicate sexual problems and a cause of worsened sexual difficulties.

Clinical studies of alcoholic women in treatment typically report elevated rates of sexual dysfunction,[109,124,125] but temporal sequences of heavy drinking and sexual problems are generally ambiguous. Our longitudinal survey data suggest that sexual dysfunction may contribute to the chronicity of women's problem drinking. Among women showing signs of problem drinking in 1981, a higher level of sexual dysfunction then was the single best predictor of continued problem drinking in 1986.[14] Furthermore, 1981 problem drinkers who divorced or separated between 1981 and 1986 were more likely to report remission of problem drinking if their 1981 marriages had been sexually dysfunctional.[55]

4.4. Violent Victimization and Women's Drinking

4.4.1. Physical and Sexual Victimization in Childhood. Recent clinical studies have found elevated rates of childhood physical and sexual abuse in histories of alcoholic women in treatment[126–128] and elevated rates of alcohol abuse and dependence in mental health clients with histories of childhood sexual abuse.[129] In one set of studies described in detail later in this volume (see Chapter 4), women treated for alcohol problems had higher rates of childhood physical and sexual abuse than either women in a general household sample or women without alcohol problems but receiving other mental health services.[130] Childhood victimization remained linked to adult alcohol abuse even after controlling for demographic characteristics and parental alcohol problems. These patterns suggest that physical and sexual victimization in childhood increase women's risks of later alcohol abuse in ways that are not explained by family histories of alcohol problems or by other background characteristics.

Data from our 1991 survey suggest that childhood sexual abuse is strongly associated with problem drinking also among women in the general population. Based on criteria for childhood sexual abuse from Russell[131] and Wyatt,[132] after controlling for age, sexual abuse before age 18 was significantly related to 1991 heavy episodic drinking, intoxication, drinking-related problems, alcohol-dependence symptoms, use of drugs other than alcohol, depression, binge eating, and vaginismus.[133,134] These nationally representative data, combined with clinical studies, support the conclusion that childhood sexual abuse may be an important risk factor for a variety of adverse long-term psychological and behavioral consequences in women.

4.4.2. Adult Relationship Violence and Victimization. Early studies of relationship violence and drinking focused on women's increased risks of victimization by intoxicated or alcoholic partners, particularly in treatment samples (e.g., of battered wives or abusive husbands).[135,136] A few clinical studies that examined women's drinking also found increased relationship violence when the woman herself was drinking and/or a problem drinker.[137] General population studies have found similar patterns for marital and other relationship violence[138,139] and for sexual assault and violent assault in general[140,141]: a woman's risks of physical or sexual assault increase when the perpetrator has been drinking *or* when the female victim herself is a problem drinker and/or has been drinking.

There are several possible reasons why women's drinking may increase their risks of victimization: (1) Men may perceive women who have been drinking as more sexually accessible and more vulnerable to dominance[142]; (2) women who have been drinking may be less alert to interpersonal cues that would ordinarily enable them to avoid or deflect conflicts with male partners; and (3) women drinking may seem to deviate from traditional femininity, and men may expect greater social tolerance for aggression toward women who are not acting conventionally feminine.[143]

Like childhood victimization, physical and sexual assault in adulthood may increase women's risks of subsequently abusing alcohol or other drugs. A recent national telephone survey asked 4009 women about their experiences of aggravated assault, sexual assault, completed rape, and homicide of a family member or a close friend.[144,145] Women with any such experiences were far more likely (6.6%) than nonvictims (1.5%) to report two or more alcohol-related problems. When victims were grouped according to whether they had ever experienced posttraumatic stress disorder (PTSD), victims of violence with PTSD were much more likely (14.5%) than nonvictims (1.5%) to report two or more alcohol-related problems. Although 54% of the victims reported a later age for their first alcohol intoxication than for their first victimization, better longitudinal research is needed to unravel the time-ordered relationships between violent victimization and women's risks of alcohol abuse.

5. Some Implications for Future Research

5.1. Time Trends in Women's Drinking

Although there is evidence that women's drinking has declined since the 1980s,[8,9,15,82] the declines seem more gradual and irregular than reported declines in per capita sales of ethanol.* This contrast may be exaggerated by inconsistencies in how surveys measured alcohol consumption and by reduced ethanol sales that are due to aging of the population and declining beverage alcohol content. If declines in women's drinking are in fact slower or more gradual than declines in men's drinking, this may suggest that changes in women's drinking depend partly on changes in men's drinking, a hypothesis consistent with the evidence on drinking influences between marital partners. Alternatively, smaller and more irregular changes in women's drinking might be the net result of two conflicting influences: (1) inhibition of women's drinking by growing health concerns, including awareness of hazards of excessive consumption; and (2) facilitation of women's drinking by expansion and diversification of women's roles, providing increased opportunities for women to drink. Careful testing of these hypotheses could help to determine to what extent the ability of educational programs to reduce women's problem drinking may be limited by environmental factors.

Any declines in women's drinking should *not* be interpreted as evidence that prevention has "succeeded" and that policy and research priorities can now be shifted to other problems. Because of persisting sexual double standards, cultural shifts in drinking attitudes and norms could carry with them

---

* Although statistical comparisons have not been made between alcohol sales data showing declining per capita sales in the 1980s[7] and declines in women's drinking as reported here, simple inspection of the patterns of change suggests that declines in women's drinking may be less consistent and more gradual than declines in alcohol sales during the same period.

decreased tolerance for women who *do* have alcohol-related problems, making it even more difficult for such women to acknowledge and overcome their problems. Thus prevention and treatment services for women could become even more badly needed if social changes make problem-drinking women increasingly deviant or isolated. Furthermore, efforts to learn more about the sociocultural *causes* of the current downturn in women's (and men's) alcohol consumption may eventually help us to control or modify rather than simply to observe long-wave cycles[146] in drinking behavior.

5.2. "Spontaneous" Changes in Women's Drinking Problems

Data from several longitudinal surveys indicate considerable fluctuation in women's problem drinking over time, with this fluctuation greatest among younger women.[1,14,15] Further longitudinal research may help identify specific factors that predict women's movement into and out of problem drinking. Such factors are likely to include changes in drinking environments, drinking partners, number and quality of social roles, and characteristics of women's marital or quasimarital relationships. Such research might be used to design specific strategies to identify and intervene with women at greatest risk for transitions *into* problem drinking and to nurture and strengthen those personal and social–environmental factors that predict movement *out of* hazardous drinking behavior.

5.3. Multiple Substance Abuse in Women

Because many women use alcohol in a context of current and past use of other substances,[14,83,88,90] it is essential to learn more about the causes and consequences of combined or sequential use of other drugs with alcohol. Women who abuse alcohol with no other drugs should be compared with women combining alcohol with psychoactive prescription drugs, and with women combining alcohol and illicit drugs such as cocaine or marijuana. Any development of gender-specific drinking measures may need research to determine whether to modify such measures to take into account effects of other drugs women are using concurrently with alcohol. Research is also needed to learn how women's habitual use of one substance may perpetuate use of another. For example, although women's concurrent use of tobacco with alcohol is well known,[88] there is little research on whether women's habitual smoking may contribute to the chronicity or relapse of women's habitual heavy drinking and vice versa.

5.4. Specific Recommendations for Future Research

Epidemiological research on women's drinking has made good progress in the past decade. Attention to gender differences in analyzing general population surveys has become routine (or nearly routine), and several large surveys have focused specifically on women or on issues specifically relevant to women (such as domestic violence).[139] Results of these studies suggest that future epidemiological research would produce the greatest benefits by focusing on three general issues: (1) subgroup differences in women's drinking, (2) how women's drinking changes and has changed over time, and (3) how women's drinking is embedded in contexts of personal relationships and psychological problems. Specific recommendations include the following:

1. Continued monitoring of *time trends* in women's drinking and drinking-related problems, to determine (a) whether the apparent recent downturn in consumption will continue, stabilize, or reverse, and (b) which specific drinking behaviors are undergoing the greatest historical changes in which subgroups of women. Research is also needed to learn (c) what societal factors have contributed to recent declines in women's alcohol consumption, and (d) what effects declining consumption patterns will have on social attitudes toward women who drink excessively.

2. Attention to unresolved questions about *how to measure women's drinking*. Such questions would include (a) to what extent gender differences in physiological alcohol effects should be incorporated into measures of alcohol consumption, and (b) to what extent measures of alcohol consumption should be adjusted for effects of simultaneous or concurrent use of other drugs.

3. Designing and analyzing survey research on women's drinking to detect potentially important *subgroup variations*, e.g., among groups defined by age, employment, marital or family status, and sexual orientation.

4. Continued attention to *ethnic variations* in women's drinking and drinking problems, including efforts to learn whether specific subgroups within ethnic populations (e.g., young Hispanic women undergoing rapid acculturation) may be at risk for increased alcohol abuse. Investigators studying ethnic minorities should be encouraged (a) to oversample heavier-drinking women within ethnic subsamples, and (b) to design strategies for obtaining representative samples of women from ethnic groups often inadequately represented in national surveys, such as American Indians and Asian-Americans.

5. Greater efforts to evaluate women's tendencies to abuse *multiple substances*. Such efforts might include (a) improved measurement of patterns of multiple substance use/abuse in both "alcohol" surveys and "drug" surveys, (b) analysis of antecedents and consequences of using specific combinations of alcohol and other drugs, and (c) increased communication and collaboration between researchers studying how to prevent alcohol abuse and researchers studying how to prevent smoking.

6. Continued research on relationships between women's drinking behavior and that of their *significant others*. Specific foci might include (a) how spouses or partners mutually influence each other's drinking, (b) discrepancies between partners' drinking patterns as a possible risk indicator for alco-

hol problems and/or relationship problems, (c) relationships between women's drinking and that of their co-workers (e.g., women in nontraditional occupations), and (d) partners' attitudes toward women's drinking-related problems.

7. Further research on associations between women's drinking and other characteristics of their *primary interpersonal relationships*, including (a) sexual adjustment and sexual satisfaction, and (b) relationship conflict and violence.

8. *Longitudinal research* on biological, psychological, interpersonal, and sociocultural predictors of when women are likely to move into and out of problem drinking behavior, with particular attention to predictors of "spontaneous" remission.

9. Use of survey methods to replicate and extend findings of *clinical research* on such possible risk factors as depression, problems of sexual adjustment, and sexual abuse.

10. Specific attention to *childhood sexual abuse* as a potential risk factor for women's problem drinking, including research on (a) possible confounding factors and mechanisms of influence, and (b) environmental and personal resilience factors that may help protect abuse victims from long-term adverse effects.

ACKNOWLEDGMENTS. Portions of this chapter are adapted from a paper, "Patterns and trends in women's drinking: Recent findings and some implications for prevention," presented to the Working Group for Prevention Research on Women and Alcohol, Prevention Research Branch, National Institute on Alcohol Abuse and Alcoholism, Bethesda, Maryland, September 13–14, 1993. The 1981–1991 national longitudinal survey reported in this chapter was supported by Research Grant No. R37AA04610 from the National Institute on Alcohol Abuse and Alcoholism. Other senior project staff are Albert D. Klassen, T. Robert Harris, and Nancy D. Vogeltanz. We are grateful for expert assistance from Perry Benson, Louise Diers, Loraine Olson, and Michelle Schumacher in the preparation of this chapter.

References

1. Fillmore KM, Hartka E, Johnstone BM, *et al*: A meta-analysis of life course variation in drinking. *Br J Addict* 86:1221–1268, 1991.
2. Fillmore KM, Golding JM, Leino EV, *et al*: Patterns and trends in women's and men's drinking, in Wilsnack RW, Wilsnack SW (eds): *Gender and Alcohol*. New Brunswick, NJ, Rutgers Center of Alcohol Studies, in press.
3. Fillmore KM: "When angels fall": Women's drinking as cultural preoccupation and as reality, in Wilsnack SC, Beckman LJ (eds): *Alcohol Problems in Women: Antecedents, Consequences, and Intervention*. New York, Guilford, 1984, pp 7–36.
4. Morrissey ER: Power and control through discourse: The case of drinking and drinking problems among women. *Contemp Crises* 10:157–179, 1986.

5. Wilsnack RW, Wilsnack SC, Klassen AD: Women's drinking and drinking problems: Patterns from a 1981 national survey. *Am J Public Health* 74:1231–1238, 1984.
6. Hilton ME: Trends in U. S. drinking patterns: Further evidence from the past 20 years. *Br J Addict* 83:269–278, 1988.
7. Williams GD, Stinson FS, Clem D, *et al*: Apparent per capita alcohol consumption: National, state, and regional trends, 1977–1990. Surveillance Report No. 23. Rockville, MD, National Institute on Alcohol Abuse and Alcoholism, December 1992.
8. Williams GD, DeBakey SF: Changes in levels of alcohol consumption: United States, 1983–1988. *Br J Addict* 87:643–648, 1992.
9. Wilsnack RW, Harris TR, Wilsnack SC: Changes in U. S. women's drinking: 1981–1991. Paper presented at the 19th Annual Alcohol Epidemiology Symposium of the Kettil Bruun Society for Social and Epidemiological Research on Alcohol, Krakow, Poland, June 1993.
10. Midanik LT, Room R: The epidemiology of alcohol consumption. *Alcohol Health Res World* 16:183–190, 1992.
11. Williams GD, Shaw-Taylor Y, DeBakey S, *et al*: Drinking status and knowledge of risks of heavy drinking: 1985 and 1990 health promotion and disease prevention questionnaire, National Health Interview Survey. Washington, DC, Alcohol Epidemiologic Data System, Cygnus Corporation, 1993.
12. Draper NR, Smith H: *Applied Regression Analysis*, 2nd ed. New York, Wiley, 1981.
13. Room R: Measuring alcohol consumption in the US: Methods and rationales, in Kozlowski LT, Annis HM, Cappell HD, *et al* (eds): *Research Advances in Alcohol and Drug Problems*, vol 10. New York, Plenum, 1990, pp 39–80.
14. Wilsnack SC, Klassen AD, Schur BE, *et al*: Predicting onset and chronicity of women's problem drinking: A five-year longitudinal analysis. *Am J Public Health* 81:305–318, 1991.
15. Caetano R, Kaskutas LA: Longitudinal changes in drinking patterns among whites, blacks, and Hispanics: 1984–1992. Paper presented at the Annual Meeting, Research Society on Alcoholism, San Antonio, TX, June 1993.
16. National Institute on Alcohol Abuse and Alcoholism: *Alcoholism and Alcohol Abuse Among Women: Research Issues*, NIAAA Research Monograph No. 1, US Department of Health, Education and Welfare Publication No. ADM 80-835. Washington, DC, US Government Printing Office, 1980.
17. Hilton ME: The demographic distribution of drinking patterns in 1984, in Clark WB, Hilton ME (eds): *Alcohol in America: Drinking Practices and Problems*. Albany, State University of New York Press, 1991, pp 73–86.
18. Popkin CL: A consideration of factors influencing drinking and driving by women. *Alcohol Drugs Driv* 9:197–210, 1994.
19. Dufour M, Colliver J, Grigson MB, *et al*: Use of alcohol and tobacco, in Cornoni-Huntley JC, Huntley RR, Feldman JJ (eds): *Health Status and Well-being of the Elderly*. New York, Oxford University Press, 1990, pp 172–183.
20. Glantz MD, Backenheimer MS: Substance abuse among elderly women. *Clin Gerontol* 8:3–26, 1988.
21. Gomberg ESL: Drugs, alcohol, and aging, in Kozlowski LT, Annis HM, Cappell HD, *et al* (eds): *Research Advances in Alcohol and Drug Problems*, vol 10. New York, Plenum, 1990, pp 171–213.
22. Rathbone-McCuan E, Triegaardt J: The older alcoholic and the family. *Alcohol Health Res World* 3:7–12, 1979.
23. Caracci G, Miller NS: Epidemiology and diagnosis of alcoholism in the elderly (a review). *Int J Geriatr Psychiatry* 6:511–515, 1991.
24. Dufour MC, Archer L, Gordis E: Alcohol and the elderly. *Clin Geriatr Med* 8:127–141, 1992.
25. Wilsnack SC, Vogeltanz ND, Diers LE, *et al*: Drinking and problem drinking in older women, in Beresford TP, Gomberg ESL (eds): *Alcohol and Aging*. London, Oxford University Press, in press.
26. Johnson PB: Sex differences, women's roles and alcohol use: Preliminary national data. *J Soc Issues* 2:93–116, 1982.

27. Parker DA, Parker ES, Wolz MW, *et al*: Sex roles and alcohol consumption: A research note. *J Health Soc Behav* 21:43–48, 1980.

28. Shore ER: Alcohol consumption rates among managers and professionals. *J Stud Alcohol* 46:153–156, 1985.

29. Shore ER: Drinking patterns and problems among women in paid employment. *Alcohol Health Res World* 16:160–164, 1992.

30. Hammer T, Vaglum P: The increase in alcohol consumption among women: A phenomenon related to accessibility or stress? A general population study. *Br J Addict* 84:767–775, 1989.

31. Shore ER, Batt S: Contextual factors related to the drinking behaviors of American business and professional women. *Br J Addict* 86:171–176, 1991.

32. Wilsnack RW, Cheloha R: Women's roles and problem drinking across the lifespan. *Soc Probl* 34:231–248, 1987.

33. Shore ER: Business and professional women: Primary prevention for new role incumbents, in Roman PM (ed): *Alcohol Problem Intervention in the Workplace: Employee Assistance Programs and Strategic Alternatives*. New York, Quorum, 1990, pp 113–124.

34. Romans-Clarkson SE, Walton VA, Herbison GP, *et al*: Alcohol-related problems in New Zealand women. *Aust N Z J Psychiatry* 26:175–182, 1992.

35. Wilsnack RW, Wilsnack SC: Women, work, and alcohol: Failures of simple theories. *Alcohol Clin Exp Res* 16:172–179, 1992.

36. Wilsnack RW, Wright SI: Women in predominantly male occupations: Relationships to problem drinking. Paper presented at the Annual Meeting of the Society for the Study of Social Problems, Cincinnati, OH, August 1991.

37. LaRosa JH: Executive women and health: Perceptions and practices. *Am J Public Health* 80:1450–1454, 1990.

38. Lennon MC: Sex differences in distress: The impact of gender and work roles. *J Health Soc Behav* 28:290–305, 1987.

39. Kubicka L, Csemy L, Kozeny J: The sociodemographic, microsocial, and attitudinal context of Czech women's drinking. Paper presented at the Symposium on Alcohol, Family and Significant Others, Social Research Institute of Alcohol Studies and Nordic Council for Alcohol and Drug Research, Helsinki, Finland, March 1991.

40. Haavio-Mannila E: Impact of colleagues and family members on female alcohol use. Paper presented at the Symposium on Alcohol, Family and Significant Others, Social Research Institute of Alcohol Studies and Nordic Council for Alcohol and Drug Research, Helsinki, Finland, March 1991.

41. Wilsnack SC, Wilsnack RW, Klassen AD: Epidemiological research on women's drinking, 1978–1984, in National Institute on Alcohol Abuse and Alcoholism: *Women and Alcohol: Health-related Issues*. NIAAA Research Monograph No. 16, Department of Health and Human Services Publication No. ADM 86-1139. Washington, DC, US Government Printing Office, 1986, pp 1–68.

42. Cahalan D, Cisin IH, Crossley HM: *American Drinking Practices: A National Study of Drinking Behavior and Attitudes*. New Brunswick, NJ, Rutgers Center of Alcohol Studies, 1969.

43. Clark WB, Midanik L: Alcohol use and alcohol problems among US adults: Results of the 1979 national survey, in National Institute on Alcohol Abuse and Alcoholism: *Alcohol Consumption and Related Problems*. Alcohol and Health Monograph No. 1, Department of Health and Human Services Publication No. ADM 82-1190. Washington, DC, US Government Printing Office, 1982, pp 3–52.

44. Darrow SL, Russell M, Cooper ML, *et al*: Sociodemographic correlates of alcohol consumption among African-American and white women. *Women Health* 18:35–51, 1993.

45. Taylor J, Jackson B: Factors affecting alcohol consumption in black women: Part I. *Int J Addict* 25:1287–1300, 1990.

46. Taylor J, Jackson B: Factors affecting alcohol consumption in black women: Part II. *Int J Addict* 25:1415–1427, 1990.

47. Health and Welfare Canada: National Alcohol and Other Drugs Survey (1989): Highlights report. Catalogue No. H39-175/1990E. Ottawa, Health and Welfare Canada, 1990.

48. Horwitz AV, White HR: Becoming married, depression, and alcohol problems among young adults. *J Health Soc Behav* 32:221–237, 1991.
49. Wilsnack SC, Wilsnack RW: Epidemiological research on women's drinking: Recent progress and directions for the 1990s, in Gomberg ESL, Nirenberg TD (eds): *Women and Substance Abuse.* Norwood, NJ, Ablex, 1993, pp 62–99.
50. Magura M, Shapiro E: Alcohol consumption and divorce: Which causes which? *J Divorce* 12:127–136, 1988.
51. Hanna E, Faden V, Harford T: Marriage: Does it protect young women from alcoholism? *J Subst Abuse* 5:1–14, 1993.
52. Temple M, Fillmore KM, Hartka E, *et al*: A meta-analysis of change in marital and employment status as predictors of consumption of alcohol on a typical occasion. *Br J Addict* 86:1269–1281, 1991.
53. Power C, Estaugh V: The role of family formation and dissolution in shaping drinking behaviour in early adulthood. *Br J Addict* 85:521–530, 1990.
54. Romelsjo A, Lazarus NB, Kaplan GA, *et al*: The relationship between stressful life situations and changes in alcohol consumption in a general population sample. *Br J Addict* 86:157–169, 1991.
55. Klassen AD, Wilsnack SC, Harris TR, *et al*: Partnership dissolution and remission of problem drinking in women: Findings from a US longitudinal survey. Paper presented at the Symposium on Alcohol, Family and Significant Others, Social Research Institute of Alcohol Studies and Nordic Council for Alcohol and Drug Research, Helsinki, Finland, March 1991.
56. Wilsnack RW: Unwanted statuses and women's drinking. *J Employee Assist Res* 1:239–270, 1992.
57. Bakan D: *The Duality of Human Existence.* Boston, Beacon Press, 1966.
58. Jordan JV, Kaplan AG, Miller JB, *et al*: *Women's Growth in Connection: Writings from the Stone Center.* New York, Guilford, 1991.
59. Colliver J, Grigson MB, Barbano H, *et al*: NHANES I Epidemiologic Follow-up Study: Methodological issues and preliminary findings, in Spiegler D, Tate D, Aitken S, *et al* (eds): *Alcohol Use Among US Minorities.* NIAAA Monograph No. 18, Department of Health and Human Services Publication No. ADM 89-1435. Washington, DC, US Government Printing Office, 1989, pp 411–423.
60. Grant BF, Harford TC, Chou P, *et al*: Epidemiologic Bulletin No. 27: Prevalence of DSM-III-R alcohol abuse and dependence: United States, 1988. *Alcohol Health Res World* 15:91–96, 1991.
61. Wilson RW, Williams GD: Alcohol use and abuse among US minority groups: Results from the 1983 National Health Interview Survey, in Spiegler D, Tate D, Aitken S, et al. (eds): *Alcohol Use Among US Ethnic Minorities.* NIAAA Monograph No. 18, Department of Health and Human Services Publication No. ADM 89-1435. Washington, DC, US Government Printing Office, 1989, pp 399–410.
62. Collins RL: Methological issues in conducting substance abuse research on ethnic minority populations. *Drugs Soc* 6:59–77, 1992.
63. Trimble JE: Ethnic specification, validation prospects, and the future of drug use research. *Int J Addict* 25:149–170, 1990–91.
64. Gilbert MJ, Collins RL: Ethnic variation in women and men's drinking, in Wilsnack RW, Wilsnack SC (eds): *Gender and Alcohol.* New Brunswick, NJ, Rutgers Center of Alcohol Studies, in press.
65. Chi I, Lubben JE, Kitano HHL: Differences in drinking behavior among three Asian-American groups. *J Stud Alcohol* 50:15–23, 1989.
66. Caetano R: Alcohol use among Hispanic groups in the United States. *Am J Drug Alcohol Abuse* 14:293–308, 1988.
67. Herd D: Drinking by black and white women: Results from a national survey. *Soc Probl* 35:493–505, 1988.
68. Herd D: The epidemiology of drinking patterns and alcohol-related problems among US blacks, in Spiegler D, Tate D, Aitken S, *et al* (eds): *Alcohol Use Among US Ethnic Minorities.*

NIAAA Monograph No. 18, Department of Health and Human Services Publication No. ADM 89-1435. Washington, DC, US Government Printing Office, 1989, pp 3–50.

69. Herd D: Drinking problems in the black population, in Clark WB, Hilton ME (eds): *Alcohol in America: Drinking Practices and Problems*. Albany, State University of New York Press, 1991, pp 308–328.

70. May PA: Alcohol abuse and alcoholism among American Indians: An overview, in Watts TD, Wright R. Jr. (eds): *Alcoholism in Minority Populations*. Springfield, IL, Charles C. Thomas, 1989, pp 95–119.

71. Leland J: Alcohol use and abuse in ethnic minority women, in Wilsnack SC, Beckman LJ (eds): *Alcohol Problems in Women: Antecedents, Consequences, and Intervention*. New York, Guilford, 1984, pp 66–96.

72. Weibel-Orlando J: Women and alcohol: Special populations and cross-cultural variations, in National Institute on Alcohol Abuse and Alcoholism: *Women and Alcohol: Health-related Issues*. Research Monograph No. 16, Department of Health and Human Services Publication No. ADM 86-1139. Washington, DC, US Government Printing Office, 1986, pp 161–187.

73. Weibel-Orlando JC: Pass the bottle, Bro!: A comparison of urban and rural Indian drinking patterns, in Spiegler D, Tate D, Aitken S, *et al* (eds): *Alcohol Use Among US Ethnic Minorities*. NIAAA Monograph No. 18, Department of Health and Human Services Publication No. ADM 89-1435. Washington, DC, US Government Printing Office, 1989, pp 259–289.

74. May PA, Smith MB: Some Navajo Indian opinions about alcohol abuse and prohibition: A survey and recommendations for policy. *J Stud Alcohol* 49:324–334, 1988.

75. Kitano HHL, Chi I, Rhee S, *et al*.: Norms and alcohol consumption: Japanese in Japan, Hawaii and California. *J Stud Alcohol* 53:33–39, 1992.

76. Caetano R, Medina Mora ME: Acculturation and drinking among people of Mexican descent in Mexico and the United States. *J Stud Alcohol* 49:462–471, 1988.

77. Caetano R: Acculturation and drinking patterns among US Hispanics. *Br J Addict* 82:789–799, 1987.

78. Caetano R: Drinking patterns and alcohol problems in a national sample of US Hispanics, in Spiegler D, Tate D, Aitken S, *et al* (eds): *Alcohol Use Among US Ethnic Minorities*. NIAAA Monograph No. 18, Department of Health and Human Services Publication No. ADM 89-1435. Washington, DC, US Government Printing Office, 1989, pp 147–162.

79. Caetano R: Findings from the 1984 National Survey of Alcohol Use among US Hispanics, in Clark WB, Hilton ME (eds): *Alcohol in America: Drinking Practices and Problems*. Albany, State University of New York Press, 1991, pp 293–307.

80. Cahalan D: *Problem Drinkers: A National Study*. San Francisco, Jossey-Bass, 1970.

81. Fillmore KM: Prevalence, incidence and chronicity among men as a function of age: A longitudinal and cohort analysis. *Br J Addict* 82:77–83, 1987.

82. Midanik LT, Clark WB: The demographic distribution of US drinking patterns in 1990: Description and trends from 1984. *Am J Pub H* 84:1218–1222, 1994.

83. Celentano DD, McQueen DV: Multiple substance abuse among women with alcohol-related problems, in Wilsnack SC, Beckman LJ (eds): *Alcohol Problems in Women: Antecedents, Consequences, and Intervention*. New York, Guilford, 1984, pp 97–116.

84. Curlee JA: A comparison of male and female patients at an alcoholism treatment center. *J Psychol* 74:239–247, 1970.

85. Mulford HA: Women and men problem drinkers: Sex differences in patients served by Iowa's community alcoholism centers. *J Stud Alcohol* 38:1624–1639, 1977.

86. Association of Junior Leagues: Summary of findings: WOMAN-TO-WOMAN Community Services Survey. New York, Association of Junior Leagues, 1988.

87. Lex BW: Women and illicit drugs: Marijuana, heroin, and cocaine, in Gomberg ESL, Nirenberg TD (eds): *Women and Substance Abuse*. Norwood, NJ, Ablex, 1993, pp 162–190.

88. Bobo JK: Nicotine dependence and alcoholism epidemiology and treatment. *J Psychoactive Drugs* 21:323–329, 1989.

89. Carmody TP, Brischetto CS, Matarazzo JD, *et al*: Co-occurrent use of cigarettes, alcohol, and coffee in healthy, community-living men and women. *Health Psychol* 4:323–335, 1985.

90. Lex BW, Griffin ML, Mello NK, et al: Concordant alcohol and marihuana use in women. Alcohol 3:193–200, 1986.
91. Carver V, Graham K, Lundy C: Older women: Their use of alcohol and other substances. Working paper prepared for Health and Welfare Canada. London (Ontario) and Toronto, Addiction Research Foundation, February 1991.
92. Graham K, Carver V, Brett PJ: Alcohol and drug use by older women: Results of a national survey. Can J Aging 14, 1995.
93. Dahlgren L: Female Alcoholics: A Psychiatric and Social Study. Stockholm, Karolinska Institute, 1979.
94. Fernandez-Pol B, Bluestone H, Missouri C, et al: Drinking patterns of inner-city black Americans and Puerto Ricans. J Stud Alcohol 47:156–160, 1986.
95. Jacob T, Bremer DA: Assortative mating among men and women alcoholics. J Stud Alcohol 47:219–222, 1986.
96. Kolonel LN, Lee J: Husband–wife correspondence in smoking, drinking, and dietary habits. Am J Clin Nutr 34:99–104, 1981.
97. Corbett K, Mora J, Ames G: Drinking patterns and drinking-related problems of Mexican-American husbands and wives. J Stud Alcohol 52:215–223, 1991.
98. Johnson RC, Nagoshi CT, Danko GP, et al: Familial transmission of alcohol use norms and expectancies and reported alcohol use. Alcohol Clin Exp Res 14:216–220, 1990.
99. Wilsnack RW, Wilsnack SC: Husbands and wives as drinking partners. Paper presented at the 16th Annual Alcohol Epidemiology Symposium of the Kettil Bruun Society for Social and Epidemiological Research on Alcohol, Budapest, Hungary, June 1990.
100. Wilsnack SC, Wilsnack RW: Marital drinking and the quality of marital relationships: Patterns from a US longitudinal survey. Paper presented at the 35th International Institute on the Prevention and Treatment of Alcoholism and Drug Dependence, International Council on Alcohol and Addictions, Berlin, Germany, June 1990.
101. Gleiberman L, Harburg E, DiFranceisco W, et al: Familial transmission of alcohol use: V. Drinking patterns among spouses, Tecumseh, Michigan. Behav Genet 22:63–79, 1992.
102. Hesselbrock MN, Hesselbrock VM: Gender, alcoholism, and comorbidity, in Wilsnack RW, Wilsnack SC, (eds): Gender and Alcohol. New Brunswick, NJ, Rutgers Center of Alcohol Studies, in press.
103. Hesselbrock M, Meyer R, Keener J: Psychopathology in hospitalized alcoholics. Arch Gen Psychiatry 42:1050–1055, 1985.
104. Midanik L: Alcohol problems and depressive symptoms in a national survey. Adv Alcohol Subst Abuse 2:9–28, 1983.
105. Hartka E, Johnstone BM, Leino V, et al: A meta-analysis of depressive symptomatology and alcohol consumption over time. Br J Addict 86:1283–1298, 1991.
106. National Institute on Alcohol Abuse and Alcoholism. Alcohol Health Res World 15:1991.
107. Goldman MS, Roehrich L: Alcohol expectancies and sexuality. Alcohol Health Res World 15:126–132, 1991.
108. Lang AR: The social psychology of drinking and human sexuality. J Drug Issues 15:273–289, 1985.
109. Wilsnack SC: Drinking, sexuality, and sexual dysfunction in women, in Wilsnack SC, Beckman LJ (eds): Alcohol Problems in Women: Antecedents, Consequences, and Intervention. New York, Guilford, 1984, pp 189–227.
110. Klassen AD, Wilsnack SC: Sexual experience and drinking among women in a US national survey. Arch Sex Behav 15:363–392, 1986.
111. Fillmore KM, Bacon SD, Hyman M: The 27-year longitudinal panel study of drinking by students in college, 1949-1976. Final report to NIAAA, Contract No. ADM-281-76-0015. Berkeley, University of California at Berkeley, School of Public Health, Social Research Group, 1979.
112. Harvey SM, Beckman LJ: Alcohol consumption, female sexual behavior, and contraceptive use. J Stud Alcohol 47:327–332, 1986.

113. Leigh BC: Alcohol consumption and sexual activity as reported with a diary technique. *J Abnorm Psychol* 102:490–493, 1993.

114. Cooper ML: Alcohol and increased behavioral risk for AIDS. *Alcohol Health Res World* 16:64–72, 1992.

115. Fifield LH, Latham JD, Phillips C: *Alcoholism in the Gay Community: The Price of Alienation, Isolation, and Oppression.* Los Angeles, Gay Community Services Center, 1977.

116. Saghir MT, Robins E: *Male and Female Homosexuality: A Comprehensive Investigation.* Baltimore, Williams & Wilkins, 1973.

117. Paul JP, Stall R, Bloomfield KA: Gay and alcoholic: Epidemiologic and clinical issues. *Alcohol Health Res World* 15:151–160, 1991.

118. McKirnan DJ, Peterson PL: Alcohol and drug use among homosexual men and women: Epidemiology and population characteristics. *Addict Behav* 14:545–553, 1989.

119. Bradford J, Ryan C: *The National Health Care Survey: Final Report.* Washington, DC, National Lesbian and Gay Health Foundation.

120. Underhill BL, Wolverton T: *Creating Visibility: Providing Lesbian-Sensitive and Lesbian-Specific Alcoholism Recovery Services.* Los Angeles, Alcoholism Center for Women, 1993.

121. Norris J: Alcohol consumption and female sexuality: A review. Paper presented to the Working Group for Prevention Research on Women and Alcohol, National Institute on Alcohol Abuse and Alcoholism, National Institutes of Health, Bethesda, MD, September 1993.

122. Hughes TL, Wilsnack SC: Research on lesbians and alcohol: Gaps and implications. *Alcohol Health Res World,* 18:202–205, 1994

123. Schilit R, Lie G, Montagne M: Substance abuse as a correlate of violence in intimate lesbian relationships. *J Homosex* 19:51–65, 1990.

124. Covington SS, Kohen J: Women, alcohol, and sexuality. *Adv Alcohol Subst Abuse* 4:41–56, 1984.

125. Schaefer S, Evans S: Women, sexuality and the process of recovery, in Coleman E (ed): *Chemical Dependency and Intimacy Dysfunction.* New York, Haworth, 1987, pp 91–120.

126. Miller BA, Downs WR: The impact of family violence on the use of alcohol by women. *Alcohol Health Res World* 17:137–143, 1993.

127. Rohsenow DJ, Corbett R, Devine D: Molested as children: A hidden contribution to substance abuse? *J Subst Abuse Treat* 5:13–18, 1988.

128. Russell SA, Wilsnack SC: Adult survivors of childhood sexual abuse: Substance abuse and other consequences, in Roth P (ed): *Alcohol and Drugs Are Women's Issues,* vol 1. New York, Women's Action Alliance, 1991, pp 61–70.

129. Pribor EF, Dinwiddie SH: Psychiatric correlates of incest in childhood. *Am J Psychiatry* 149:52–56, 1992.

130. Miller BA, Downs WR, Testa M: Interrelationships between victimization experiences and women's alcohol use. *J Stud Alcohol* Suppl 11:109–117, 1993.

131. Russell DEH: The incidence and prevalence of intrafamilial and extrafamilial sexual abuse of female children. *Child Abuse Negl* 7:133–146, 1983.

132. Wyatt GE: The sexual abuse of Afro-American and white women in childhood. *Child Abuse Negl* 9:507–519, 1985.

133. Wilsnack SC, Klassen AD: Childhood sexual abuse and problem drinking in a US national sample of women. Paper presented at the Women's Issues Related to Alcohol Abuse and Violence Conference, University of Illinois at Chicago, College of Nursing, September 1992.

134. Wilsnack SC, Vogeltanz ND, Klassen AD, Harris TR: Childhood sexual abuse and women's substance abuse: National survey findings. Paper presented at the American Psychological Association Conference, Psychosocial and Behavioral Factors in Women's Health: Creating an Agenda for the 21st Century. Washington, DC, May 1994.

135. Frieze IH, Schafer PC: Alcohol use and marital violence: Female and male differences in reactions to alcohol, in Wilsnack SC, Beckman LJ (eds): *Alcohol Problems in Women: Antecedents, Consequences, and Intervention.* New York, Guilford, 1984, pp 260–279.

136. Leonard KE, Jacob T: Alcohol, alcoholism, and family violence, in Van Hasselt VB, Morrison RL, Bellack AS, et al (eds): *Handbook of Family Violence*. New York, Plenum, 1988, pp 383–406.
137. Miller BA, Downs WR, Gondoli DM: Spousal violence among alcoholic women as compared to a random household sample of women. *J Stud Alcohol* 50:533–540, 1989.
138. Amaro H, Fried LE, Cabral H, *et al*: Violence during pregnancy and substance use. *Am J Public Health* 80:575–579, 1990.
139. Kaufman Kantor G, Asdigian NL: Gender differences in alcohol-related spousal agression, in Wilsnack RW, Wilsnack SC (eds): *Gender and Alcohol*. New Brunswick, NJ, Rutgers Center of Alcohol Studies, in press.
140. Fillmore KM: The social victims of drinking. *Br J Addict* 80:307–314, 1985.
141. Martin SE: The epidemiology of alcohol-related interpersonal violence. *Alcohol Health Res World* 16:230–237, 1992.
142. George WH, Gournic SJ, McAfee MP: Perceptions of postdrinking female sexuality: Effects of gender, beverage choice, and drink payment. *J Appl Soc Psychology* 18:1295–1317, 1988.
143. Miller BA: Women's alcohol use and the connections to violent victimization. Paper presented to the Working Group for Prevention Research on Women and Alcohol, National Institute on Alcohol Abuse and Alcoholism, National Institutes of Health, Bethesda, MD, September 1993.
144. Kilpatrick DG: Violence as a precursor of women's substance abuse: The rest of the drugs–violence story. Paper presented at Topical Mini-Convention on Substance Abuse and Violence, 98th Annual Convention, American Psychological Association, Boston, August 1990.
145. Kilpatrick DG, Edmonds CN, Seymour AK: *Rape in America: A Report to the Nation*. Arlington VA, National Victim Center, 1992.
146. Room R: Cultural changes in drinking and trends in alcohol problems indicators, in Clark WB, Hilton ME (eds): *Alcohol in America: Drinking Practices and Problems*. Albany, State University of New York Press, 1991, pp 149–162.

3

Older Women and Alcohol
Use and Abuse

Edith S. Lisansky Gomberg

Abstract. Although estimates of elderly problem drinkers and alcohol-related health problems among the elderly are approximate, there does appear to be a decline in the number of drinkers and the number of heavy drinkers. As with all age groups, there are fewer women who drink than men and fewer women problem drinkers. Moderate social drinking varies with health and income. Among older women, there may well be more problematic use of prescribed psychoactive drugs than alcohol.

In the few studies of older problem drinkers available, there are gender differences: Older men are more likely to be married, divorced, or separated, but older women problem drinkers show a high rate of widowhood; onset is more recent for older women than for older men; older women are more problematic users of prescribed psychoactive drugs; and the prevailing comorbidity among older women alcohol abusers is probably depressive disorder.

1. Introduction

The definition of "older women" to be described here will be 65 and over. The US Social Security system defines pensioners as 65 and over, and 65 has been traditionally the age of retirement. As is true of all population samples defined by age, however, there is a good deal of heterogeneity among older people. They vary in age; they may be young-old, old-old, or frail elderly.[1] They vary in health status,[2] marital status, income, and subcultural affiliation.[3,4]

There are also significant gender differences in the older population.

Edith S. Lisansky Gomberg • Department of Psychiatry, Alcohol Research Center, University of Michigan, Ann Arbor, Michigan 48104.

Recent Developments in Alcoholism, Volume 12: Women and Alcoholism, edited by Marc Galanter. Plenum Press, New York, 1995.

Women have a longer life expectancy than men. More than 75% of older men are married compared with 40% of women in the same age group.[5] There are more widows in the older population than there are widowers. More older women live alone than do older men. Older women have higher rates of poverty than older men.[6]

Older women who are not in the workplace and those who are working outside the home continue to have domestic role responsibilities. Such responsibilities include not only household maintenance but a continued role as caretaker of the sick and disabled.[7] Elderly women themselves may need care that may be given by a spouse, though it is more likely to be given by a younger female relative. Among women 65 to 74, 14% need assistance in self-care and home management; this increases to 26% in the next decade, 75 to 84, and to 48% of those 85 and older.[5]

To what extent are social networks and social supports significantly related to health and well being among older people? One social network index[8] includes marriage, contact with extended family and close friends, church membership, and other group affiliations, and Berkman[8] reports that the relationship between lack of social networks and heavy drinking is clearer among men than among women. In general, the repertoire of emotional responses among older people does not appear to be very different from that in other age groups; there are, however, indications that older people show higher levels of arousal when confronted with novel, stress-inducing situations, and take longer to return to baseline.[10] But there is little evidence of universal specific age-related crises.[11]

2. Use of Alcohol

By and large, the evidence is that social drinking diminishes, heavy drinking diminishes, and abstinence increases as people age. From the earlier surveys[12] to the most recent ones,[13] men and women are less likely to drink when they reach their 50s and 60s. In the 1984 survey reported by Hilton,[14] men and women drop in percentage of "drinkers" when they reach 60 and over; heavier drinking also diminishes and this appears somewhat earlier with women—in their 50s—than with older men. These population surveys have been cross-sectional but the same trend appears with longitudinal surveys; Fillmore and her colleagues[15] analyzed results of 39 longitudinal surveys from 15 countries and reported alcohol consumption to be lower for older people than for younger ones and lower for older women than for older men. A recent survey conducted by the University of North Dakota research group[16] shows 74% of women 21 to 34 to be drinkers; 64% of women 35 to 49; 52% of women 50 to 64; and 29% of women 65 and older.

There have been both epidemiological and clinical research challenges to the frequently reported findings of decline in drinking among older people. Glynn and his colleagues,[17] in a longitudinal study of male drinkers over a 9-year period, report that drinking habits remained quite stable over time. Their data indicate that while older men drank less than younger men, ". . . As the men in their fifties moved into their sixties, they did not reduce their alcohol consumption to amounts similar to the amounts consumed by men over 60 in the 1973 (first) survey." [17](p 110)

A community survey of healthy older people, 65 to 74 years of age, in northern California[18] found 90% to be "drinkers." Note that (1) this is a sample of young-old elderly, and (2) "drinkers" include people who had one drink in that last half year. The California investigators further report no association between gender and alcohol or psychoactive drug use; such association disappeared when analyses included simultaneously income, marital status, education, and gender.

2.1. Who Drinks?

Among older men and women, who is likely to participate in social drinking? Several studies show a relationship among the elderly of good health, social contacts, adequate income, and a sense of well-being with moderate alcohol use.[19–22] Older people living alone are likely to be abstainers, but it is also true that heavy/problem older drinkers are likely to be living alone.[23] It has been suggested that older women living alone are likely to be the abstainers and that older men who have alienated family and are living alone are likely to be the problem drinkers. But this is speculative: Some older problem drinkers are isolates, while others are embedded in groups of family or friends. The natural history of alcoholism must also be considered and the question raised: Was it isolation/loneliness that preceded the heavy drinking or did the drinking produce increasing distance from social networks?

Understanding the alcohol consumption behaviors of older people necessitates knowledge about the biological effects of alcohol on aging organisms. Similar amounts of alcohol produce higher blood alcohol concentrations in older persons than in younger ones.[24,25] The absorption and elimination rates are not affected by age, but the decrease in volume of body water does affect blood alcohol levels.[25] Some investigators describe a "greater sensitivity" among elderly drinkers but the conclusion of Dufour et al. is that ". . . old age per se is not a contradiction to moderate alcohol consumption." [24](p 138)

There is speculation about the increase in abstinence among older men and women.[26] Some reasons given:

1. A unique cohort effect, possibly experience with Prohibition and the Depression years, producing more abstemious behaviors. The fact that current aging persons show a higher proportion of drinkers than was true in the past gives some support to this explanation.
2. Effects of alcohol, for example, heightened sensitivity, discourages drinking among older persons.
3. Older subgroups are more characterized by the presence of acute and chronic illness which may discourage alcohol intake.

4. The drop in percentage of drinkers could be related to lower income, but this is difficult to separate from the fact that the elderly in poverty are very likely to be women who are less likely to be drinkers than men.

The question as to why women drink less than men, in smaller percentages and smaller amounts, is also open to speculation. Why do older women drink less than older men and less than younger women? One hypothetical explanation could rest on employment outside the home; the weakness of this explanation lies in the disagreements about women working outside the home and housewives and the relationship to drinking.[27] A more adequate explanation may lie in sex role acceptance. Older women are more likely to accept the traditional sex roles of wife and mother and, while the traditional role contains frustrations and distresses, it is true that it is less ambiguous and in some ways less strainful. There is still another possible explanation that could relate the smaller percentage of drinkers among older women to biological factors—to body distribution of water, to hormones, to biological vulnerability.

In one of the early national surveys of drinking, Cahalan et al.[28] pointed out that younger people tended to drink in larger quantities but less often and older people tend to drink more frequently but in less quantities. While this observation related to both sexes, a recent analysis does suggest that older women who do drink are likely to drink more frequently after age 40.[15] This is not an indicator of more heavy, problematic drinking but rather a shift in daily patterns of drinking. Younger women, involved in the dating/mating scene are more likely to be drinking at bars, parties, cocktail lounges, on dates, and so forth; older women who do drink are more likely to have 1–2 drinks daily.

2.2. Ethnicity

In spite of the multiethnic character of American society, little attention has been paid to ethnic subgroups and differing norms. A report of drinking by black and white women[29] shows a considerably higher percentage of abstainers among black women in all age groups by 30–39 (there are still more black abstainers in this age group but the black/white difference is modest). There is a sharp increase in abstinence among black women 40 years and older; a similarly large increase in abstinence occurs among white women who are 60 and older. Aggregate results show white women drinking more frequently and in higher quantities than black women; heavy drinking is significantly greater among white women under the age of 49, and after that the proportion of heavy drinkers is very low and similar for both groups. We know something of the history of alcohol use by the black population of the United States, but study of the norms and attitudes about drinking in black and white communities are lacking. Are differences to be explained by socioeconomic differences, by patterns of religious participation, or by regional variations?

There is some available information about ethnic minority use of alcohol[30] and some recent reviews about minority women.[31],[32] Of some interest is a report about Chinese-Americans[33] that suggests that they are more permissive about drinking among the elderly. Among Chinese older men, 51% reported lifetime abstinence; among old Chinese women, the percentage was 57%. Drinking by older persons, however, is tolerated ostensibly for health reasons. Yu *et al.* states that ". . . It may well be that at younger ages Chinese women do not drink, but at older ages the social acceptability of drinking makes many of them drink moderately for health reasons." [33(p 338)] It is possible that these norms will shift with assimilation. It is important, nonetheless, to understand that cultural values and family organizations are different in the many American subpopulations and that these values will influence drinking behaviors. Some subgroups are more permissive rather than less permissive about elderly drinking.

2.3. Summary

The evidence is strong that social drinking and heavy drinking diminishes as people get older, and the evidence comes from both cross-sectional and longitudinal study.[15,34] The extent of alcohol use among older people seems to vary with the state of health and income, and the evidence suggests that healthier, more affluent people are more likely to continue drinking as they get older. Such moderate drinking is likely to be social,[35] and the use of alcohol as escape from stress or a coping mechanism is not relevant for most older drinkers. Ethnic differences in norms about drinking need to be considered.

3. Use of Psychoactive Drugs

Are older women prescribed psychoactive drugs (sedatives, tranquilizers, etc.) more often than men? Are older women more frequent users of such drugs than older men? For more than 20 years, we have known that the answer was yes.[36] As summarized recently by Graham *et al.*[37] from a Canadian national survey, ". . . older women drink less alcohol, smoke less and use less illicit drugs than other age-gender groups. . . . older women reported the highest rate of psychoactive prescription drug use of all groups." (p 1) There are gender differences, too, in the source of psychoactive drugs: women receive more prescriptions; more men than women obtain such drugs from nonmedical sources.[38] It is of some interest that young women are likely to use these drugs nonmedically; among men, it is older males who are likely to use drugs nonmedically obtained.

It is believed that older people are more "sensitive" to psychoactive medication[39]; for example, the half-lives of most psychoactive drugs are extended. Of medications prescribed for older persons, most reports suggest that cardiovascular preparations and analgesics head the list, with sedatives and tranquilizers next in frequency of prescription. Although the older population constitutes 12% of the US population, they receive 30% of prescriptions. Problems do arise: drug interactions, noncompliance, and adverse reactions. Older patients are more likely than younger ones to experience adverse drug reactions, but it is not clear whether this is because of the multiplicity of drugs prescribed, relatively poorer health, or their increased susceptibility to adverse drug effects.[40]

Regardless of whether more older men or older women use psychoactive drugs, there is clear evidence that psychoactive drug use is more of a problem for older women. Older women are more likely than older men to be long-term users.[41] Data from the Drug Abuse Warning Network[42] indicate that people 60 and older are most likely to appear in emergency rooms in difficulty with nonbarbiturate sedatives, tranquilizers, barbiturate sedatives, and antidepressants; on all counts, the percentage of women appearing in emergency rooms is greater than the percentage of men. It is not only an issue for older women; at all points in the life span, women are reported as more likely to be users and abusers of psychoactive drugs. Use of psychoactive drugs among older women tends to be associated with widowhood, less education, greater religiosity, poorer health, higher stress, lower income, and less social support.[37] Substance abuse personnel need to be aware of at least two problems: the older woman who presents with the psychoactive drugs as her primary drug of abuse, and the older woman who may be abusing alcohol and who uses tranquilizers and sedatives in addition. A community study of women who used psychoactive drugs alone, alcohol alone, both drugs and alcohol, and abstainers who used neither found alcohol users and drugs users to be quite different populations: ". . . Psychotrope users . . . [are] subjectively more anxious, depressed, ill, and under greater stress than alcohol users."[43(p 998)] The same research group reports psychoactive drug users to be older, in poorer health, and less educated than abstainers.[44]

There are a number of associated sociopolitical issues. It is possible that physicians respond differently in prescribing for older men and older women, that the gender difference in health-seeking behavior becomes less as people age, or it may be that older men appear with depression and anxiety disorders more than do older women.[45] Older women are viewed at greater risk for iatrogenic drug abuse involving psychoactive drugs.[46] A study of the correlates of long-term regular use of anxiolytics showed regular users to be predominantly older women with ". . . high levels of emotional distress and chronic somatic health problems."[41(p 375)] A recent comparison of older men and women alcoholics (see Section 4.1) showed that when asked about heavy use of drugs like sedatives and tranquilizers, the women reported more dependence, more tolerance, and more withdrawal effects.

4. Abuse of Alcohol

On the basis of epidemiological and clinical evidence, it is generally accepted that older women are less likely to be heavy/abusive drinkers than men in the same age group or than younger women. Two questions are raised: (1) are we underestimating the extent to the problem among older women, and (2) what can be predicted for future cohorts? For the first question there is no clear answer, but there are hints that older women may be the most in-the-closet group of alcohol abusers. A recent report of male/female differences in liver cirrhosis mortality over a 25-year period[47] found increasing divergence in mortality rates by gender under the age of 55 but a trend toward convergence in those 55 and older. Estimated prevalence of histories of alcohol abuse are high for hospitals and nursing homes and examination/screening for women in these sites is needed. The interpretation is unclear, but in the clinical research on older men and women alcoholics described in Section 4.1, the easiest group to find were the elderly women who described a *past* history of alcohol abuse but had maintained sobriety for at least 1 year; the alcoholics in treatment were the next easiest group to find; and elderly women who were alcohol abusers but *not* in treatment were most difficult to find. As with all alcoholic populations, the prevalence will vary with the site: hospital, outpatient services, mental health facilities, senior services, nursing homes, and so forth. As for the question about prediction of future cohorts, it is a long distance from young adulthood to old age, but the fact that there has been an increase in the proportion of women who drink during the last decades leads many to predict future large numbers of older women alcohol abusers. The crystal ball is clouded, however.

A report of an epidemiological community survey[48] examined the relationship of the marital status, educational achievement, and income of 4600 respondents 60 and older:

1. Marital status. Alcohol abuse was highest among older men who were divorced or separated, i.e., who manifested marital disruption; for the older women, however, alcohol abuse was highest among the married. This seems at first glance to be contradicted by clinical reports.[49,50] Schuckit and his colleagues in an early study found 37% of older alcoholic women in a detoxification center to be widowed.[49] The Michigan study reported in Section 5 found 51% of the older alcoholic women in treatment to be widowed; in that sample almost twice as many older men reported marital disruption as older women alcohol abusers. There is a pattern that needs more research investigation of older women who drink with a spouse or companion, whose drinking continues when the spouse or companion die, and whose drinking is discovered at this point.

2. Educational achievement. In the community survey,[48] elderly alcohol abuse is reported to be associated with lower educational achievement.

3. Income. Elderly alcohol abuse is reported to be associated with low income. It is of interest that older men still in the workplace manifest more alcohol abuse than those not working; among older women, the rate appears to be higher among those not working—again the pattern of drinking at home with spouse or companion is suggested.

A recent survey of alcohol and drug use by older women in Canada[37] has some interesting findings on the reason given for drinking by current drinkers 65 and older. From most frequently cited to least, they include: to be sociable, to add to the enjoyment of meals, to help you relax, to feel good, to forget worries, and to feel less inhibited or shy. For women aged 20 to 64, the order is almost the same, but younger women more frequently cited the relaxing and "feel good" effects of alcohol, feeling less inhibited or shy, or forgetting worries. When queried about harmful consequences of alcohol, women of all ages cite physical health consequences most frequently, the younger women almost 2.5 times more frequently than the older ones. Negative effects on family and social life rank next, then effect on one's finances, and last, effect on employment. In all instances, negative consequences are reported by a considerably higher proportion of the women 20 to 64 than 65 and older.

While the percentage of drinkers and of heavy drinkers drops with age, those are aggregate findings. Some individuals maintain the same level of drinking, others may drink more. A number of investigations[51–53] have shown that for a modest proportion of elderly people there will be an increase in drinking (almost 4% of Akers and LaGreca's respondents and an additional 1.1% who first began drinking after age 60).[53]

This brings us to a critical issue: the question of early versus late onset. There is no other age group for whom this looms as a major classification of problem drinkers. There are controversies about the role or nonrole of "stress," about the therapies and prognosis for elderly problem drinkers who are early onset, i.e., have a long history of problem drinking extending back to their 20s, 30s, and 40s, and elderly problem drinkers who have manifested late onset. The term *recent onset* may be preferable because a 65-year-old client who began heavy drinking in his/her 40s has a 25-year history. In the research study described in the next section, we have defined "recent-onset drinkers" as those whose problem dates back 10 years or less. The relevance of early versus late onset for older women is evident in the general agreement that there are relatively more women problem drinkers of recent onset than men. This is consistent with a general finding about all male/female comparisons of problem drinkers: onset for females of all ages tends to be later than it is for the males of the same ages. This often appears in the literature as "shorter drinking histories" for women.

4.1. Abuse of Alcohol: Men versus Women

Schuckit et al.[49] compared 30 women, mean age 60.8, who were admitted to a detoxification center, and 44 men, mean age 58.7, admitted to an inpatient treatment program in a veterans' hospital. Comparing these two groups, the authors conclude:

> . . . many more men were currently married than were women. There was also a tendency for older women, as compared to men, to use more drugs especially . . . barbiturates, stimulants, and opiates. . . . the men tended to have an older age of onset for many alcohol problems than the women did. (p. 411)

The last finding was attributed to differences in the samples: for the older women, the first alcohol-related problems were public drunkenness and being fired from a job, suggesting a high degree of public visibility.

A more recent study[55] compared community residents between ages 55 and 65 who had recent contact with local medical centers. There were 509 men and 195 women, mean age for both genders 61.0, who reported one or more current drinking problems in initial assessment. Differences between the older men and women were: (1) the women consumed less alcohol and reported fewer alcohol-related drinking problems; (2) the women reported more recent onset; 46% of the women and 28% of the men reported their drinking problems to have begun within the past two years; (3) the women reported more psychoactive medication use, particularly antidepressants and tranquilizers; (4) the women were more depressed; and (5) the women were less likely to seek alcohol treatment.

5. The Michigan Study

The Alcohol Research Center of the University of Michigan School of Medicine is mandated for research on alcohol and aging. In connection with a study of factors that facilitate older alcoholics' entry into treatment,[54] data were collected from both male and female older alcoholics in a number of different treatment facilities. The question raised was whether the gender differences between male and female alcoholics in younger age groups occur or disappear when an *older* sample is compared.

Subjects. The respondents were men and women, 55 and older, currently diagnosable as alcohol abusers or as alcohol dependent. In this clinical study, subjects were recruited from a variety of sources: (1) referrals from substance abuse treatment facilities, (2) recruitment from a university hospital and veterans' hospital wards, (3) recruitment at meetings of Alcoholics Anonymous (particularly for a subgroup of older persons with a past history of alcohol abuse, currently maintaining sobriety), and (4) advertising and mailings to senior citizen groups and seniors housing.

Measures. Preliminary screening involved the use of a mini–mental status examination, a brief medical and a psychiatric inventory, and administration of the CAGE[56] and the MAST,[57] both widely used screening instruments. If there were indications of current/recent alcohol abuse, the screening was followed by two interviews, the Diagnostic Interview Schedule and an interview designed specifically for this research, covering life events, social networks, leisure time activities, drinking history, religious participation, and so forth.[58] Subjects who were alcohol abusers were interviewed, whether in treatment or not in treatment, but for present purposes only men and women alcohol abusers *in treatment* were compared.

The male/female differences noted in other age groups of alcoholics:

1. Demographics of education, employment, income, and marital status.
2. Report of a family history positive for alcoholism.
3. Drinking history: first drink, first intoxication, first problem (age at onset).
4. Heavy/problem drinking in a significant other, most frequently the spouse.
5. Report of a specific stressful event as precipitant.
6. Drinking at home and drinking in public places.
7. Reported marital disruption.
8. Subjective effects of drinking: alcohol response.
9. Use and abuse of drugs other than alcohol.
10. Comorbidity patterns.

A discussion of the differences between male and female alcoholics appears in a current review[59] and the background of comparison for the older alcoholics in treatment presented here is drawn from this review.

5.1. Results

The mean age of the 83 males interviewed was 64.0; of the 41 women interviewed, 66.2. The difference was nonsignificant.

1. *Demographics.* Average educational achievement for the men was 12.6 grades, for the women 12.9 grades. The difference is nonsignificant, but it should be noted that it is more usual for women, particularly older women, to report lower educational achievement than men. Employment status differed significantly because twice as many men were working or temporarily laid off than women (28% and 12%) and almost one third of the women described themselves as "homemakers" (29%). Information on income was not available but there was a significant difference in current marital status: more older men reported themselves as married or separated/divorced. The first difference (more men married) probably relates to difference in life expectancies and the second difference (more men separated/divorced) to the longer drinking histories of men. Of some interest is the fact that almost three times as many women are widowed (51% of women, 18% of men). Although marital disruption is reported more frequently by all age groups of women in

treatment than by men, the patterns of marital disruption are different for the older population, modified by differences in the life span, by duration of drinking history, and possibly by gender difference in availability of remarriage.

2. *Report of a family history positive for alcoholism.* In clinical populations, women alcoholics report positive family history more frequently than do male alcoholics.[60],[61] In the older sample of alcoholics in treatment, gender differences are not significant but the women report more drinking problems among fathers, mothers and siblings:

Drinking problems	Men	Women
Fathers	26%	36%
Mothers	2%	12%
Siblings	33%	49%

3. *Drinking history.* Consistent with observations made in all age groups of alcoholics,[62],[63] the older women report their first drink at 16.9 years, the men at 13.6 years; the difference is significant ($p = 0.007$). Age at which first problem appears is also significantly different and consistent with the literature on all age groups: 46.2 for the older women and 27.0 for the older men ($p = 0.0001$). This indicates that women alcoholics in *all* age groups present for treatment with a shorter duration of alcohol abuse.

Gender difference in the age of onset among older problem drinkers has a number of important implications (Table I). In gerontological alcohol studies, the debate about early versus later development of problem drinking has not touched upon possible gender differences in such development. There is an accumulating body of evidence that later onset is more characteristic of older women problem drinkers, e.g., the national epidemiological study that includes the diagnosis of current and lifetime alcohol abuse and depen-

Table I. Older Male and Female Alcoholics in Treatment: Gender Comparison[a]

	Male ($n = 83$)	Female ($n = 41$)	p
Age at first drink	13.6 years	16.9 years	0.007
Age at first problem	27.0 years	46.2 years	0.0001
Onset before age 30	70%	17%	
Onset age 40 or older	12%	71%	
Problem onset within the last 10 years	4%	38%	<0.005

[a]NIAAA Grant 1P50 AA07378.

dence[67] presents the percentage of late- versus early-onset drinkers among elderly respondents and notes,

> . . . Among elderly alcoholics reporting problems within the last six months, less than a third of the males reported onset at age 40 or later. In contrast, more than half the females reported late onset. (p 235)

4. *Heavy problem drinking in a significant other.* The likelihood that problem-drinking women will have a spouse/lover who is a heavy problem drinker is greater than the likelihood for men and this has been demonstrated in both epidemiological[64] and clinical populations.[65] Differences between the older female and male sample in the current study are quite large: 36% of the older currently married women and 27% of those currently divorced, separated, or widowed report the spouse to have had a drinking problem. The figures for the older men are 16% and 6%, respectively. Gender differences are significant: for the currently married, $p = 0.034$, for those who are divorced, separated, or widowed, $p = 0.001$.

5. *Report of a specific stressful event as precipitant.* The information is ambiguous. Although early literature cited specific trauma as more frequently mentioned by women alcoholics than men,[62] this has been questioned.[66] There are other problems: the question of definition/measurement of elderly stress is not resolved,[68] and the trend of reports about the elderly is to negate a major role of stressful events as precipitants for elderly heavy drinking.[9] The question is an open one, but the high frequency of widowhood should be noted; an earlier study[49] reported 37% of older women alcoholic respondents to be widowed, the present study found 51% of the women to be widows, and the patterns of drinking with spouse followed by exacerbation of the problem after the husband dies has been described.[69]

6. *Drinking at home and in public places.* Since women are more likely to be at home, it is hardly surprising that more women alcoholics drink at home and that more men drink in public places. Of the older women in our sample, 29% reported themselves to be "homemakers." When older men and older women are compared, there are small nonsignificant differences in the proportion who report drinking at home and drinking alone: 89% of the men and 95% of the women drink at home and 52% of the men and 66% of the women report drinking alone. The differences in the report of drinking in public places are larger: 51% of the men and 27% of the women report drinking in bars ($p = 0.012$); 37% of the men and 5% of the women report drinking in cars ($p = 0.000$), and 24% of the men and 7% of the women report drinking in the workplace ($p = 0.024$). The gender difference in private/public context of the drinking seems to hold throughout the life span.

7. *Reported marital disruption.* As discussed above, the literature reports marital disruption more frequent among women in treatment than by men in treatment. There has been some speculation about whether the drinking or the marital disruption comes first. A recent epidemiological report[70] finds that

among women identified as problem drinkers in a 1981 survey, divorce or separation was followed by a reduction in problem drinking when the women were reinterviewed 5 years later. When we compare the clinical sample of elderly men and women alcoholics in treatment, almost twice as many men report divorce or separation than women (31% and 17%). It is in the status of widowhood that the women exceed the men (51% and 18%). We have suggested that the pattern of marital disruption is different among older people than those 60 and younger; the relatively higher mortality of males in the young-old group and the potential for remarriage are two significant influences and might produce a higher degree of marital disruption, defined broadly, among older women than among older men. The 1985 statistical reports show 77% of older men married compared with 40% of older women.[5] The term *marital disruption* needs redefinition and perhaps modification for different age groups.

8. *Subjective effects of drinking: alcohol response.* There are differences in the report of alcohol effects by the older men and women. By and large, women report becoming more depressed when drinking and the men are more likely to report positively about alcohol effects (Table II). Interestingly, the older men say they get on better with "people" when drinking but they also report more family conflict. The lack of gender difference in expression of anger is of interest: both older men and older women report losing temper and fighting in similar numbers.

9. *Use and abuse of drugs other than alcohol.* In the discussion in Section 3 about the use of psychoactive drugs, the point was made that such use is more of a problem for older women than for older men. The present data bear this out. The use of marijuana and other illegal substances is very limited in the sample of older alcoholics but within these small numbers, there are more males (Table III). When it comes to legal, prescribed substances, women present more drug problem. It is of interest that when asked whether a physi-

Table II. Older Male and Female Alcoholics in Treatment: Gender Comparison[a]

Effects of drinking: Self report	Male ($n = 83$)	Female ($n = 41$)	p
Feel miserable	22%	39%	<0.05
Get more depressed	37%	56%	<0.05
Feel increasingly lonely	47%	61%	
Falls/hurt myself	49%	71%	<0.05
Get along better with people	57%	30%	<0.01
Quarrels with family	57%	37%	<0.05
Lose my temper	30%	34%	
Get into fights	10%	10%	

[a]NIAAA Grant 1P50 AA07378.

Table III. Older Male and Female Alcoholics in Treatment: Gender Comparison for Drugs Other Than Alcohol[a]

	Male (n = 50)	Female (n = 23)	p
1. Have you ever used a tranquilizer every day for two weeks or more?	38%	74%	0.003
2. Felt dependent, unable to keep from using them	23%	53%	0.041
3. Tolerance, needed larger amounts to get effect	7%	37%	0.013
4. Been high on drugs while working or taking care of children	0	11%	0.085

[a]NIAAA Grant 1P50 AA07378.

cian had prescribed a tranquilizer, sedative, pain pill, antidepressant, or headache medicine, exactly the same proportion of men and women replied that they had had such prescriptions: 70%. Whatever the reasons for the female heavier use of prescribed psychoactive drugs, gender difference in physicians' prescription does not appear to be an explanation. Heavier and more problematic use of such prescribed drugs appears in a significantly larger proportion of users among women, and signs of drug dependence are reported by significantly more women than men. The sample size is small but the results are consistent with national survey data; the report of Mellinger et al[41] in 1984 was of "long-term regular use of anxiolytics," and the authors reported a preponderance of women who were long-term regular users: ". . . [they] tend to be older persons with high levels of emotional distress and chronic somatic health problems" (p 375). This survey concluded that most long-term users were being monitored by their physicians; but whether that applies to older men and women alcoholics is a question.

10. *Comorbidity patterns.* There are two questions: gender differences in the presence of comorbidity and gender differences in codiagnoses. The trend of evidence is that, other things being equal, women problem drinkers show a diagnosable psychiatric disorder more often than men, and one study reports 44% of the male alcoholics with a second diagnosis compared with 65% of female alcoholics.[71] The reports on diagnosis are consistent: affective disorder occurs more frequently among female alcoholics and antisocial personality occurs more frequently among male alcoholics.[59]

While the data on the older men and women alcoholics do not include an official codiagnosis, there are many indications that the same gender differences in comorbidity appear in the older group: (1) the older women subjects describe the effects of alcohol as making them feel "more depressed," and (2) if antisocial personality is defined, in part by early onset, the men's report of first problem with alcohol appearing for 26% during adolescence (ages 13 to 18) and another 44% during their 20s certainly suggests alcohol-related and possibly other deviance difficulties early in life.

5.2. Discussion

Two studies that have compared older men and women alcoholics[49],[55] may be compared with present findings and there are several points on which there is good agreement:

1. Older women are more likely to be using psychoactive drugs (in addition to alcohol) and in larger quantities; the women's report of dependence symptoms confirms this as a problem to be considered in dealing with older female problem drinkers.

2. Two of the three studies agree in reporting more of the older men as currently married, divorced, or separated from a spouse; older women alcoholics who reach treatment seem more likely to be widowed: 37% of the Schuckit, Morrissey, and O'Leary[49] sample and 51% of the respondents in the Michigan study.[54] For the elderly women studied in alcoholism treatment settings, there appears to be a distinguishable pattern that suggests drinking with a spouse or significant other, to widowhood, after which the drinking continues or increases.

3. Two of the three studies agree in reporting more recent onset for older women alcoholics than for men. Since that finding is also supported by epidemiological data,[67] it is recommended that prevention strategies directed toward older problem drinkers should be targeted to women in their 50s and 60s.

4. Two of the three studies suggest that the major comorbidity of older women problem drinkers is depressive disorder. This is consistent with other age groups of women problem drinkers.

6. Conclusions

The size of the problem, that is, the number of older problem drinkers in the population is, at best, an estimate. Numbers will vary tremendously depending on whether one looks at a general population sample or hospital wards. The Epidemiological Catchment Area studies of the National Institute of Mental Health reported a lifetime prevalence of alcohol abuse and alcoholism in men 60 and older to be 3.3% and in women of the same age 0.4%.[67] Often reported, particularly in the popular literature is between 2 and 10% apparently derived from a mix of community surveys and institutional studies.[72] A recent analysis of alcohol-related hospitalizations of elderly people points up the fact that although elderly use and abuse of alcohol declines, rates of alcohol-related diagnoses among hospitalized persons remain high in the elderly group. [73(p 1224)]

Some of the common symptoms of alcohol problems in the elderly are described in a discussion of evaluation.[74] There are screening instruments, both old and new, but for those dealing with elderly persons, indicators of health problems, behavior changes, confusion, and falls suggest a need for evaluation. Withdrawal and self-neglect also suggest problems.

Finally, when the effects of alcohol on the elderly organism are considered, is it advisable for older persons to drink at all? The general consensus of those who report on alcohol and the elderly is to advise moderate intake,[74],[75] and indeed, as Lamy comments, "Reasonably small and controlled alcohol intake may be of benefit to the elderly, as it may stimulate appetite, increase socialization, and may play a "protective" role against coronary artery disease." [75(p 10)]

References

1. Neugarten BL: The psychology of aging: An overview. Journal Supplement Abstract Service of the American Psychological Association, MS 1340, 1976.
2. Rowe JW, Kahn RL: Human aging: Usual and successful. *Science* 237:143–148, 1987.
3. Jackson JJ: Race, national origin, ethnicity and aging, in Binstock RH, Shanas E (eds): *Handbook of Aging and the Social Sciences*, 2nd ed. New York: Van Nostrand, 1985, pp 000.
4. Gelfand DE, Barresi CM (eds): *Ethnic Dimensions of Aging*. New York: Springer, 1987.
5. *A Profile of Older Americans*. Program Resources Department, American Association of Retired Persons and the Administration on Aging. HHS PF 3049 (1086) D 996, 1986.
6. *Old, Alone and Poor: A Plan for Reducing Poverty among Elderly People Living Alone*. Baltimore: The Commonwealth Fund Commission on Elderly People Living Alone, 1987.
7. Exploding the Myth: Caregiving in America. Study of the Subcommittee on Human Services of the Select Committee on Aging. House of Representatives, One Hundredth Congress, Publ. No. 99-611. 1987.
8. Berkman LF: Stress, social networks and aging, in Gottheil E, Druley KA, Skoloda TE, Waxman HM (eds): *The Combined Problems of Alcoholics, Drug Addiction and Aging*. Springfield, IL: Thomas, 1985, pp 14–35.
9. Welte JW, Mirand AL: Alcohol use by the elderly: Patterns and correlates. A Report on the Erie County Elder Drinking Survey Buffalo: Research Institute on Addictions, 1992.
10. Schultz R: Emotion and affect, in Birren JE, Schaie KW (eds): *Handbook of the Psychology of Aging*. New York, Van Nostrand, 1985, pp 531–543.
11. Costa PT Jr, McCrae RR: Still stable after all these years: Personality as a key to some issues in adulthood and old age, in Baltes PB, Brim OG (eds): *Life-Span Development and Behavior*. New York: Academic Press, 1980, pp 000.
12. Riley JW Jr, Marsden CF: The social pattern of alcoholic drinking. *Q J Stud Alcohol* 8:265–273, 1947.
13. Clark WB, Hilton ME (eds): *Alcohol in America, Drinking Practices and Problems*. Albany, NY: State University of New York Press, 1991.
14. Hilton ME: The demographic distribution of drinking patterns in 1984, in Clark WB, Hilton ME (eds): *Alcohol in America, Drinking Practices and Problems*. Albany, NY: State University of New York Press, 1991.
15. Fillmore KM, Hartka E, Johnstone BM, *et al*: A meta-analysis of life course variation in drinking. *Br J Addict* 86:1221–1268, 1991.
16. Wilsnack SC, Vogeltanz ND, Diers LE, Wilsnack RW: Drinking and problem drinking in older women, in Beresford TP, Gomberg ESL (eds): *Alcohol and Aging*. New York: Oxford University Press, forthcoming.
17. Glynn RJ, Bouchard GR, Locastro JSM, Hermos JA: Changes in alcohol consumption behaviors among men in the normative aging study, in Maddox G, Robins LN, Rosenberg N (eds): *Nature and Extent of Alcohol Problems among the Elderly*, Monograph 14, Washington, DC: NIAAA, 1984, pp 101–116.
18. Huffine C, Folkman S, Lazarus RS: Psychoactive drugs, alcohol, and stress and coping processes in older adults. *Am J Drug Alcohol Abuse* 15:101–113, 1989.

19. Johnson LA, Goodrich CH: *Use of Alcohol by Persons 65 Years and Over*. New York: Mt. Sinai School of Medicine, City University of New York, 1974.
20. Goodwin JS, Sanchez CJ, Thomas P, *et al*: Alcohol intake in a healthy elderly population. *Am J Public Health* 77:173–176, 1987.
21. Guttman D: *A Study of Legal Drug Use by Older Americans*. Washington, DC: National Institute on Drug Abuse, 1977.
22. Branch LG, Jette AM: Personal health practices and mortality among the elderly. *Am J Public Health* 74:1126–1130, 1984.
23. Monk A, Cryns AG, Cabral R: Alcohol consumption and alcoholism as a function of adult age. *Gerontologist* 17:101–106, 1977.
24. Dufour MC, Archer L, Gordis E: Alcohol and the elderly. *Clin Geriatr Med* 8:127–141, 1992.
25. Vogel-Sprott M, Barrett B: Age, drinking habits and the effects of alcohol. *J Stud Alcohol* 45:517–521, 1984.
26. Gomberg ESL: Alcohol use and alcohol problems among the elderly. Alcohol and Health Monograph 4. *Special Population Issues*. Washington, DC: National Institute on Alcohol Abuse and Alcoholism. DHHS Publ. No. (ADM) 82-1193, 263-290, 1982.
27. Wilsnack RW, Wilsnack SC: Women, work and alcohol: Failure of simple theories. *Alcohol Clin Exp Res* 16:172–179, 1992.
28. Cahalan D, Cisin IG, Crossley HM: *American Drinking Practices*. New Haven: College & University Press, 1969.
29. Herd D: Drinking by black and white women: Results from a national survey. *Soc Prob* 15:493–505, 1988.
30. Spiegler D, Tate D, Aitken S, Christian C (eds): *Alcohol Use among US Ethnic Minorities*. NIAAA Research Monograph 18. DHHS Publ. No. (ADM) 89-1435. Washington, DC: Government Publishing Office, 1989.
31. Liepman MR, Goldman RE, Monroe A, *et al*: Substance abuse by special populations of women, in Gomberg ESL, Nirenberg TD (eds): *Women and Substance Abuse*. Norwood, NJ: Ablex, 1993, pp 214–257.
32. Gomberg ESL: Drinking practices and problems of women: The life span and ethnic groupings. Proceedings of the NIAAA conference on Women and Alcohol, 1993. Washington, DC: US Government Printing Office, forthcoming.
33. Yu ESH, Liu WT, Xia Z, Zhang N: Alcohol use, abuse and alcoholism among Chinese Americans: A review of the epidemiologic data, in Spielger D, Tate D, Aitken S, Christian C (eds): *Alcohol Use among US Ethnic Minorities*. NIAAA Research Monograph 18. DHHS Publ. No. (ADM) 89-1435. Washington, DC: Government Printing Office, 1989, pp 329–342.
34. Adams WL, Garry PJ, Rhyne R, *et al*: Alcohol intake in the healthy elderly. Changes with age in a cross-sectional and longitudinal study. *J Am Geriatr Soc* 38:211–216, 1990.
35. Busby, WJ, Campbell AJ, Borrie MJ, Spears GFS: Alcohol use in a community-based sample of subjects aged 70 years and older. *J Am Geriatr Soc* 36:301–305, 1988.
36. Parry HJ, Balter MB, Mellinger GD, *et al*: National patterns of psychotherapeutic drug use. *Arch Gen Psychiatry* 28:769–784, 1973.
37. Graham K, Carver V, Brett PJ: Alcohol and drug use by older women. Results of a national survey. *Can J Aging*, forthcoming.
38. Robbins C, Clayton RR: Gender-related differences in psychoactive drug use among older adults. *J Drug Issues* 19:207–219, 1989.
39. Kekich WA: Psychotropic medication and the elderly. *Top Geriatr Rehab* 2:45–53, 1987.
40. Stewart RB: Drug use and adverse drug reactions in the elderly: An epidemiologic perspective. *Top Geriatr Rehab* 2:1–11, 1987.
41. Mellinger GD, Balter MB, Uhlenhuth EH: Prevalence and correlates of the long-term regular use of anxiolytics. *J Am Med Assoc* 251:375–379, 1984.
42. *Drug Abuse Warning Network Annual Data*. Rockville, MD: National Institute on Drug Abuse, 1989.
43. Pihl RO, Murdoch D, Lapp JE, Marinier R: Psychotrope and alcohol use by women: One or two populations. *J Clin Psychol* 42:991–999, 1986.

44. Marinier R, Pihl RO, Wilford C, Lapp J: Psychotropic drug usage by women: Demographics, lifestyle and personality correlates. *Drug Intell Clin Pharm* 19:40–45, 1985.
45. Gomberg ESL: Men, women and prescribed psychoactive drugs, in Seeman MV (ed): *Gender and Psychopathology.* Washington, DC: American Psychiatric Association Press, forthcoming.
46. Glantz MD, Backenheimer MS: Substance abuse among elderly women. *Clin Gerontol* 8:3–24, 1988.
47. Hasin DS, Grant B, Harford TC: Male and female differences in liver cirrhosis mortality in the United States, 1961–1985. *J Stud Alcohol* 51:123–129, 1990.
48. Holzer CE III, Robins LN, Myers JK, *et al*: Antecedents and correlates of alcohol use and dependence in the elderly, in Maddox GL, Robins LN, Rosenberg N (eds): *Nature and Extent of Alcohol Problems among the Elderly.* Washington, DC: NIAAA, 1984, pp 217–244.
49. Schuckit MA, Morrissey ER, O'Leary MR: Alcohol problems in elderly men and women. *Addict Dis* 3:405–416, 1978.
50. Gomberg ESL, Nelson BW: Gender differences among older alcoholics in treatment. Presentation at Research Society on Alcoholism symposium, Alcohol and Aging, San Diego, CA, June 1992.
51. Dunham RG: Aging and changing patterns of alcohol use. *J Psychoactive Drugs* 13:143–151, 1981.
52. Alexander F, Duff RW: Drinking in retirement communities. *Generations* XII:58–60, 1988.
53. Akers RI, LaGreca AJ: Alcohol use among the elderly: Social learning, community context, and life events, in Pittman DJ, White HR (eds): *Society, Culture, and Drinking Patterns Reexamined.* New Brunswick, NJ: Rutgers Center of Alcohol Studies, 1991, pp 242–262.
54. Gomberg ESL, Nelson BW, Iacob A, Young J: Elderly male alcoholics: Who enters treatment? *Alcohol Clin Exp Res* 17:490, 1993.
55. Brennan PL, Moos RH, Kim JY: Gender differences in the individual characteristics and life contexts of late-middle-aged and older problem drinkers. *Addiction* 88:781–790, 1993.
56. Ewing JA: Detecting alcoholism: The CAGE questionnaire. *J Am Med Assoc* 252:1905–1907, 1984.
57. Selzer ML: The Michigan Alcoholism Screening Test: The quest for a new diagnostic instrument. *Am J Psychiatry* 127:1653–1658, 1971.
58. *The Coping Strategies of Older People, MRC 2.* Interview Schedule. Ann Arbor, MI: University of Michigan Alcohol Research Center, unpublished, 1988.
59. Gomberg ESL: Female drinking patterns in the United States, in Pittman DJ, White HR (ed): *Society, Culture and Drinking Patterns Reexamined.* New Brunswick, NJ: Rutgers Center of Alcohol Studies Press, 1991, pp 263–284.
60. Armor DJ, Polich JM, Stambul HB: *Alcoholism and Treatment.* New York: Wiley, 1978.
61. Bissell L, Haberman PW: *Alcoholism in the Professions.* New York: Oxford University Press, 1984.
62. Lisansky ES: Alcoholism in women: Social and psychological concomitants. I. Social history data. *Q J Stud Alcohol* 18:588–623, 1957.
63. Ross, HE: Alcohol and drug abuse in treated alcoholics: A comparison of men and women. *Alcohol Clin Exp Res* 13:810–816, 1989.
64. Wilsnack RW, Wilsnack SC, Klassen AD: Women's drinking and drinking problems: Patterns from a 1981 national survey. *Am J Public Health* 74:1231–1238, 1984.
65. Hesselbrock MN, Hesselbrock VM, Babor TF, *et al*: Antisocial behavior, psychopathology and problem drinking in the natural history of alcoholism, in Goodwin DW, Van Dusen KT, Mednick SA (eds): *Longitudinal Research in Alcoholism.* Boston, Kluwer-Nijoff, 1984, pp 197–214.
66. Allan CA, Cooke DJ: Stressful life events and alcohol misuse in women: A critical review. *J Stud Alcohol* 46:147–152, 1985.
67. Holzer CE, Robins LN, Myers JK, *et al*: Antecedents and correlates of alcohol abuse and dependence in the elderly, in *Nature and Extent of Alcohol Problems among the Elderly.* NIAAA Research Monograph 14, DHHS (ADM) 84-1321, Washington, DC: US Government Printing Office, 1984, pp 217–244.

68. Lazarus RS, DeLongis A: Psychological stress and coping in aging. *Am Psychol* 38:245–254, 1983.
69. Hubbard RW, Santos JF, Santos MA: Alcohol and older adults: Overt and covert influences. *Soc Casework* 60:166–170, 1979.
70. Wilsnack SC, Wilsnack RW: Epidemiology of women's drinking. *J Subst Abuse* 3:133–158, 1991.
71. Helzer JE, Pryzbeck TR: The co-occurrence of alcoholism with other psychiatric disorders in the general populations and its impact on treatment. *J Stud Alcohol* 49:219–224, 1988.
72. Whittington FJ: Making it better: Drinking and drugging in old age. Generations, Quarterly Journal of the American Society on Aging XII:5-8, 1988.
73. Adams WL, Yuan Z, Barboriak JJ, Timm AA: Alcohol-related hospitalizations of elderly people. *J Am Med Assoc,* 270(10): 1222–1225, 1993.
74. Willenbring M, Spring WD: Evaluating alcohol use in elders. Generations *Q J Am Soc Aging* XII:27–31, 1988.
75. Lamy PP: Actions of alcohol and drugs in older people. *Generations Q J Am Soc Aging* XII:9–13, 1988.

4

Violent Victimization among Women with Alcohol Problems

Brenda A. Miller and William R. Downs

Abstract. Empirical evidence regarding the role of childhood victimization in the development of women's alcohol problems is examined in this chapter. In particular, childhood sexual abuse and father-to-daughter violence are found to predict later alcohol problems. Key variables that link experiences of childhood victimization and the development of adult alcohol problems are identified. Strengths and weaknesses of the research provide a better assessment of our confidence in the empirical evidence to date. Possible explanations for how and why the experiences of violent victimization may lead to women's alcohol problems are presented. Finally, important directions for policymakers, clinicians, and researchers are discussed.

1. Introduction

Despite several years of increased attention to women with alcohol problems, there has been relatively little information about the contexts of the violence that surround women's lives and why these experiences may be important to the development of women's alcohol problems. Violence that occurs in childhood is particularly troublesome as we develop more knowledge about the sequelae of events that follow childhood trauma.[1–4] Experiences of being physically abused or the target of verbal aggression by a parent comprise one series of victimization that children may experience. Childhood sexual abuse, including sexual molestation of children, is another form of violent victimization that children experience. Not only may parents be perpetrators of childhood sexual abuse, but also other relatives, family friends, and adults trusted

Brenda A. Miller • Research Institute of Addictions, Buffalo, New York 14203.   **William R. Downs** • Center for the Study of Adolescence, University of Northern Iowa, Cedar Falls, Iowa 50614.

Recent Developments in Alcoholism, Volume 12: Women and Alcoholism, edited by Marc Galanter. Plenum Press, New York, 1995.

by children (e.g., teachers, priests, or club leaders). Childhood sexual abuse may also be perpetrated by a stranger.

Revealing the relationships between childhood victimization and the development of women's alcohol problems is important to develop relevant public policy, respond to treatment needs of women, and to prevent further victimization and alcohol problems for women. Public policy makers can develop more efficient and effective systems with knowledge about these relationships. Responding to the long-standing trauma and pain of victimization experiences in legislation and public policy provides a more rational and humane response to the complex set of problems women experience. Understanding how and why childhood victimization becomes connected to later development of alcohol problems is important to those who provide services to victims. Providers in treatment settings can more appropriately deliver services and facilitate the healing and recovery process for women. Preventing children who have been victimized from experiencing long-term consequences, such as alcohol problems, is also possible with the knowledge of these connections.

In this chapter, we review existing studies that suggest a significant and important link between childhood victimization and the later development of women's alcohol problems. A brief review of methodological issues is provided for assessing the empirical evidence to date. Explanations for how and why these events are linked provide a framework for understanding how intervention and prevention programs might benefit from this knowledge. Finally, the importance of this work for policy, planning, delivery of treatment, prevention, and future research is discussed.

2. Empirical Evidence Linking Childhood Victimization and the Development of Alcohol Problems in Women

2.1. Empirical Evidence

Beginning in the mid 1980s, a series of studies were initiated at the Research Institute on Addictions to investigate the links between childhood victimization and the development of alcohol problems in women. In our first study, in-depth interviews were conducted with 45 women who were currently receiving alcoholism treatment or had received alcoholism treatment previously and were still involved in Alcoholic's Anonymous groups in the Western New York area.[5,6] In addition, 40 women without alcohol problems were drawn from the community using random digit dialing methods to obtain the sample.* This research assessed more than one type of childhood victimization, relied on in-depth face-to-face interviews to assess victimization, used

---

* Women were excluded from the community sample if they had alcohol-related problems during lifetimes.

multiple questions to assess childhood sexual abuse, and assessed mother and father moderate and severe verbal violence. Measures of childhood sexual abuse include a range of experiences from exposure and invitations to do something sexual (e.g., taking pictures in the nude), physical touching (e.g., rubbing the breast or buttocks), and penetration (e.g., vaginal or anal intercourse).[†] These events occurred prior to 18 years of age for the woman. To ensure that childhood sexual abuse did not include exploratory play by children, perpetrators were defined as individuals 5 or more years older than the child. Any relative was defined as a perpetrator regardless of age differences. Thus, the perpetrators included parental figures, relatives, family friends, individuals in authority (e.g., teacher), and strangers. To further limit the measure to the most potentially harmful sexual experiences, we excluded any boyfriend experience that was defined as consensual by the woman, even if the boyfriend was more than 5 years older.[‡] Parental violence was assessed by measuring verbal aggression (e.g., threatening to hit or to throw something), moderate physical violence (e.g., slapping or spanking), and severe physical violence (e.g., beating up, using knife or gun).[§] Measures of mother-to-daughter violence and father-to-daughter violence were both assessed. If more than one mother and/or father figure were present during the woman's childhood, the parental figure that was predominant (longest duration) was used in these analyses. Further, there were assessments of other important family background characteristics such as parental alcohol problems, number of changes in the family structure (e.g., divorces, death) and socioeconomic status of childhood family.

Comparisons were made between alcoholics who had received treatment ($n = 45$) and women from the community who did not have alcohol problems ($n = 40$) for rates of father-to-daughter violence, mother-to-daughter violence, and childhood sexual abuse.[5,6] Findings from this first study revealed that alcoholic women (67%) were 2.5 times more likely to report childhood sexual abuse than nonalcoholic women (28%).[5] Alcoholic women also reported approximately twice the levels of father-to-daughter verbal aggression and moderate violence and approximately four times the level of father-to-daughter severe violence than nonalcoholic women.[6] For example, alcoholic women experienced an average of 1.21 different severe violent acts in their childhood compared with an average of 0.32 for the household sample. Interestingly, there were no significant mother-to-daughter differences in any of the parental violence scales. The differences in women's experiences of childhood sexual abuse and violence by fathers remained significant, even when parental alcoholism, number of changes in the family structure, age, and present

[†] Measures of childhood sexual abuse were based on earlier work of Finkelhor[81] and Sgroi.[82]

[‡] A few incidents that were described as not traumatic and that were qualitatively different were also excluded, for example, playing doctor with brothers and sisters and showing genitalia to each other or experiencing a flasher out on the streets as a teenager.

[§] The measures of childhood physical violence were based on the Conflict Tactics Scale.[83]

income source variables—which differed between the two groups—were controlled.

Moreover, the differences in the rates of childhood victimization were substantial, suggesting a link between childhood victimization and development of women's alcohol problems. However, several questions remained: (1) Can these findings be replicated with a larger sample? (2) Are differences in childhood victimization rates for alcoholic and nonalcoholic women an artifact of the help–seeking behavior of alcoholic women? (3) Would other women who are seeking treatment for problems other than alcoholism have similar rates and types of childhood victimization? (4) Are rates of childhood victimization greater for women who drink heavily but are not yet alcoholic or only for women with substantial alcohol problems?

In a subsequent study, conducted in the late 1980s, 472 women were interviewed to determine rates of childhood victimization as measured by childhood sexual abuse, father-to-daughter violence, and mother-to-daughter violence, thus, replicating the measures of the first study.* Samples of women were drawn from five different populations in Western New York: women from outpatient alcoholism clinics ($n = 98$); women attending drinking and driving classes following conviction for a driving while intoxicated offense (DWI), hereafter referred to as the DWI sample ($n = 100$); women receiving services from shelters or support groups for women experiencing partner violence ($n = 97$); women in outpatient mental health clinics ($n = 77$); and women from households obtained through random digit dialing and who did not have alcohol problems ($n = 82$), hereafter referred to as the community sample.[7]

The first set of comparisons were between women in the alcoholism clinics, DWI, and community samples to determine if the rates of childhood victimization are higher for all women with heavy drinking patterns or only for women who seek treatment. In fact, alcoholic women were more likely to report being sexually abused as a child (66%) compared with either the women in the DWI (21%) or the community women (35%).[7] Not only were these differences significant, they were also substantial; women in alcoholism treatment were three times more likely than DWI women and at almost two times more likely than the community women to report experiences of sexual abuse.† Furthermore, alcoholic women were significantly more likely to have experienced all three types of sexual abuse (exposure, touching, penetration) compared with women in the DWI and community samples. For example,

* Our most recent work was funded by the National Institute on Alcoholism and Alcohol Abuse, R01AA07554. For further information on the methodology of this study, see Miller and colleagues.[7]

† Rates of childhood sexual abuse are lower for women in the DWI sample than for women in the community sample. This may be explained in part by the different sociodemographic characteristics in the two groups. Women in the DWI sample were more likely to be white, have higher socioeconomic status, and were younger than women in the general population.[7]

when experiences of penetration (the most physically intrusive type of sexual abuse) were compared for the three samples, alcoholic women were nearly seven times more likely (47%) to experience sexual abuse that involved penetration than the DWI sample (7%) and over five times more likely than the household sample (9%). These differences remained significant when personal and family background characteristics (i.e., race, age, childhood socioeconomic status, parental alcoholism, and number of changes in the childhood family structure) were controlled. Controlling for these variables is critical because differences in rates of childhood victimization may be due to these personal or family background characteristics. When these variables are controlled and differences between groups are still found, evidence for the relationship between childhood victimization and the development of women's alcohol problems proves to be very strong.

Similar results were found for father-to-daughter violence. Alcoholic women were significantly more likely to report father-to-daughter verbal aggression (71%) and severe violence (45%) than either the DWI (verbal, 43%; severe, 18%) or household (verbal, 31%; severe, 13%) samples.[7] These differences also remained significant when personal characteristics and family background characteristics were controlled. However, while some significant differences were found between groups for levels of mother-to-daughter violence, none of these differences remained significant when personal and family background characteristics were controlled.

To address whether victimization in childhood has a unique connection to the later development of alcohol problems or is merely an artifact of treatment seeking, women who were in various treatment settings (alcoholism, mental health, and partner violence services) were divided into two groups. Groups consisted of women with (n = 178) and without (n = 92) alcohol problems. These groups were compared for their rates of childhood victimization. Women in treatment with alcohol problems were significantly more likely to report sexual abuse experiences (70%) than women in treatment without alcohol problems (52%).[7] Moreover, women with alcohol problems were significantly more likely to report both touching and penetration as specific types of sexual abuse. For example, women with alcohol problems experience significantly more penetration than women without alcohol problems (44% vs. 27%, respectively). These differences remained significant, controlling for parental alcoholism—the only personal or family background characteristic that differed between these groups. Women in treatment with alcohol problems were significantly more likely to report verbal aggression by fathers (67%) compared with women in treatment without alcohol problems (49%); however, neither moderate nor severe violence were significantly different.[7] As with childhood sexual abuse, rates of father verbal aggression remained significantly higher for women with alcohol problems even when parental alcoholism was controlled. In another test of the strength of this relationship, when controlling for parental alcohol problems as well as the woman's current level of psychiatric symptomology, women with alcohol problems experienced significantly greater father verbal aggression regardless of the whether or not they experienced severe partner violence.[8]

Other studies provide support for connections between childhood victimization and the development of alcohol problems in women. In studies of adults, Briere and Runtz[9] found that women receiving crisis services who suffered sexual abuse as children were approximately ten times more likely to have a drug addiction history and greater than two times more likely to have an alcoholism history than female crisis clients who had not been sexually abused. Using a random sample, Peters[10] found childhood sexual abuse to be related to the development of alcohol abuse and other drug abuse for women. Methodologically weaker studies have shown no connection between childhood victimization and alcohol problems for women. For example, studies using only one or two questions to assess victimization, studies that failed to report results by gender of respondent, and studies with small sample size do not find relationships between childhood victimization and women's alcohol problems.[11-13]

Research conducted with adolescents has not yielded consistent findings on the relationship between childhood victimization and alcohol abuse, although connections have been found with various indicators of problem drinking (e.g., drunkenness). For example, a study with male and female adolescents in detention by Dembo and colleagues[14-16] found that sexual abuse in childhood had a direct effect on illicit drug use for both males and females. However, no association was found between childhood sexual abuse and alcohol use for either males or females.[15] Dembo and colleagues[14-16] also reported that experiences of nonsexual physical abuse had a strong direct effect on illicit drug use for both male and female adolescents. However, physical abuse had no direct effect on alcohol use for either males or females.[15] In a later replication study, the sample size was insufficient to test their models for females, using structural equation modeling.[17] However, the authors reported few significant correlations between childhood physical and sexual abuse and other variables among girls in the study.

Connections between childhood victimization and alcohol abuse for women may not be evident in the adolescent years. In Dembo and colleague's work, this may be an artifact of the sample. Adolescents in detention may be more likely to show involvement in drugs rather than in alcohol. Another possible explanation for these contradictory results with adolescents is that sexually or physically abused adolescents are no more likely to consume alcohol than nonabused adolescents, but are more likely to use drugs, drink at an earlier age, or drink abusively than nonabused adolescents. For example, Singer, Petchers, and Hussey[18] found that psychiatric inpatient adolescents (64 females and 32 males) with a history of childhood sexual abuse reported more frequency of intoxication and more times high on drugs than adolescents without a history of childhood sexual victimization. Also, in a study of chemically dependent adolescents (51% female), Cavaiola and

Schiff[19] found that adolescents with a history of physical or sexual abuse began alcohol and drug use earlier than nonabused adolescents.

Alcohol problems also may require more time to emerge than other substance abuse problems. Our inquiries with the alcoholic and heavy drinking women, along with this additional information from studies on adolescents, suggest that experiences of childhood victimization may not be connected to heavy drinking in later life but rather be linked to drinking problems of sufficient severity to warrant a diagnosis of alcohol dependence—a diagnosis that may take several years to develop.

2.2. Key Variables

2.2.1. Time-Ordering of Events. In assessing the nature of the relationship, it is essential to know whether childhood victimization occurs prior to the establishment of drinking patterns that may lead to later alcohol problems. The first drinking experience, the first intoxication experience, the emergence of a heavy drinking pattern, and/or the first drinking problems are possible measures for assessing the temporal ordering of events. In inquiries with adolescents, Dembo and colleagues[14] found that only 13% of the sample reported first substance use prior to sexual victimization. In our interviews with 472 women from five samples, virtually all of the women who experienced childhood victimization did so prior to heavy drinking. (Heavy drinking was defined as drinking six or more drinks per drinking occasion or four–five drinks four or more days per week.) Ninety-two percent had experienced childhood sexual abuse and 98% had experienced severe parental violence prior to their first heavy drinking pattern. In this same study, for women with alcohol problems in treatment the average age of the first experience of severe violence (e.g., beaten up with fists or object to cause severe injury, used knife or gun on child) by a parent was 7 years of age. The average age of the first experience of sexual abuse was 10 years of age. The onset of heavy drinking did not occur until an average age of 19 years old. Although these age differences indicate the *direction* of the relationship, the number of years between these incidents underlines the importance of intervening events in plotting the path from childhood victimization and to the development of women's alcohol problems.

2.2.2. Characteristics of the Perpetrator. Across the five samples of women ($n = 472$) in Western New York, one of the most dramatic finding is that the experiences of victimization that are most linked to the development of women's alcohol problems are perpetrated by men. However, perpetrators of childhood sexual abuse are generally not the father. Instead, the perpetrators were most likely to be an adult male relative or male family friend. For example, only 4% of all women reported either a biological or adoptive father as the sexual abuse perpetrator. Strangers are not likely to be the perpetrators either; only 9% reported a stranger as a perpetrator of childhood sexual abuse. Neither are women likely to perpetrate childhood sexual abuse: 3% reported a female perpetrator. For these types of perpetrators women receiving outpatient alcoholism services did not differ from the women in the DWI or from the community samples. Significant differences did emerge between groups when other father figures (e.g., grandfathers, uncles, mother's boyfriends who also were defined as serving in the role of father) are added to the biological or adoptive fathers. Women in alcoholism treatment were 5 times more likely to have reported a father figure as a perpetrator of childhood sexual abuse than women in the DWI sample and 19 times more likely to have reported father figures than women in the community sample.* Similarly, a much higher percentage of women in the alcoholism treatment sample reported sexual abuse or molestation by any male relative (father, father figures, uncles, grandfathers, cousins, brothers) (40%) than either the DWI (9%) or community (13%) samples. A significantly higher percentage of the women in the alcoholism treatment sample reported a male family friend as a perpetrator (37%) than either the DWI (12%) or community samples (16%).

Even when women in various forms of treatment (i.e., alcoholism, mental health, partner violence) with and without alcohol problems are compared, a significantly higher percentage of the women in treatment with alcohol problems reported a male relative as a perpetrator (44%) than women in treatment without alcohol problems (33%). A higher percentage of the women in treatment with alcohol problems also are more likely to experience sexual abuse by a male family friend (38%) than women in treatment without alcohol problems (27%).

2.2.3. Experiences of Multiple Victimization. Finally, based on the five samples of women in Western New York, women receiving services from outpatient alcoholism treatment were significantly more likely to have experienced *both* severe parental violence and childhood sexual abuse (45%) than women in the DWI (11%) or community (14%) samples. They were also significantly less likely to have escaped childhood sexual abuse or severe parental violence. Only 13% of the women in alcoholism treatment compared with 57% of the DWI sample and 41% of the community sample escaped these severe forms of victimization.[7] Again, when women in treatment from various types of treatment sources with and without alcohol problems were compared, significant differences were found in comparing the percentage of women who escaped any form of severe parental violence or sexual abuse as a child. Only 12% of the women in treatment with alcohol problems did not have one of the forms of victimization compared with 28% of the women without alcohol problems.[7]

---

* Father figures were defined as the man who took care of the respondent between the ages of 7 and 18, and could have been the natural or adoptive father, stepfather, mother's boyfriend, uncle, grandfather, brother, or foster father. Women could have more than one perpetrator and therefore may have reported an experience with a perpetrator in several different categories.

2.3. Summary of Empirical Evidence

To date, empirical evidence strongly suggests that experiences of childhood victimization are significantly related to the development of alcohol problems in women. As evidenced in the lack of findings for violence by the mother relating to the development of women's alcohol problems, there is a need to separate the types of violent victimization experiences according to type of perpetrator. In addition, it is important to control for personal and family background characteristics when examining these relationships. Methodologically stronger studies have yielded the most consistent positive support for the connection between experiences of childhood victimization and the development of women's alcohol problems in adulthood. Whereas studies of adolescents have shown mixed results between the connections of childhood victimization and alcohol use by females, stronger results have been shown for indicators of alcohol problems in adult women.

3. Importance of Methodological Issues

3.1. Retrospective Recall

To date, most studies examining the relationship between childhood victimization and the development of women's alcohol problems have relied on retrospective methodologies. Retrospective reports are a reliable and valid means of collecting information on violence occurring in families, drinking behavior, consequences of alcohol abuse, and women's alcohol problems.[20–22] The use of standardized interviews with clear multiple questions, follow-up questions that clarify the responses more clearly, time frames and other important events (e.g., Christmas) to clarify recall, and memory aids such as time lines has improved the reliability and validity of self-report retrospective data on alcohol use.[23] Multiple, specific questions also aid memory for sexual abuse events.[24] Nevertheless, retrospective accounts of childhood sexual and physical abuse have been questioned as to the accuracy of their recall.[25] Problems with retrospective recall may include false-negative (failure to report childhood victimization when it had, in fact, occured) or false–positive reports (reports of childhood victimization when none occurred) of childhood sexual or physical abuse, inaccurate recall of specific abuse-related events, and differential recall of abuse across different samples.[25–27]

The inability to recall experiences of childhood sexual abuse has been extensively discussed in the literature.[28,29] In one of the most recent and extensive studies completed, Williams reinterviewed 129 adults for whom contact sexual abuse was both reported and substantiated by trained professionals 17 years earlier.[27] Over one third (38%) of the abused women *did not* report childhood sexual abuse documented 17 years earlier. Studies have noted that nonrecall was related to younger age at the time of abuse, abuse by a family member, and also intensive levels of physical violence.[27–29]

While the problem of false-positive reports has received considerable media attention recently, the available empirical evidence suggests that its is a relatively rare event. The most reliable estimates are that from 2% to 8% of childhood sexual abuse reports are false, with the highest rates of false reporting for adolescents.[30]

A major concern in examining the relationships between childhood victimization and the development of women's alcohol problems is that there may be differential rates of recall among women in alcoholism treatment compared with women in other groups. While acknowledging the importance of women's perceptions to the consequences that are evident in their lives, unacknowledged events also can have negative consequences. However, Williams found that nonrecall was unrelated to past treatment for alcohol abuse or drug abuse.[27] Further, the perspectives and memories of childhood events that are reported by adults may be more accurate, more meaningful, and may more closely mirror the truth than those perspectives held as children.[3,31,32] The elements of secrecy that accompany childhood sexual abuse and the child's definitions of what happened are likely to undergo transformation as the child develops. What individuals recall about important events in their lives has as much value for understanding the long-term consequences of negative events as more objective accounts that might be obtained from multiple observers of these events.[33–38]

Despite the controversy over accuracy of recall,[39,40] retrospective studies of adults provide the best data available on unreported and untreated cases of childhood sexual abuse and child abuse.[41] This is particularly true for studying alcohol problems as a long-term consequence of early victimization. Alcohol problems can take years to develop and longitudinal studies may not show effects for years. Retrospective data identify relationships found between childhood victimization and the development of women's alcohol problems in a time frame that allows more meaningful and timely services and interventions to women.

3.2. Prospective Studies

The strengths of prospective studies can be used to complement findings from retrospective studies. Longitudinal designs can provide data on the course of symptomatology over time as it occurs, without relying on retrospective accounts for the time-ordering of events. In addition, prospective studies can provide data on factors that facilitate recovery as recovery proceeds.[4] Time between the event and the reporting of that event is decreased, with a corresponding increase in the accuracy of the self-report data.

Prospective research designs also may be limited with regard to generalizability to reported cases of abuse. Straus and Gelles[42] estimated that from 70% to 95% of annual childhood physical abuse cases are unreported. Using very conservative assumptions, Finkelhor[41] estimates that less than half of the annual childhood sexual abuse cases are officially identified. Another disadvantage of a prospective study is that cases of child abuse or childhood sexual abuse that are identified within a sample of minors would require intervention, eliminating the possibility of studying long-term consequences that occur without identification. From an ethical standpoint, a study of the natural history of childhood victimization is simply not feasible.

Prospective studies based on found cases also have the problems of both false-negative and false-positive reports of childhood victimization. Official reports depend on the veracity of the data obtained by the investigating worker as well as the validity of that worker's judgments regarding that data. In the absence of physical evidence of abuse, child protective service (CPS) workers rely on self-report data to verify that child abuse has occurred, specifically self-report data obtained under conditions in which a crime has been alleged and investigated. Further, Everson and Boat[30] found that a subset of CPS workers were predisposed *not* to believe childrens' reports of sexual abuse, a subjective bias that resulted in underreporting of abuse in official records. At best, then, found cases of abuse represent only a small proportion of true cases.

3.3. Other Methodological Considerations

In addition to the overall design questions of retrospective versus prospective data, there are a number of other methodological considerations. Sex of the interviewer, training given to the interviewer, placement of the questions in the interview instrument, types of questions, and how the interviews are conducted are all critical to the design of the study.[37]

Given the range and extent of methodological restrictions of various research paradigms, what is needed are studies using various methodologies.[26,33,37,43] There is also a need to improve existing methodology. For example, Martin and colleagues[44] report a two-stage methodology using both self-report questionnaire as well as in-person interviews to examine childhood sexual abuse, retrospectively. Each technique discovered cases *excluded* by the other technique. This illustrates the need to use multiple techniques to minimize retrospective recall bias. Multiwave panel studies of adults provide the opportunity to reexamine the issue of childhood sexual abuse and child abuse at each wave, thus increasing the potential for enhancing the recall of these events.

Specific questions on both child abuse and childhood sexual abuse are superior to single, more generic questions about victimization in obtaining disclosure of victimization.[24,26,32] Reading a list of types of experiences (e.g., fondling your breasts) also allows the researcher to gather data and make determination of criteria without asking the woman to label herself as sexually or physically abused. Further, knowledge of the specific nature of traumatic events does not predict responses of individuals.[45] Therefore, information about short- and long-term consequences needs to be assessed. Given the findings on male perpetrators, characteristics of the perpetrator must be clarified, including measures of the perpetrator's sex, age, and relationship to the woman.

4. Connecting Victimization Histories with the Development of Women's Alcohol Problems

In this section, three different explanations are suggested for connecting childhood victimization to the later development of women's alcohol problems: (1) Alcohol use provides a coping mechanism for handling negative feelings toward the self that are generated by the experiences of victimization. (2) Victimization leads to identification with peer groups involved in delinquency, heavy drinking, and drug use. (3) Alcohol is used to numb and block psychological pain, thereby allowing women to dissociate from the memories of childhood victimization. These explanations are supported, in part, by similarities in the consequences of childhood victimization and the precursors' to women's drinking. For example, Hurley[46] lists 15 profile comparisons found in the literature that are similar for the incest survivors and women with alcohol problems. Both immediate and long-term effects have been consistently identified as associated with childhood victimization, particularly childhood sexual abuse, including increased risk for alcohol and drug abuse.[1,9]

4.1. Alcohol as a Coping Mechanism

Negative psychological consequences resulting from childhood victimization may contribute to the later development of women's alcohol problems. Women alcoholics are commonly identified as having a poor self-esteem and feelings of inadequacy.[47–49] A number of different studies have reported that women with alcohol problems are more likely to suffer from depression.[49–51] Although these assessments of women with alcohol problems cannot clarify when the negative self-images occur (before or after drinking problems), these same negative views of self are generated by experiences of childhood victimization.

Using a nationwide random sample, Straus[52] found that corporal punishment from both mothers and fathers during adolescence was related to depression and suicidal ideation for both females and males. Kazdin et al.[53] found that physically abused children had lower self-esteem and were more depressed compared with a group of psychiatrically disturbed children who had not been abused. Sexual abuse in childhood is also likely to contribute to psychological consequences such as low self-exteem, depression, guilt, feelings of inferiority, and anxiety.[1,3,4,9] Studies also have supported a connection between childhood victimization and self-destructive behavior.[9,12,13] For example, Lanktree et al.[54] compared children in outpatient treatment, with and without histories of childhood sexual abuse, and found abuse history to be related to a greater likelihood of and a greater number of suicide attempts and diagnosis for major depression. In a study of male and female adolescents in inpatient treatment for substance abuse, girls who were victims of sexual abuse were more likely than nonvictims to attempt suicide in the past year (42% vs. 20%).[55]

Although Kaplan's[56] theory of self-esteem and self-derogation was developed to explain drug abuse, it provides some understanding of how and why women's experiences of childhood victimization might be connected to subsequent alcohol use. Experiences that produce self-devaluation, create a situation which is almost impossible to defend against, present a situation requiring coping skills that are, at best, beyond the scope of a child's ability, can set the stage for drug (or alcohol) use. According to Steffenhagen,[57] low self-esteem results in poor coping mechanisms in the face of stress, leading to drug use as an alternative coping strategy. According to Harrison and colleagues,[55] sexual abuse victims reported use of substances to mediate distress and to escape family problems. Similarly, Rohsenow et al.[58] propose that drinking may provide the victim of childhood sexual abuse with a way to control emotional and interpersonal consequences of the abuse. From the same five samples of women in Western New York presented earlier, women reported significantly more self-stigmatization if they had histories of childhood victimization during their adolescent years.* Women in the alcoholism treatment sample reported a significantly greater level of self-stigmatization than women in the DWI and community samples. Also, women with alcohol problems in treatment reported a significantly greater level of negative self-stigmatization than women in treatment without alcohol problems.

4.2. Identification with Deviant Peer Groups

Kaplan[56] proposes a connection between low self-esteem, rejection of others, ineffectual coping mechanisms, and identity with peer groups that do not conform to societal norms (e.g., peer groups involved in drugs, delinquency). In his three-wave panel study of junior high school students, Kaplan and co-workers[59] tested the model that self-derogation leads to drug use. Using a path model, their findings indicated that self-derogation predicts drug use due to the loss of motivation to conform to more normative peer groups. This may lead to associations with more deviant peers and adoption of their behaviors.

---

* Women reported whether they had ever used a list of negative words to describe or think of themselves. Items included such pejorative labels as bitch, whore, and bad mother. A total of 14 stigmatizing labels were used.

Given that women who have been victimized may develop negative views of themselves, feel rejected by others, and be unsuccessful in coping with the severity of the trauma they have experienced, deviant peer groups may provide a more comfortable and accepting context for them than other peer groups who have different histories. Watt and Ellis[60] expressed the view that unhappy children seek out others who are unhappy and together they use drugs. Thus, there is a type of social support and solace that may be engendered in the peer culture that keeps a survivor of victimization linked to a group, even if this link encourages the development of drinking or drug problems. Over time, involvement in a substance-using peer group can lead to peer relations based on mutual needs for procuring and using drugs and or alcohol.

When adolescents join peer groups involved in delinquent activity, including heavy drinking and drug use, the adolescent is unlikely to develop the social skills and experience to reenter more normative contexts. Use of substances may cause the adolescent to regress and to give up age-appropriate responsibilities and tasks.[56] Further, substance-using peer groups typically reject involvement with peer groups who do not use drugs.

Empirical studies have also identified a risk of delinquent and aggressive behavior following experiences of childhood victimization.[9,61] Theft and vandalism are sometimes correlated highly with sexual abuse histories.[60] A comparison of female adolescents in inpatient treatment for substance abuse with and without sexual abuse histories found that sexually abused victims were more likely to have been arrested (43% vs. 33%), more likely to be arrested prior to age 14 years (16% vs. 6%), and more likely to have been in detention (18% vs. 6%).[55] These histories of delinquency must be taken in the context that abused adolescents may leave home at an early age and their delinquent involvement occurs in an effort to support themselves.

Alcoholic women have reported delinquency and status offenses during adolescence, specifically stealing and running away from home, more often than a community sample.[62] Further, our sample of women in treatment with alcohol problems were significantly more likely (56%) than women in treatment without alcohol problems (25%) or women in the community population (5%) to have belonged to peer groups involved in delinquent activities. Among women in treatment with alcohol problems, sexual abuse was significantly related to membership in a group that rejected traditional ways and more involved in delinquency and drug or alcohol use; 61% had been involved in such a group compared with 44% of the women not sexually abused.

4.3. Use of Alcohol to Numb Psychological Pain

Recently, the construct of Posttraumatic Stress Disorder (PTSD) has received attention for its applicability to women and children who have been sexually or physically assaulted.[63–66] As described in the *Diagnostic and Statis-*

tical Manual of Disorders, Fourth Edition, this disorder occurs after exposure to extreme traumatic stressors such as

a. personal experiences that threaten death, serious injury, or personal integrity in some other manner, or

b. witnessing or learning about another family member's or close associate's unexpected death, serious injury, or threat to personal integrity.

The individual's response to the event must involve intense fear, helplessness, or horror. Such experiences can trigger symptoms characteristic of PTSD:

1. A persistent reexperiencing of the trauma (e.g., recurrent distressing dreams of the event),

2. avoidance of the associated stimuli (e.g., efforts to avoid activities, places, or people that arouse recollections of the trauma), as well as a numbing of the general responsiveness (e.g., feelings of detachment or estrangement from others), and

3. persistent symptoms of increased arousal (e.g., hypervigilance, startle response).

These symptoms must be present for more than 1 month and create significant distress or impairment in social, occupational, or other important areas of functioning for a diagnosis of PTSD.

The relevance of PTSD for women with histories of violent victimization is undergoing considerable rethinking at this point.[66,68,69] Herman[69] has proposed an additional diagnosis of complex posttraumatic stress disorder (CPTSD) for individuals who have experienced prolonged periods of totalitarian control and great stress.[69] This diagnosis would include symptoms of alterations in consciousness (e.g., reliving experiences), alterations in self-perception (e.g., sense of defilement or stigma), alterations in perception of perpetrator (e.g., acceptance of belief system or rationalizations of perpetrator), alterations in relations with others (e.g., isolation and withdrawal), and alterations in systems of meaning (e.g., sense of hopelessness and despair)—all characteristics commonly noted in victims of childhood sexual abuse.[64]

Women experiencing symptoms of PTSD or CPTSD may also seek chemical relief through alcohol (or other drugs). More specifically, there is evidence that women's experiences of violent victimization are followed by symptoms of PTSD and that victimization, PTSD, and alcohol problems are linked for women. Using a nationwide telephone sample of youth aged 10 to 16, Boney-Mccoy and Finkelhor[70] found that being victimized by both a sexual assault and parental violence was related to PTSD symptomatology for both male and female adolescents. In the National Women's Study, a strong interrelationship between victimization, alcohol problems, and PTSD symptomology was found.[71] Two or more alcohol problems were significantly more likely among women who had been victimized and who had PTSD symptoms (14.5%)

compared with women who had been victimized but did not experience PTSD symptoms (3.9%) and women who had not been victimized (1.5%).

To ease the impact of child abuse, alcohol may be consumed to produce chemical dissociation (disturbance in the individual's ability to integrate identity, memory, or consciousness), a more difficult task for adults compared with children.[9,18,60] In her book on traumatized individuals, Herman[69] proposes that using alcohol or narcotics can help the individual produce the numbing effects that some traumatized individuals are unable to do spontaneously through dissociation. Women's own stated motives for drinking provide some support for this connection. When asking women why they drink, the stated motives for drinking are often related at least in part to their desire to relieve unpleasant feelings.[72–74]

5. Implications of Findings

Empirical evidence on the relationship between childhood victimization and later development of alcohol problems in women is sufficiently strong and important to warrant action by policymakers, clinicians, and researchers. Policymakers can provide structures to encourage coordinated and cooperative models of working together among those engaged in providing services for alcohol problems, family violence, and, more generally, mental health. As managed health care dominates the provision of services for the future, policymakers need to ensure that the relationships between victimization and alcohol problems is understood, covered, and effectively treated in our systems of service delivery. As new legislation to address social and legal issues such as women who drink and/or use drugs during pregnancy, children and teenagers who run away, or families who experience violence within the home is proposed, understanding the relationship between childhood victimization and later development of alcohol problems is critical. Not only can this lead to more humane responses, this understanding is key to the development of successful approaches to complex problems.

Clinicians providing alcoholism and other drug treatment services need to recognize that childhood victimization is an important experience for most women. Screening for childhood experiences of physical and sexual abuse as well as adult experiences of victimization should occur. Failure to address the importance and meaning of these experiences for women in treatment may contribute to relapse. If women have used alcohol as a way of coping with negative feelings generated toward self or as a way of numbing pain and images of victimization, removal of the alcohol must be accompanied by support in healing from these traumatic experiences. For many treatment programs, the expertise and experience to provide this type of counseling may not be readily available within the program. Training of personnel and/or collaborating with family violence and other victimization service providers may be necessary. Standard practices of having women and men together in treatment settings, particularly in group sessions, also may not work well for women who have experienced repeated physical and sexual assault from adult males in childhood. These settings are particularly inappropriate for encouraging the recall and discussion of childhood experiences, especially abuse by adult male perpetrators. Establishing and nurturing an atmosphere for discussing childhood victimization experiences is important to treatment. However, treatment providers need to recognize that each woman has the right to control when she wants to reveal her personal experiences and to whom. Treatment settings that "schedule" when certain issues should be discussed in the course of treatment take control away from women. This lack of control occurred during the abusive experience and if repeated in treatment can make the treatment experience uncomfortably similar to the victimization experience.

Screening for alcohol and drug problems needs to occur in treatment and intervention settings that provide services for family violence or more general victim services. Since women sexually victimized as children are thought to be at increased risk for adult victimization,[69] this screening needs to occur in services for family violence where adult women are found. Service providers for family violence have sometimes excluded women who have alcohol and/or drug problems because they felt that they could not adequately address the dual problems of addiction and victimization.[75] Increasingly, there is a growing awareness that a large portion of victimized women are also struggling with alcohol problems. For some, the recognition of alcohol and/or drug problems among women who have been victimized will be threatening because of the concern that women will be blamed for their victimization. Clearly, a woman's alcohol problems do not give license for another individual to victimize her. Furthermore, our fears that women may not be seen as a "pure" victim reflect our unrealistic understanding of human beings. Acknowledging the links between victimization and alcohol/drug use should be seen as providing information that empowers women.

Finally, researchers need to continue exploration of the connections between childhood victimization and the development of women's alcohol problems. Additional populations of women can provide better information on the extent to which these relationships exist across different groups of women. The relationships need to be tested for women at different developmental stages and for women who are at various stages of alcohol problems. Especially valuable would be to determine whether the links hold for women in different geographic regions, from various cultural backgrounds, and from more diversified socioeconomic backgrounds. Careful testing of the models for how and why childhood victimization can lead to women's alcohol problems is needed. Finally, the question of whether this same relationship exists for men should be a focus of inquiry.

ACKNOWLEDGMENT. The authors wish to express their thanks to Dr. Angela Browne for her comments and editorial assistance.

References

1. Browne A, Finkelhor D: Impact of child sexual abuse: A review of the literature. *Psychol Bull* 99:66–77, 1986.
2. Beitchman JH, Zucker KJ, Hood JE, *et al:* A review of the short-term effects of child sexual abuse, *Child Abuse Negl* 15:537–556, 1991.
3. Beitchman JH, Zucker KJ, Hood JE, *et al:* A review of the long-term effects of child sexual abuse. *Child Abuse Negl* 16:101–118, 1992.
4. Kendall-Tackett KA, Meyer Williams L, Finkelhor D: Impact of sexual abuse on children: A review and synthesis of recent empirical studies. *Psychol Bull* 113(1):164–180, 1993.
5. Miller BA, Downs WR, Gondoli DM, Keil A: The role of childhood sexual abuse in the development of alcoholism in women. *Violence Vict* 2(3):157–172, 1987.
6. Downs WR, Miller BA, Gondoli DM: Childhood experiences of parental physical violence for alcoholic women as compared with a randomly selected household sample of women. *Violence Vict* 2(4):225–240, 1987.
7. Miller BA, Downs WR, Testa M: Interrelationships between victimization experiences and women's alcohol/drug use. *J Stud Alcohol Suppl* 11:109–117, 1993.
8. Downs WR, Miller BA, Testa, M, Panek, D: Long-term effects of parent-to-child violence for women. *J Interpers Violence* 7(3):365–382, 1992.
9. Briere J, Runtz M: Post sexual abuse trauma: Data and implications for clinical practice. *J Interpers Violence* 2:367–379, 1988.
10. Peters SD: Child sexual and later psychological problems, in Wyatt GE, Powell GJ (eds): *Lasting Effects of Child Sexual Abuse.* Newbury Park, CA, Sage, 1988, pp 101–118.
11. Bryer JB, Nelson BA, Miller JB, Krol PA: Childhood sexual and physical abuse as factors in adult psychiatric illness. *Am J Psychiatry* 144(11):1426–1430, 1987.
12. Brown GR, Anderson BA: Psychiatric morbidity in adult inpatients with childhood histories of sexual and physical abuse. *Am J Psychiatry* 148(1):55–61, 1991.
13. Briere J, Zaidi LY: Sexual abuse histories and sequelae in female psychiatric emergency room patients. *Am J Psychiatry* 146:1602–1606, 1989.
14. Dembo R, Derke M, LaVoie L, *et al:* Physical abuse, sexual victimization and illicit drug use: A structural analysis among high risk adolescents. *J Adolesc* 19:13–33, 1987.
15. Dembo R, Dertke M, Borders S, *et al:* The relationship between physical and sexual abuse and tobacco, alcohol, and illicit drug use among youths in a juvenile detention center. *Int J Addict* 23(4):351–378, 1988.
16. Dembo R, Williams L, Wish ED, *et al:* The relationship between physical and sexual abuse and ilicit drug use: A replication among a new sample of youths entering a juvenile detention center. *Int J Addict* 23(11):1101–1123, 1988.
17. Dembo R, Williams L, Schmeidler J, *et al:* A structural model examining the relationship between physical child abuse, sexual victimization, and marijuana/hashish use in delinquent youth: A longitudinal study. *Violence Vict* 7(1):41–62, 1992.
18. Singer MI, Petchers MK, Hussey D: The relationship between sexual abuse and substance abuse among psychiatrically hospitalized adolescents. *Child Abuse Negl* 13:319–325, 1989.
19. Cavaiola AA, Schiff M: Self-esteem in abused chemically dependent adolescents. *Child Abuse Negl* 13:327–334, 1989.
20. Straus MA, Gelles RJ, Steinmetz SK: *Behind Closed Doors: Violence in the American Family.* Garden City, NJ, Anchor Books, 1980.
21. Sobell LC, Sobell MB, Riley DM, *et al:* The reliability of alcohol abusers' self-reports of drinking and life events that occurred in the distant past. *J Stud Alcohol* 49:225–232, 1988.

22. Wilsnack RW, Klassen AD, Wilsnack SC: Retrospective analysis of lifetime changes in women's drinking behavior. *Adv Alcohol Subst Abuse* 5:9–26, 1988.
23. Babor TF, Stephen RS, Marlatt GA: Verbal report methods in clinical research on alcoholism: Response bias and its minimization. *J Stud Alcohol* 48:410–424, 1987.
24. Peters SD, Wyatt GE, Finkelhor D: Prevalence, in Finkelhor D (ed): *A Sourcebook on Child Sexual Abuse.* Newbury Park, CA, Sage, 1986, pp 15–59.
25. Widom CS: Child abuse and alcohol use. Prepared for the Working Group on Alcohol-Related Violence: Fostering Interdisciplinary Perspectives, convened by the National Institute on Alcohol Abuse and Alcoholism, Washington, DC, 1992.
26. Briere J: Methodological issues in the study of sexual abuse effects. *J Consult Clin Psychol* 60:196–203, 1992.
27. Williams LM: Recall of childhood trauma: A prospective study of women's memories of child sexual abuse. *J Consult Clin Psychol* 62:1167–1176, 1994.
28. Briere J, Conte J: Self-reported amnesia for abuse in adults molested as children. *J Traum Stress* 6(1):21–31, 1993.
29. Herman JL, Schatzow E: Recovery and verification of memories of childhood sexual trauma. *Psychoanal Psychol* 4(1):1–14, 1987.
30. Everson MD, Boat BW: False allegations of sexual abuse by children and adolescents. *J Am Acad Child Adolesc Psychiatry* 28(2):230–235, 1989.
31. Beutler LE, Hill CE: Process and outcome research in the treatment of adult victims of childhood sexual abuse: Methodological issues. *J Consult Clin Psychol* 60(2):204–212, 1992.
32. Russell, DE: *The Secret Trauma: Incest in the Lives of Girls and Women.* New York, Basic Books, 1986.
33. Babor TF, Brown J, Del Boca FK: Validity of self-reports in applied research on addictive behaviors: Fact or fiction. *Behav Assess* 12(1):5–31, 1990.
34. Maisto SA, Connors GJ: Using subject and collateral reports to measure alcohol consumption, in Litten RZ, Allen JP (eds): *Measuring Alcohol Consumption: Psychosocial and Biochemical Methods.* Totowa, NJ, Humana Press, 1992, pp 73–76.
35. Midanik LT: Validity of self-reported alcohol use: A literature review and assessment. *Br J Addict* 83(9):1019–1029, 1988.
36. Sobell LC, Sobell MB: Self-report issues in alcohol abuse: State of the art and future directions. *Behav Assess* 12(1):77–90, 1990.
37. Miller BA: Investigating links between childhood victimization and alcohol problems, in Martin SE (ed): *Alcohol and Interpersonal Violence: Fostering Multidisciplinary Perspectives.* National Institute on Alcohol Abuse and Alcoholism Monograph 24 (NIH Publication No. 93-3496), Rockville, MD, US Government Printing Office, 1993, pp 315–323.
38. Schumm WR: Evolution of the family field: Measurement principles and techniques, in Touliatos J, Perlmutter BF, Straus MA (eds): *Handbook of Family Measurement Techniques.* Newbury Park, CA, Sage, 1990, pp 23–36.
39. Widom CS: Child abuse and alcohol use and abuse, in Martin SE (ed): *Alcohol and Interpersonal Violence: Fostering Multidisciplinary Perspectives.* National Institute on Alcohol Abuse and Alcoholism Monograph 24 (NIH Publication No. 93–3496) Rockville, MD, US Government Printing Office, 1993, pp 315–323.
40. Yarrow MR, Campbell JD, Burton RV: Recollections of childhood: A study of the retrospective method. *Monogr Soc Res Child Dev* 35(5, Serial No. 138), 1970.
41. Finkelhor, D: Answers to important questions about the scope and nature of child sexual abuse. Unpublished manuscript, Durham, University of New Hampshire, Family Research Laboratory, 1993.
42. Straus MA, Gelles RJ: How violent are American families? Estimates from the National Family Violence Resurvey and other studies, in Straus MA, Gelles RJ (eds): *Physical Violence in American Families: Risk Factors and Adaptions to Violence in 8,145 Families.* New Brunswick, NJ, Transaction Publishers, 1990, pp 95–112.
43. Cicchetti D: How research on child maltreatment has informed the study of child development: Perspectives from developmental psychopathology, in Cicchetti D, Carlson V (eds):

Child Maltreatment: Theory and Research on the Causes and Consequences of Child Abuse and Neglect.
New York, University Press, 1989, pp 377–431.

44. Martin J, Anderson J, Romans S, *et al:* Asking about child sexual abuse: Methodological implications of a two stage survey, *Child Abuse Negl* 17:383–392, 1993.
45. McCann L, Pearlman LA, Sakheim DK, Abrahmson DJ: Assessment and treatment of the adult survivor of childhood sexual abuse within a schema framework, in Sgroi SM (ed): *Evaluation and Treatment of Sually Abused Children and Adult Survivors: Vulnerable Populations.* Lexington, MA, Lexington Books, DC Heath, 1990, vol 11, pp 77–101.
46. Hurley DL: Women, alcohol and incest: An analytical review. *J Stud Alcohol* 52(3):253–268, 1991.
47. Beckman LJ: Perceived antecedents and effects of alcohol consumption in women. *J Stud Alcohol* 41:518–530, 1980.
48. McLachlan JFC, Walderman RL, Birchmore DF, Marsden LR: Self-evaluation, role satisfaction, and anxiety in the woman alcoholic. *Int J Addict* 14:809–832, 1979.
49. Gomberg ES, Lisansky, JM: Antecedents of alcohol problems in women, in Wilsnack SC, Beckman LJ (eds): *Alcohol Problems in Women.* New York, Guilford Press, 1987, pp 233–259.
50. Wilsnack SC, Klassen AD, Schur BE, Wilsnack RW: Predicting onset and chronicity of women's problem drinking: A five-year longitudinal analysis. *Am J Publ Health* 81(3):305–317, 1991.
51. Schuckit MA, PItts FN, Jr, Reich T, *et al:* Alcoholism I. Two types of alcoholism in women. *Arch Gen Psychiatry* 20:301–306, 1969.
52. Straus MA: Depression and sucide, in *Beating the Devil out of Them: Corporal Punishment in American Families.* New York, Leington/Macmillan, 1994, pp 67–79.
53. Kazdin AE, Moser J, Colbus, D, Bell R: Depressive symptoms among physically abused and psychiatrically disturbed children. *J Abnorm Psychol* 94:298–307, 1985.
54. Lanktree C, Briere J, Zaidi L: Incidence and impact of sexual abuse in a child outpatient sample: The role of direct inquiry. *Child Abuse Negl* 15:447–453, 1991.
55. Harrison PA, Hoffmann NG, Edwall GE: Sexual abuse correlates: Similarties between male and female adolescents in chemical dependency treatment. *J Adolesc Res* 4(3):385–399, 1989.
56. Kaplan HB: Self-esteem and self-derogation theory of drug abuse, in Lettieri DJ, Sayers M, Pearson HW (eds): *Theories on Drug Abuse.* NIDA Monograph Series. 1980, vol 30, pp 128–131.
57. Steffenhagen RA: Self-esteem theory of drug abuse, in Lettieri DJ, Sayers M, Pearson HW (eds): *Theories on Drug Abuse.* NIDA Monograph Series, 1980, vol 30, pp 128–131.
58. Rohsenow DJ, Corbett R, Devine D: Molested as children: A hidden contribuition to substance abuse? *J Subst Abuse Treat* 5(1):13–18, 1988.
59. Kaplan HB, Martin SS, Robins C: Pathways to adolescent drug use: Self-derogation, peer influence, weakening of social controls, and early substance use. *J Health Soc Behav* 25:270–289, 1984.
60. Watts WD, Ellis AM: Sexual abuse and drinking and drug use: Implications for prevention. *J Drug Educ* 23(2):183–200, 1993.
61. Wolfe DA: *Child Abuse: Implications for Child Development and Psychopathology.* Newbury Park, CA, Sage, 1987.
62. Miller BA, Downs WR, Gondoli DM: Delinquency, childhood violence, and the development of alcoholism in women. *Crime Delinquency* 35(1):94–108, 1989.
63. Terr, LC: Childhood trauma: An outline and overview. *Am J Psychiatry* 148:10–20, 1991.
64. Browne A: Family violence and homelessness: The relevance of trauma histories in the lives of homeless women. *Am J Orthopsychiatry* 63:370–384, 1993.
65. Davidson LM, Baum A: Post traumatic stress in children following natural and human-made trauma, in Davidson LM, Baum A (eds): *Handbook of Developmental Psychopathology.* New York, Plenum Press, 1990, pp 251–259.
66. Steketee G, Foa E: Rape victims: Post-traumatic stress responses and their treatment: A review of the literature. *J Anxiety Dis,* 1:69–86, 1987.

67. American Psychiatric Association: *Diagnostic and Statistical Manual of Mental Disorders*, Fourth Edition. Washington, DC, APA, 1994.

68. Brown A: Violence against women by male partners: Prevalence, outcomes, and policy implications. *Am Psychol* 48(10):1077–1087, 1993.

69. Herman JL: *Trauma and Recovery*. New York, Basic Books, 1992.

70. Boney-McCoy S, Finkelhor D: The psychosocial impact of violent victimization on a national youth sample. Unpublished manuscript, Durham, University of New Hampshire, Family Research Laboratory, 1993.

71. Crime Victims Research and Treatment Center: *Rape in America: A Report to the Nation*. Arlington, VA, National Victim Center, 1992.

72. Edwards G, Hensman C, Peto J: A comparison of female and male motivation for drinking. *Int J Addict* 8:577–587, 1973.

73. Fillmore KM: Drinking and problem drinking in early adulthood and middle age. *Q J Stud Alcohol* 35:819–840, 1974.

74. Fillmore KM: Relationships between specific drinking problems in early adulthood and middle age. *J Stud Alcohol* 36:882–907, 1975.

75. Miller BA, Downs WR, Joyce K: Victimization of drug women. Paper presentation at the Fourth International Conference on the Reduction of Drug related Harm in Rotterdam, the Netherlands, 1993.

76. Robins L, Helzer J, Cottler L, Goldring E: *NIMH Diagnostic Interview Schedule:* Version III Revised (DIS-III-R), St Louis, MO, Washington University, 1989.

77. Selzer ML: The Michigan Alcoholism Screening Test: The quest for a new diagnostic instrument. *Am J Psychiatry* 127:1653–1658, 1971.

78. Skinner HA: *Lifetime Drinking History: Administration and Scoring Guidelines*. Toronto, Addiction Research Foundation, 1979.

79. Wilsnack SC: Sexuality and women's drinking: Findings from a US national study. *Alcohol Health Res World* 15:147–150, 1991.

80. Wilsnack RW, Klassen AD, Wilsnack SC: Retrospective analysis of lifetime changes in women's drinking behavior. *Adv Alcohol Subst Abuse* 5(3):9–26, 1986.

81. Finkelhor D: *Sexually Victimized Children*. New York, Free Press, 1979.

82. Sgroi SM: *Handbook of Clinical Intervention in Child Sexual Abuse*. Lexington, MA, Lexington Books, 1982.

83. Straus, MA: Measuring intrafamily conflict and violence: The Conflict Tactics (CT) Scales. *J Marriage Fam* 41:75–88, 1979.

84. Loftus EF: The reality of repressed memories. *Am Psychol* 48(5):518–537, 1993.

Women, Alcohol, and Driving

Patricia F. Waller and Frederic C. Blow

Abstract. Alcohol-related crashes and fatalities have shown a dramatic decrease over the last decade. While males continue to account for most alcohol-related crashes, females are an increasing proportion of alcohol-involved drivers in both fatal and nonfatal crashes. Although most research has not addressed the possibility of gender differences in the effects of alcohol on driving performance, available evidence suggests that such differences may exist. Alcohol appears to have greater effects on females in terms of biomedical damage and impaired performance, although these effects have not been systematically investigated in relation to driving. Effective prevention programs for women require more focused research to understand gender-related factors in the effects of alcohol on driving.

1. Motor Vehicle Crash Casualties Predominantly Male

Motor vehicle crashes, and especially serious or fatal motor vehicle crashes, remain very much a male phenomenon[1-4] (see Fig. 1). In 1990, the rate of male drivers' fatal crash involvement per 100,000 population was about 4.5 times that for female drivers.[4]

Males are also overrepresented in the population of drinking drivers, particularly those with higher blood alcohol concentrations (BACs).[5,6] Studies of high school and college students regularly report higher rates of driving after drinking for males.[7-10] In 1989, overall alcohol-related mortality for males in California, including alcohol-related medical problems as well as alcohol-related injuries, showed more than three times the rate for females.[11]

Patricia F. Waller • University of Michigan Transportation Research Institute, Ann Arbor, Michigan 48109-2150.   **Frederic C. Blow** • University of Michigan Alcohol Research Center, Ann Arbor, Michigan 48108–3318.

Recent Developments in Alcoholism, Volume 12: Women and Alcoholism, edited by Marc Galanter. Plenum Press, New York, 1995.

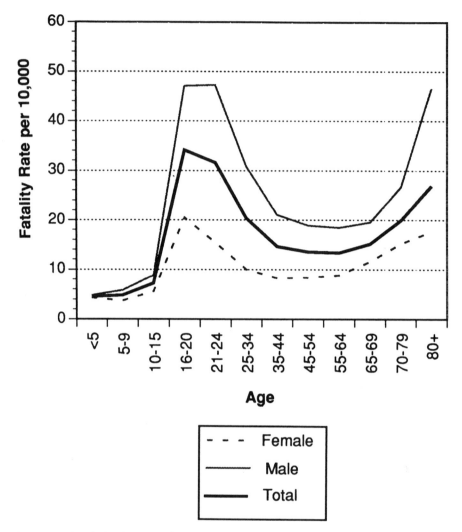

Figure 1. Crash fatality rate for males and females by age group. (From National Highway Transportation Safety Administration, 1983.[12])

2. Drunken Driving Decreasing

However, there is striking evidence that both the rate and the incidence of drunken driving have decreased. Beginning in the late 1970s and early 1980s, citizen action groups became a catalyst for energizing the public concerning the hazards posed by drinking and driving. Based on data from the Fatal Accident Reporting System (FARS), from 1982 to 1991 the proportion of fatal-crash-involved drivers at or above BAC 0.10% dropped from 30% to

24%. Drivers involved in fatal crashes who had any detectable alcohol also decreased from 39% to 31% during the same period.[12]

Because there is no national database for total crashes comparable to FARS (a standard national reporting system that includes all motor vehicle crashes occurring on public roads and that involve at least one fatality), data from two states were analyzed to estimate changes in drinking and driving for the full range of reported crashes. Crash data from Michigan were examined from 1982 through 1991. For these analyses, only drivers of cars, vans, utility vehicles, light trucks, and motorcycles were included. This limitation was imposed so that the focus would be on vehicles that are most widely used. Large trucks were omitted because they are used largely for commercial purposes and are driven primarily by males who rarely are using alcohol. If they were included, it may distort the gender comparisons for alcohol use and driving.

Nonfatal crashes involving alcohol have also decreased. In Michigan, police-reported crashes for drivers of cars, vans, light trucks, and motorcycles increased almost 27% between 1982 and 1991. During this same period, the absolute number of such drivers identified as had been drinking (HBD) decreased more than 36%. In 1982, HBD crashes represented more than 10% of all reported crashes but were only 5.2% in 1991. Washington State showed similar reductions, with an absolute increase in total crashes but a decrease in the number of HBD crashes. Generally, it appears that drinking and driving has definitely declined, and this decline has probably been a significant factor in the overall decrease in traffic fatalities nationwide.

3. Gender Differences and Drinking and Driving Trends

While males still account for most drinking and driving, and while there has been an overall decrease in both the rate and the incidence of alcohol-related driving, the changes that are occurring appear to differ by gender. This gender difference has been observed worldwide. In an international conference on women, alcohol, drugs, and traffic held in 1989, increases in the rate or proportion of women drinking drivers were reported from Canada,[13] Finland,[14] Germany,[15-18] New Zealand,[19] Sweden,[20] and the United States.[21] Fell[22] had previously reported that young females (aged 21–24) were not showing the same level of decrease in drinking and driving as evidenced by their male counterparts, based on drivers in fatal crashes from 1982 to 1985.

How should these changes over time be interpreted? In Michigan, from 1982 to 1991, there have been marked increases in total drivers in crashes for both males and females, with females showing much greater increases (47% versus 16% for males). However, for both genders there have been decreases in HBD crashes, both in proportion of total crashes and absolute number of HBD crashes. The decrease for males has been greater (37%) than for females (29%), but both are sizable.

When national data (FARS) for drivers in fatal crashes are considered (1982–1991), females show greater reductions than males in the proportion of those who are legally intoxicated (28% reduction for females vs. 17% for males). In this comparison it appears that women have shown greater reductions than men. However, because women drivers have increased their numbers since 1982 as drivers in fatal crashes, the reduction in absolute number of those in fatal crashes who are legally intoxicated is only 13.7% compared to a 23.9% reduction for male drivers in fatal crashes. These seemingly paradoxical findings are accounted for by the fact that male drivers in fatal crashes have decreased in number over the time period from 1982 to 1991 (8%), while female drivers in such crashes have increased by 20%.[12] Thus, even though the females showed a greater drop in the proportion who are legally intoxicated, because so many more women are drivers in fatal crashes, the decrease in absolute number of legally intoxicated female drivers is much less than that for males.

When total reported crashes in Michigan are considered, the picture is slightly different, although the gender relationships remain similar. Because of the increased efforts in recent years to combat drinking and driving in youth, drivers aged 16 through 20 were analyzed separately. In Fig. 2 it can be seen that HBD crashes have shown marked reductions from 1982 to 1991, with much greater reductions for drivers age 20 and under. Young males have also shown a slight decrease in total crashes, while all other groups have shown increases. Females, particularly those aged 21 and older, have shown dramatic increases in their crash involvement, probably reflecting marked increases in driving exposure.

While the proportion of female drivers in crashes has increased overall, the rate of change is not the same across age groups. Furthermore, there are important differences in the rate of change in total crashes versus the rate of change in HBD crashes. Figures 3 and 4 illustrate these changes for all reported crashes in Michigan (Fig. 3) and for fatal crashes nationwide (Fig. 4).

The data shown were derived by comparing the proportion of female drivers in each category in 1982 and in 1991 and calculating the percentage change in the proportion. For example, in 1982 females aged 16 through 20 represented 16% of the total HBD crashes for drivers in that age group. In 1991, they represented 17%. The difference translates into a 6.2% increase in their proportion of HBD crashes for drivers aged 16 through 20. Similar calculations were made for each group shown, for HBD and total crashes, for Michigan and for FARS.

Overall, the rate of increase in total crashes exceeds the rate of change for HBD crashes, but there are two notable exceptions. In both data sets (Michigan and FARS), female drivers aged 30 through 39 show greater rates of increases in HBD crashes than in total crashes. Possible explanations for this finding need to be explored and might include a cohort phenomenon in that this age group experienced the reduction in the legal drinking age at a time when women's roles were rapidly changing.

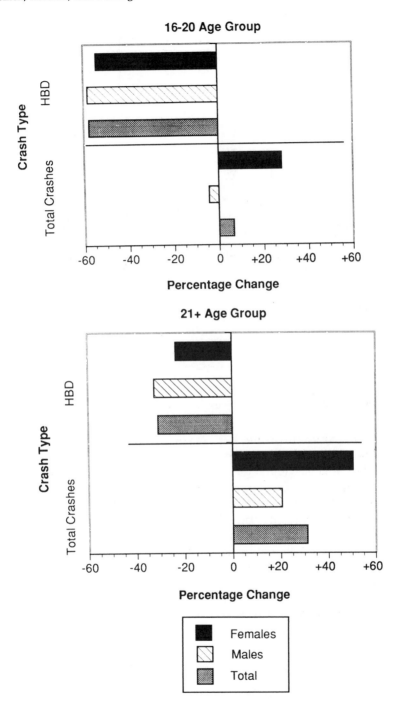

Figure 2.   Rate of change (in percent) of number of drivers in crashes by age, had been drinking (HBD) status, and gender; Michigan, 1982–1991.

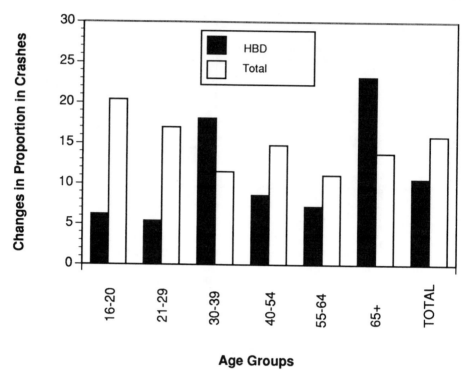

Age Groups

Figure 3. Rate of change (in percent) of female drivers in had been drinking (HBD) and total of crashes by age; Michigan, 1982–1991.

A perhaps more surprising finding concerns older women drivers, aged 65 and older. Although this group represents relatively small numbers, they are sufficiently large to suggest that the increase in HBD crashes that exceeds the corresponding increase in total crashes reflects major changes in drinking and driving practices in this cohort. Again, the finding obtains in both data sets.

In the FARS data (Fig. 4), a third age group shows disproportionate increases in HBD crashes in relation to total crashes, namely, female drivers aged 21 through 29. It should be noted that this finding is in marked contrast to the immediately younger group, where female drivers show much smaller relative increases in HBD crashes. One hypothesis is that this change is related to changes in the legal drinking age. Whether this shift will persist as the present cohort of teenage drivers moves into their 20s remains to be seen. It should also be noted that this phenomenon does not occur in the Michigan data.

4. Gender Differences in Treatment of Drivers

Questions have been raised as to whether women may be underrepresented in some of the data reported because of differences in how police

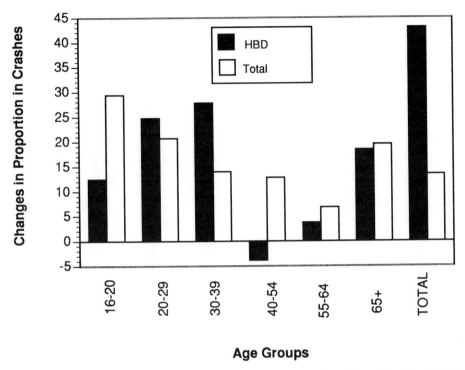

Figure 4.   Rate of change (in percent) of female drivers in had been drinking (HBD) and total fatal crashes, by age; FARS, 1982–1991.

officers deal with male and female offenders. Argeriou and Paulino[23] conclude that police are less likely to arrest women driving under the influence (DUI) because of erratic driving alone. Rather, women's arrests are more likely to result from involvement in a crash. The authors interpret these findings as indicating "unequal treatment of men and women by the police." Vingilis, Adlaf, and Chung[24] compared findings from roadside surveys and arrest data, in which arrest data showed an underrepresentation of women (6%) compared to their presence in the driving population based on roadside surveys (18%). It is suggested that females are less likely to be suspected of DWI and hence less likely to be arrested. However, the authors express caution in interpreting the findings in that there was a very small sampling in the roadside survey.

Franklin[25] has also reported that, in Indiana, law enforcement personnel "admitted to differential arrest practices for women." The male officers contend that because female offenders are more difficult to handle, they tend to avoid arresting them. However, this explanation contrasts with a hypothesis offered by Vingilis et al.,[24] whereby police reported that they are more likely to arrest drivers who do not handle themselves as well when stopped. The study by Argeriou and Paulino[23] suggests that women who physically or verbally abuse the arresting officer increase their likelihood of arrest.

In a recent study in Western Australia, Lang and Stockwell[26] compare findings from random breath tests, roadside tests administered by routine traffic patrols, and breath tests following a traffic crash. They found essentially no differences between the proportion of females arrested as a result of a crash versus those arrested as a result of random breath testing or routine traffic patrols. In fact, male drivers were slightly more likely than females to be detected as a result of a crash, suggesting that police were not showing any bias in favor of females during routine patrols.

It has long been speculated that in our society women manage to hide their alcohol problems more effectively than men, and that police are likely to excuse women for behavior for which they arrest a man. To what extent such differential treatment occurs cannot be determined in the absence of more precise data, but when objective measures are available (e.g., blood alcohol tests on deceased drivers), the persistent preponderance of males indicates that, at least for fatalities, the gender differences are marked. Likewise, the alcohol-related mortality data show consistently high male-to-female ratios. Nevertheless, if there are differences in the way in which police deal with female and male drivers who have been drinking, such differences need to be investigated and addressed.

5. Gender Differences in Recidivism

Several studies have reported lower recidivism of female offenders than for males. Indeed, their low rate of recidivism has been used as a reason for excluding them from outcome studies, since it would be difficult to evaluate the effectiveness of interventions on subsequent infractions.

Shore et al.[27] examined women arrested for DUI in Wichita, Kansas, over a 5-year period. They found that arrest appeared to have a differential impact on women versus men, with women showing a much lower rate of rearrest. This finding is consistent with that of Argeriou and Paulino,[23] who found that women offenders were much less likely than men to have prior arrests for DUI. Wells-Parker and colleagues[28] conducted a prospective study for female offenders in Mississippi in which they found that female DUI offenders were less likely to have prior DUI arrests and less likely to recidivate. Snow et al.[29] also reported lower recidivism rates for female offenders in Mississippi. Bailey[19] found much lower recidivism rates for female offenders in Wellington, New Zealand (13.3% vs. 48.5% for men). However, he noted that rates were more comparable for men and women in Auckland, where enforcement is higher.

What these differences in recidivism rates mean is difficult to determine. Because men have higher DUI rates to begin with, it would be anticipated that they would be more likely to be detected a second time. At least one study has suggested that the much lower rate of DUI arrest for women works against them in that it reduces the opportunity to identify a potential alcohol problem and channel the offender into appropriate treatment.[23]

Prevention programs focused on drinking driver, including DUI arrests, need to take into account what appears to be a much lower incidence of drinking and driving for women. Consequently, the same recidivism criteria applied to male offenders are not likely to be appropriate for women.

6. Gender Differences in Behavior

Gender differences have been noted in the tendency to engage in behaviors that are considered high risk, including high-risk driving. For example, Adebayo[30] describes a survey of a Canadian urban population ranging in age from 18 to over 35 (an upper limit is not given) in which males were much more likely to report driving while alcohol-impaired. Based on interviews with high school age drivers, Farrow[31] found that boys reported much more high-risk behavior, including using an automobile to race, "driving daredevil," using an automobile to "get high," and driving after drinking.

A survey of college students reports more frequent drinking and heavier drinking among males than females.[23] For both genders, those who reported frequent heavy drinking also reported more frequent stops by police for moving violations. While females were much less likely to be heavy drinker, those who were showed driving patterns similar to male heavy drinkers. Interestingly, the proportion of frequent drinkers among students who planned to join fraternities or sororities was twice that found for students not planning to join.

Gender differences have also been reported for aggressive behavior. Milgram[33] cites the frequently observed relationship between alcohol and behavior that may be considered aggressive in nature, including accidents. Generally, males are more likely to report problems associated with drinking, such as DUI, fights, and vandalism. White et al.[34] reported a longitudinal study of alcohol and aggression in young people. The low base rates of aggressive behavior among the females, however, precluded the possibility of examining its occurrence in relation to alcohol use. For the males, it was found that the aggressive behavior precedes the alcohol use; that is, young males who display more aggressive behavior are more likely subsequently to use alcohol and to display alcohol-related aggression. Gomberg[35] reviewed the literature on alcohol, women, and aggression and concluded that the findings are mixed. Women may be as likely as men to express aggression, depending on the circumstances.

Nevertheless, it is likely that there are gender differences in the predisposition toward aggression, and that gender differences observed in drinking and driving may reflect, to some extent, some of the differences in basic tendencies toward aggression. There are studies suggesting that women and men differ in their preception of risk in regard to the use of alcohol. Spigner et al.[36] reported that women undergraduates view the use of alcohol and drugs as posing greater risk of harm to themselves than do men. In the Netherlands, a higher proportion of women report a greater perceived chance of being stopped by the police and tested for alcohol consumption.[37] Based on surveys of high school sophomores, Farrow and Brissing[38] found that the female students reported more use of alcohol and drugs and had more disturbed family background than the males. However, the attitudes of the females toward DUI were more socially acceptable than those of the males. The females were more realistic in assessing the hazards of drinking and driving. Such differences in attitudes may relate to the gender differences observed in the driving behavior of adolescents. Such differences could account for why females are underrepresented in arrests for DUI in the absence of a crash.

7. Women's Changing Patterns of Behavior

Over the past two decades women have experienced marked changes in their lifestyles. They have entered the labor force in record numbers and achieved an unprecedented economic independence. The age at marriage has increased, so that many more women are living independently. These changes have been accompanied by increasing rates of driver licensure[39] and motor vehicle ownership. It was recently reported that female auto buyers bought 49% of all new cars in 1991 versus 36% in 1980.[40] Corresponding changes have occurred in their driving behavior. Women are increasingly represented in total mileage accumulated on our highways.[39]

Women's changing roles and their relationship to alcohol use are reviewed by Fillmore,[41] who questions whether women's alcohol use has changed as much as is sometimes purported. She points out the differences in what is considered deviant drinking for men versus women, as well as inconsistencies from one study to another in definitions used for heavy drinking. Also noted is the frequency with which studies report difficulties in identifying enough female heavy drinkers to enable meaningful analyses of data. In examining several longitudinal studies covering different cohorts of women, she found heavy frequent drinking is rare in both young and old age but seems to peak in the middle years. On the other hand, rates of abstention appear to increase with age. Despite similarities across cohorts, Fillmore concludes that there may be major changes occurring among younger cohorts; that is, heavy frequent drinking is more common in younger age females today than was true for older cohorts when they were the same age.

Whether and how changes in women's employment affects alcohol use have been reviewed recently by Wilsnack and Wilsnack,[42] who conclude that whatever relationships may exist are not clear-cut. However, one dimension that was not addressed in either review is how employment may relate to the amount of driving engaged in by women. It is reasonable to assume that increased financial independence is related to increased motor vehicle ownership, and that increased employment would be associated with increased driving. Even if employment has no effect on alcohol use per se, if driving increases, then to the extent that alcohol is used at all there is increased opportunity for alcohol use to be combined with driving.

8. Gender Differences in Crash Risk

As early as the Grand Rapids study,[43] it was reported that female drivers ran a higher risk of crash at a given level BAC. Although the crash risk for males at a 0.08% BAC was about twice the risk at zero BAC, the risk for females was increased ninefold, or 4.5 times that of the male. These early findings were attributed, at least in part, to the relative inexperience of women in driving compared with men. However, more recent studies report elevated crash risk for women who drink and drive. Zador[44] analyzed the alcohol-related risk of fatal driver injury by driver age and sex. Comparing data on fatal crashes with driver exposure data based on a national roadside breath-testing survey, he concluded that at least in the 0.05–0.09% BAC range, females have a higher relative risk of driver fatality than males. Jones *et al.*[20] found that of DUIs in Sweden, the females were more likely to be apprehended because of a crash. Although at high BACs (above 0.15) almost all of both genders were judged by a physician as unfit to drive, at lower BACs (<0.05%) a higher proportion of women were so judged.

Biecheler-Fretel *et al.*[45] studied a sample of French drivers. Although women had fewer crashes than men, when the mileage driven was considered, the reverse was true. The largest gender differences were found for the mileage-related crash rates for a driver who combined drinking with nighttime driving, with women experiencing much higher crash risk. However, Beirness[13] in Canada compared BACs from roadside survey data with the proportion of fatally injured impaired drivers and found no gender differences.

Relative performance by gender can be studied under more controlled conditions in a laboratory setting. Several studies suggest that there may be gender differences in performance in relation to alcohol ingestion. Erwin *et al.*[46] studied alcohol-induced drowsiness and vigilance performance. Using one placebo and three alcohol conditions (about 0.03% BAC, 0.06% BAC, and 0.095% BAC), they presented visual stimuli, only some of which required a response. The men performed better under all conditions, including placebo, and were less affected by the low and medium levels of alcohol. Gender differences were minimal at the high BAC. The authors conclude that "the greatest sex-related difference in performance was observed at the low and medium doses of alcohol, suggesting a sensitivity toward sedative effects of alcohol in these women" (p512).

A laboratory study of performance on an electronic grid board manual assembly task also showed gender differences in relation to alcohol.[47] Subjects were college students in their early 20s. Target BACs were zero (placebo), 0.05% BAC, 0.07% BAC, and 0.09% BAC. The assembly tasks were performed under both paced and unpaced conditions. The performance of the females was more affected by the alcohol than was that of the males. The authors interpreted the differences as attributable to gender differences in the speed–accuracy trade-off.

Niaura et al.[48] found that females recovered memory functioning more slowly on the descending limb of the blood alcohol curve than did males. Differences were not found for measures of divided attention, body sway, or pursuit tracking ability. The authors suggest that females remain sensitive to the intoxicating effect of alcohol longer than males, and that this effect may reduce their further consumption of alcohol during drinking episodes.

Another study examined the effects of alcohol on the speed of accessing long-term memory.[49] Forty-four college students served as subjects. Under the sober condition they showed no gender differences in response time, but in the alcohol condition the female subjects responded significantly more slowly. However, it should be noted that alcohol was administered as a function of body weight, and there is no indication that allowances were made for gender differences in body composition.[50] Because the actual BAC reached was not measured, it may be that the female subjects were at a higher BAC than the males.

Finally, a report by Avant[51] suggests that alcohol has a greater effect on the visual functioning of females than males. Using simulated traffic signs presented on slides, he found that alcohol affects the ability to detect the presence or absence of a sign, and that females are more affected by alcohol than males.

Each of these laboratory studies has shortcomings, and none is precisely analogous to the driving task. Nevertheless, the laboratory studies suggest that there may be gender differences in how alcohol affects performance. If this is so, it may be anticipated that driving performance might likewise show differential effects of alcohol as a function of gender. Although precision is not possible in calculations of on-road risk of crash, the repeated observation that women may be at higher risk of crash at a given BAC at least indicates a need for more careful investigation of this possibility. In addition to the interest in understanding any underlying mechanisms involved, the data would be of value in health education programs for women.

9. Alcohol Effects on Injury

Alcohol affects not only the initial risk of crash involvement, but also the injury consequences. There is evidence that both chronic and acute use of alcohol can affect the extent of injury experienced from a given impact. Alcohol use over time modifies the body so that a traumatic impact is more likely to inflict lasting damage, and so that recovery from injury may be impaired. Studies have shown that prolonged use of alcohol reduces bone strength, making bones more vulnerable to fracture from a given traumatic impact.[52,53]

Furthermore, alcohol is known to affect the immune system, and liver damage resulting from alcohol can interfere with the body's recovery from trauma.[54] Alcohol also appears to affect wound healing.[55]

Alcohol increases the amount of damage resulting from a given impact or insult to the body. Even in the absence of prior chronic use, alcohol has immediate consequences that render an organism more vulnerable should an injury occur. Carefully controlled laboratory studies based on animal models identify three areas in which these potentiating effects of alcohol on injury have been observed.[56] These include:

1. Myocardial contusion. In the presence of alcohol, a standardized non-penetrating blow to the chest was found to greatly increase the probability of death in laboratory animals as compared to the same blow in the absence of alcohol.[57,58]
2. Hemorrhagic shock. Alcohol reduces tolerance to hemorrhagic shock. Laboratory studies show that animals treated with alcohol experience shock in response to loss of smaller quantities of blood than animals not so treated.[59,60]
3. Central nervous system damage. Studies examining the effect of injury to the brain and spinal cord show that in the presence of alcohol, a controlled blow results in much more extensive damage, including hemorrhaging.[61–63] In the case of spinal cord injury, given the same impact, the likelihood of permanent paralysis increases greatly if alcohol is present.[64] These effects of alcohol on injury are evidenced in motor vehicle crash injuries.[56]

10. Gender Differences in the Effects of Chronic Alcohol Use on Injury

Gender differences in vulnerability to injury as a result of alcohol use have not been systematically investigated. However, there is sufficient evidence from related research to suggest that women may be at higher risk than men for the potentiating effects of alcohol on injury. It is known that women are more vulnerable to biomedical damage from alcohol, particularly in relation to liver function and bone density. Women develop liver damage over a shorter period of time and in response to lower quantities of consumption.[65] Consequently, to the extent that liver functioning affects the body's recovery from injury, it may be anticipated that women will show greater impairment. When death does not occur shortly after injury, delayed deaths are usually associated with secondary sepsis, a condition related to the robustness of the immune system. Although it is known that alcohol impairs the immune response and hence may interfere with recovery from injury, to what extent such impairment is related to gender has not been determined.

There may also be gender differences related to the effects of chronic use of alcohol on bone strength. A prospective study of over 84,000 women found that moderate consumption of alcohol was associated with an increased risk of both hip fractures and forearm fractures.[66] Because fractures associated with high-impact trauma were excluded (e.g., motor vehicle crashes, recreational activities such as roller-skating or skiing), the study included only injuries sustained under conditions not likely to result in injury, such as slipping on a level surface. Women who were identified as moderate drinkers were compared with those who did not consume alcohol. After adjusting for potential confounding variables, it was found that the risk of hip fractures was more than twice as high for those consuming alcohol. The risk of forearm fracture was also elevated but not so greatly.[66]

It is known that alcohol leaches calcium from the bones, reducing bone strength, and that women have smaller bones than men. This alcohol-related osteopenia is particularly relevant for women, who are at higher risk for age-related bone changes. Thus women have less bone mass to lose before they reach a critical level of bone strength. It may be expected that, on the whole, women consuming alcohol would be more vulnerable to fractures than men consuming alcohol.

11. Gender Differences in the Potentiating Effects of Acute Administration of Alcohol on Injury

The question of whether there may be gender differences in the effects of acute administration of alcohol on injury is less clear, in large part because there have been no carefully controlled studies. However, recent research suggests that there are gender differences in the metabolism of alcohol[66] that contribute to higher BACs in women than those found for men. It had been assumed in the past that the gender differences observed in BACs resulting from the same dose of alcohol for body weight were related to differences in volume of distribution. Because women usually have a higher fat-to-muscle ratio than men and because muscle has a higher water content than fat, for a given body weight women will have less muscle and therefore less water in which to dissolve the alcohol and hence will reach a higher BAC from a given dose. However, Frezza and colleagues[67] found that no such gender differences occur in response to a controlled amount of alcohol administered intravenously, a result that would be anticipated if differences were attributable simply to differences in volume of distribution. They conclude that there are gender differences in the way in which the alcohol is metabolized upon oral administration but not in response to intravenous administration. Although the underlying mechanisms are not clear, what is clear is that women cannot rely on existing guidelines for quantities of alcohol consumption per given body weight. This should be taken into account for prevention programs directed at drinking and driving for women.

12. Implications for Prevention of Drinking and Driving for Women

12.1. Women Must Be Informed

Women are not being adequately equipped with the information they need to understand the peculiar risks they confront in relation to alcohol. Without such information they cannot make informed, intelligent decisions. Information that must be communicated includes the following:

1. While drunken driving has been and remains predominantly a male problem, females are increasing their total involvement in crashes, as well as representing an increasing proportion of drunken driving crashes.

2. Women cannot use available guidelines for estimating either BAC or the effects of a given BAC. The charts do not take into account, first, the fact that for a given weight women will generally reach a higher BAC, and second, for a given BAC the performance of women may be more impaired.

3. Women are more vulnerable to the biomedical effects of alcohol. In comparison to men, women develop liver damage and become alcoholic over a shorter period of time and in response to the consumption of lower quantities of alcohol.

4. Women, as well as men, need to know that alcohol, even if it is not used chronically or in large amounts, makes the body more vulnerable to injury in case of a motor vehicle crash or other mishap. Thus, it is not enough to have a designated driver who is sober. A designated driver may do everything right, but if someone else runs a traffic signal and crashes into the designated driver's vehicle, passengers are more likely to be more injured if they have been drinking than if they have not. Thus, in any situation that poses a hazard, alcohol increases the potential injury risk.

5. Women are being targeted by the alcohol industry, and messages are tailored to appeal especially to women.[68] These messages do not include information on the greater vulnerability of women to alcohol, both in terms of performance and in terms of biological effects. Women must be equipped to withstand these pressures. Women are socialized to be more compliant and cooperative. As society is changing there are increasing pressures, both subtle and otherwise, to encourage women to consume more alcohol. While males have always been subjected to pressures to drink, and have certainly demonstrated their vulnerability to such pressures, women are experiencing similar pressures at an unprecedented rate.

6. Although men with alcohol problems usually begin drinking heavily at an early age, the onset of heavy drinking in women may occur at any stage of life. It appears that problem drinking in women may be more likely to be precipitated by a specific event, such as a death or a divorce.[69] It is also known that at least some life stresses, such as divorce, are associated with

increased risk of motor vehicle crash.[70] To what extent such increased crash risk is associated with alcohol use has not been investigated. In at least some situations that may precipitate increased alcohol use and/or crash risk, a representative of the larger society is in the picture, e.g., a divorce attorney. Intervention efforts could include training such professionals to be alert to incipient alcohol problems and to serve as referral agents. Particular emphasis may be placed on the hazards of combining alcohol with driving. Young women, including children in school, should be informed about the effects of alcohol in the individual, the family, and the larger society.

12.2. Targeting Women

Women should be recognized as a special target population in regard to potential alcohol problems, not because women are more important but because women are different. Programs should be designed specifically for this population, taking into account both their special vulnerabilities and their special needs. Countermeasures for drunken driving have been designed in the absence of special attention to women. Efforts must be directed toward greater understanding of how women develop alcohol problems and how they are affected by alcohol. Efforts must include research, communication of information, development and implementation of interventions, and careful evaluation of programs that lead to revisions based on new knowledge.

12.3. Gender Equality

Finally, it must be recognized by women, as well as men, that equality is not synonymous with identity. True liberation includes the right to say no, to refuse to adopt carte blanche the model that society has imposed on the male. Women must create their own models, taking into consideration both their special strengths and their vulnerabilities, so that they can capitalize on their strengths and minimize any adverse consequences resulting from their vulnerabilities. When it comes to alcohol, women are different from men, and women need to know what these differences are and how to cope with them.

12.4. Future Research Needs

Although there has been much progress in the overall reduction of both alcohol-related fatalities and HBD driving arrests during the last two decades for women and men, much of the reduction has resulted from prevention efforts directed primarily at drunken driving by men. Research on the prevention of alcohol-related driving problems for women needs to focus, first, on the identification of gender-specific risk factors, and, second, on implementation of targeted prevention strategies taking these unique aspects of women's drinking and driving into account. More specifically, the following issues should be considered in pursuing a research agenda:

• Are the trends observed in reductions in drunken driving reflecting real changes in cultural norms that will persist regardless of special measures to combat this behavior?

• While both males and females have reduced their alcohol involvement in fatal crashes, the relative reduction for females has been greater (although they have increased in absolute numbers of drivers in fatal crashes). What are the factors underlying this gender difference?

• Women age 30 through 39 and 65 and older are not showing the same reductions in drunken driving seen in other age and gender groups. What are the factors underlying this phenomenon? Are they the same for both cohorts or are the older women responding to different factors?

• It has long been contended that women are treated differentially when alcohol-related infractions occur. Objective evidence is difficult to obtain. Nevertheless, if women are less likely to be prosecuted for a drunken driving offense, they are also less likely to come to the attention of the authorities and thus become eligible for intervention. Consequently, it is important to establish whether women offenders are experiencing differential consequences.

• Because drunken driving occurs at lower rates for women as compared to men, there is a need to develop appropriate criteria for measuring the effectiveness of intervention approaches. Recidivism is not sufficiently sensitive to provide a valid outcome evaluation.

• Laboratory studies suggest the possibility that women are more sensitive than men to the effects of alcohol on tests of performance. Epidemiological studies of crash involvement are consistent with these findings. However, in terms of driving performance, virtually nothing is known about how alcohol affects which driving behaviors.

• Drinking behavior in relation to changing patterns of motor vehicle use need to be studied in women. There is a need for a comprehensive analysis of what kinds of trips pose greatest risk and how lifestyles may be modified to reduce risk while maintaining mobility.

• There is a need for good information on history of alcohol use and how it may be associated with extent of injury experienced from a given motor vehicle crash. Injury types should be of particular interest in that the effects of alcohol on bone density may be expected to increase vulnerability to fracture.

• No research has been conducted to determine whether there are any gender differences in the potentiating effects of acute administration of alcohol.

• Research is needed to determine the characteristics of women who are at greatest risk of drinking/driving and the circumstances contributing to risk.

• There is a need for basic information on what women believe in regard to alcohol use and driving, including what they know about BAC limits, and how women may differ from men in the effects of alcohol dosage in relation to weight.

• Materials need to be developed and evaluated for educating women concerning their greater biological vulnerability to the effects of alcohol use.

13. Conclusion

Alcohol-related driving has shown dramatic decreases in recent years. Initial concerns about the apparent increased involvement of women in alcohol-related driving appear to be partially confirmed by some age groups. However, young drivers, both male and female, below age 21, have shown remarkable decreases in alcohol-related driving. Women of all ages have increased their crash involvement, although they have increased their driving exposure even more. While, on the whole, women appear to have responded favorably to efforts to reduce alcohol-related driving, two age groups have not shown such positive effects. Women aged 30 through 39 and age 65 and older may be in special need of attention.

Although research evidence is limited, it appears that alcohol may have differential effects on women compared with men. Women appear to be more vulnerable to physiological damage from prolonged alcohol use. They may also be more vulnerable to impairment of performance from low doses of alcohol. Such differential effects of alcohol may affect both driving performance and injury resulting from motor vehicle crashes. Gender-specific research is critical to understanding the role of alcohol in driving behavior.

References

1. Warren RA, Simpson HM: Exposure and alcohol as risk factors in the fatal nighttime collisions of men and women drivers. *J Safety Res* 12:151–156, 1980.
2. Soderstrom CA, Arias JD, Carson SL, Cowley RA: Alcohol consumption among vehicular occupants injured in crashes. *Alcohol Clin Exp Res* 8:269–271, 1984.
3. Simpson HM, Mayhew DR: The hard core drinking driver. Ottawa, Traffic Injury Research Foundation of Canada, 1991, p 26.
4. Cerrelli EC: Crash data and rates for age–sex groups of drivers—1990. Research note. Washington, DC, National Highway Traffic Safety Administration, 1992.
5. Traffic Injury Research Foundation of Canada: Characteristics of drivers involved in traffic crashes: Gender and age in *Drinking and Driving in Ontario—Statistical Yearbook 1988–89.* Toronto, Drinking/Driving Counter measures Office, Ministry of the Athorney General, 1991, p. 6.
6. Meyers AR, Perrine MW, Foss RD: Roadside surveys of nocturnal drinking drivers in Ohio, in *Alcohol, Drugs and Traffic Safety,* T92. Cologne, TUV Rheinland, pp 1104–1109.
7. US Centers for Disease Control: *Preventing Injuries.* Atlanta, GA, US Department of Health and Human Resources, 1983.
8. Williams AF, Lund AK, Preusser DF: Drinking and driving among high school students. *Int J Addict* 21:643–655, 1986.

 9. Smith PF, Remington PL: The epidemiology of drinking and driving: Results from the behavioral risk factor surveillance system, 1986. *Health Educ Q* 16:345–358.
10. Johnston LD: Statement of Lloyd D. Johnston, Ph.D., Program Director, Institute for Social Research, University of Michigan. Made before the Subcommittee on Select Education and Civil Rights of the House Education and Labor Committee in hearings on the reauthorization of The Drug-Free Schools and Communities Act, March 1993, Washington, DC.
11. Sutoky JW, Shultz JM, Kizer KW: Alcohol-related mortality in California, 1980 to 1989. *Am J Publ Health* 83:817–823, 1993.
12. National Highway Traffic Safety Administration: *Fatal Accident Reporting System 1991.* Washington, DC, NHTSA, 1993.
13. Beirness, DJ: Female drivers in Canada: Trends in accident involvement, in Valverius MR (ed): *Women, Alcohol, Drugs and Traffic: Proceedings of the International Workshop*, 1988, Stockholm, Sweden Stockholm, Almquist and Wiksell, 1989, pp 23–31.
14. Pikkarainen J, Penttila A: Women arrested for drunken driving in Finland during 1967–1987, in Valverius MR (ed): *Women, Alcohol, Drugs and Traffic, Proceedings of the International Workshop*, Sept 29, Stockholm, Sweden. Stockholm, DALCTRAF, 1989, pp 129–132.
15. Puschel K, Janssen W, Schmutte P, Jansen R: Comparison of female and male drunken drivers in hamburg 1970–1987, in Valerius MR (ed): *Women, Alcohol, Drugs and Traffic: Proceedings of the ICADTS International Workshop*, 1988, Stockholm, Sweden Stockholm, Almquist and Wiksell, 1989, pp 59–62.
16. Freudenstein P, Schmidt P, Wolfgang B: Female DWI offenders: The situation in Dusseldorf, in Valerius MR (ed): *Women, Alcohol, Drugs and Traffic: Proceedings of the ICADTS International Workshop*, 1988, Stockholm, Sweden. Stockholm, Almquist and Wiksell, 1989, pp 63–64.
17. Erkens M: Involvement of drunken women in road traffic, in Valverius MR (ed): *Women, Alcohol, Drugs and Traffic: Proceedings of the International Workshop*, Sept 29, Stockholm, Sweden. Stockholm: DALCTRAF, 1989, pp 65–71.
18. Gruner O, Bilzer N, Frevel HF: Drinking and driving women/Schlewsing–Holstein between 1977–1987, in Valverius MR (ed): *Women, Alcohol, Drugs and Traffic, Proceedings of the International Workshop*, Sept 29, Stockholm, Sweden. Stockholm, DALCTRAF, 1989, pp 101–107.
19. Bailey JPM: Female drinking drivers in New Zealand, in Valerius MR (ed): *Women, Alcohol, Drugs and Traffic: Proceedings of the ICADTS International Workshop*, 1988, Stockholm, Sweden. Stockholm, Almquist and Wiksell, 1989, pp 73–81.
20. Jones W, Holmgren P, Andersson E: FEmale drinking drivers in Sweden, in Valerius MR (ed): *Women, Alcohol, Drugs and Traffic: Proceedings of the ICADTS International Workshop*, 1988, Stockholm, Sweden. Stockholm, Almquist and Wiksell, 1989, pp 43–51.
21. Popkin CL: Drinking and driving by young females. *Accid Anal Prev* 23(1): 37–44, 1991.
22. Fell JC: Alcohol involvement rates in fatal crashes: A focus on young drivers and female drivers, in *31st Proceedings of the American Association for Automotive Medicine*. Des Plaines, IL: American Association for Automotive Medicine, 1987, pp 1–30.
23. Argeriou M, Paulino D: Women arrested for drunken driving in Boston. *J Stud Alcohol* 37(5):648–657, 1976.
24. Vingilis E, Adlaf EM, Chung L: Comparison of age and sex characteristics of police-suspected impaired drivers and roadside-surveyed impaired drivers. *Accid Anal Prev* 14:425–430, 1982.
25. Franklin S: Demographic and diagnostic characteristics of 108 women convicted of driving while intoxicated in Allen County, Indiana, in Valerius MR (ed): *Women, Alcohol, Drugs and Traffic: Proceedings of the International Workshop*, 1988, Stockholm, Sweden. Stockholm, Almquist and Wiksell, 1989, pp 157–164.
26. Lang E, Stockwell T: Drinking locations of drunk-drivers: A comparative analysis of accident and nonaccident cases. *Accid Anal Prev* 23:573–584, 1991.
27. Shore ER, McCoy ML, Toonen LA, Kuntz EJ: Arrests of women for driving under the influence. *J Stud Alcohol* 49(1):7–10, 1988.
28. Wells-Parker E, Pang MG, Anderson BJ, *et al*: Female DUI offenders: A comparison to male counterparts and an examination of the effects of intervention on women's recidivism rates. *J Stud Alcohol* 52(2):142–147, 1991.

29. Snow RW, Anderson BJ, Landrum JW: *The life activities inventory as a DUI countermeasure: An attempted replication*, Social Science Research Center (Ed). Mississippi State: Mississippi State University, 1993, p 7.

30. Adebayo A: Factors antecedent to impaired driving in an Canadian urban sample. *Int J Addict* 26:897–909, 1991.

31. Farrow JA: Drinking and driving behaviors of 16 to 19 year-olds. *J Stud Alcohol* 46:369–374, 1985.

32. Canterbury RJ, Gressard CF, Vieweg WVR, *et al*: Risk-taking behavior of college students and social forces. *Am J Drug Alcohol Abuse* 18:213–222, 1992.

33. Milgram GG: Adolescents, alcohol and aggression. *J Stud Alcohol* 11:53–61, 1993.

34. White HR, Brick J, Hansell S: A longitudinal investigation of alcohol use and aggression in adolescence. *J Stud Alcohol* 11:62–77, 1993.

35. Gomberg ESL: Alcohol, women and the expression of aggression. *J Stud Alcohol* 11:89–95, 1993.

36. Spigner C, Hawkins W, Loren W: Gender differences in perception of risk associated with alcohol and drug use among college students. *Women Health* 20:87–97, 1993.

37. Weseman P: Drinking and driving: No longer "only for men," in Valerius MR (ed): *Women, Alcohol, Drugs and Traffic: Proceedings of the ICADTS International Workshop*, 1988, Stockholm, Sweden. Stockholm, Almquist and Wiksell, 1989, pp 83–90.

38. Farrow JA, Brissing P: Risk for DWI: A new look at gender differences in drinking and driving influences, experiences, and attitudes among new adolescent drivers. *Health Educ Q* 17:213–221, 1990.

39. Federal Highway Administration: Highway Statistics, 1993.

40. Belton, B: Automakers come a long way, baby. *USA Today*, 27 Jan: 1A, final edition, 1992.

41. Fillmore KM: "When angels fall": Women's drinking as cultural preoccupation and as reality, in Wilsnack SC, Beckman LJ (eds): *Alcohol Problems in Women: Antecedents, Consequences, and Intervention*. New York, Guilford Press, 1984, pp 7–36.

42. Wilsnack RW, Wilsnack SC: Women, work, and alcohol: Failures of simple theories. *Alcohol Clin Exp Res* 16:172–179, 1992.

43. Borkenstein RF, Crowther RF, Shumate RP, *et al*: *The Role of the Drinking Driver in Traffic Accidents*. Bloomington, IN, Department of Police Administration, 1964.

44. Zador PL: Alcohol-related risk of fatal driver injuries in relation to driver age and sex. *J Stud Alcohol* 52:302–310, 1991.

45. Biecheler-Fretel MB, Danech-Pajouh M, El Quadrani A: Drinking and driving. A typological approach comparing men and women, in Valerius MR (ed): *Women, Alcohol, Drugs and Traffic: Proceedings of the International Workshop*, 1988, Stockholm, Sweden. Stockholm, Almquist and Wiksell, 1989, pp 119–127.

46. Erwin CP, Wiener EL, Linnoila MI, Truscott TR: Alcohol-induced drowsiness and vigilance performance. *J Stud Alcohol* 39(3):505–516, 1978.

47. Price DL, Radwan MAE, Tergou DE: Gender, alcohol, pacing and incentive effects on an electronics assembly task. *Ergonomics* 29(3):393–406, 1986.

48. Niaura RS, Nathan PE, Frankenstein W, *et al*: Gender differences in acute psychomotor, cognitive, and pharmacokinetic response to alcohol. *Addict Behav* 12:345–356, 1987.

49. Haut JS, Beckwith BE, Petros TV, Russell S: Gender differences in retrieval from long-term memory following acute intoxication with ethanol. *Physiol Behav* 45:1161–1165, 1989.

50. Moscowitz H, Burns M: Effects of alcohol on driving performance. *Alcohol Health Res World* 14(1):12–14, 1990.

51. Avant LL: Alcohol impairs visual presence/absence detection more for females than for males. *Percept Psychophysiol* 48(3):285–290, 1990.

52. Saville PD: Alcohol-related skeletal disorders. *Ann NY Acad Sci* 25(252):287–291, 1975.

53. Peng TC, Garner SC, Frye GD, Crenshaw MA: Evidence of a toxic effect of ethanol on bone in rats. *Alcohol Clin Exp Res* 6(1):96–99, 1982.

54. Sherlock S: Liver disease in women. Alcohol, autoimmunity, and gallstones. *West J Med* 149(6):683–686, 1988.

55. Benveniste K, Thut P: The effect of chronic alcoholism on wound healing. *Proc Soc Exp Biol Med* 166(4):568–575, 1981.
56. Waller, PF, Steward JR, Hansen AR, *et al:* The potentiating effects of alcohol on driver injury. *J Am Med Assoc* 256(11):1461–1466, 1986.
57. Liedtke AJ, DeMuth WE: Effects of alcohol on cardiovascular performance after experimental nonpenetrating chest trauma. *Am J Cardiol* 35(2):243–250, 1975.
58. Nicholas GG, DeMuth WE Jr: Blunt cardiac trauma: The effect of alcohol on survival and metabolic function. *J Trauma* 20(1):58–60, 1980.
59. Malt SH, Baue AE: The effects of ethanol as related to trauma in the awake dog. *J Trauma* 11(1):76–86, 1971.
60. Garrison HG, Hansen AR, Cross RE, Proctor HJ: Effect of ethanol on lactic acidosis in experimental hemorrhagic shock. *Ann Emerg Med* 13(1):26–29, 1984.
61. Flamm ES, Demopoulos HB, Seligman ML, *et al:* Ethanol potentiation of central nervous system trauma. *J Neurosurg* 46(3):328–335, 1977.
62. De Crescito V, Demopoulos HB, Flamm ES, Ransohoff J II: Ethanol potentiation of traumatic cerebral edema. *Surg Forum* 25:438–440, 1974.
63. Anderson TE: Effects of acute alcohol intoxication on spinal cord vascular injury. *J Neurotrauma* 3(3):183–192, 1986.
64. Brodner RA, Van Gilder JC, Collins WF Jr.: Experimental spinal cord trauma: Potentiation by alcohol. *J Trauma* 21(2):124–129, 1981.
65. Blume SB: Alcohol problems in women. *NY State J Med* 82(8):1222–1224, 1982.
66. Hernandez-Avila M, Colditz GA, Stampfer MJ, *et al:* Caffeine, moderate alcohol intake, and risk of fractures of the hip and forearm in middle-aged women. *Am J Clin Nutr* 54:157–163, 1991.
67. Frezza M, Di Padova C, Pozzato G, *et al:* High blood alcohol levels in women: The role of decreased gastric alcohol dehydrogenase activity and first-pass metabolism. *N Engl J Med* 322(2):95–99, 1990.
68. Minkler M, Wallack L, Madden P: Alcohol and cigarette advertising in *Ms.* magazine. *J Publ Health Policy* 8(2):164–179, 1987.
69. Temple MT, Fillmore DM, Harka E, *et al:* A meta-analysis of change in marital and employment status as predictors of alcohol consumption on a typical occasion. *Br J Addict* 86(10):1269–1281, 1991.
70. McCormack A: Risk for alcohol-related accidents in divorced and separated women. *J Stud Alcohol* 46(3):240–243, 1985.

6

Employed Women with Alcohol Problems Who Seek Help from Employee Assistance Programs

Description and Comparisons

Terry C. Blum, Paul M. Roman, and Eileen M. Harwood

Abstract. After a brief description of employee assistance programs (EAP), we present data collected from 6,400 employees from 84 worksites who used the services of EAPs, a portion of whom were assessed by the EAP as having alcohol-related problems and/or recieved scores on the Alcohol Dependence Scale (ADS) indicative of a potential alcohol–related problem. In addition, data were collected at intake from the EAP administrators, and employment status of the employee clients was assessed 18 to 24 months later. These data indicate that EAPs are effective in sustaining the employment of most women with alcohol-related problems who seek services from EAPs and that EAPs' goal of early intervention is especially realized among women with alcohol problems. Other conclusions include: women with alcohol problems do not enter EAPs through routes that are strikingly different from those of men; many of the gender differences that are revealed are associated with job status differences; employed women with alcohol problems are detached from nuclear families, with markedly low rates of current marriage; even when married, spouses are less likely to play a role in the referral of women with alcohol problems than the spouses of the men; and, there is no clear indication that women are the target of any form of discrimination in the process of EAP utilization. However, women are considerably more likely to have less adequate insurance coverage, according to the EAP administrators' assessment reported at client intake, than their male counterparts, leading to treatment choices that may be less than appropriate.

Terry C. Blum • School of Management, Georgia Institute of Technology, Atlanta, Georgia 30332-0520.   **Paul M. Roman and Eileen M. Harwood** • Institute for Behavioral Research, University of Georgia, Athens, Georgia 30602-2401.

Recent Developments in Alcoholism, Volume 12: Women and Alcoholism, edited by Marc Galanter. Plenum Press, New York, 1995

1. Introduction

The increased rate of employment of women in the United States over recent decades is a dramatic and far-reaching social change. It is a fundamental socioeconomic impact, affecting women's well-being and behavior, relations between the genders, and the emergence of an extremely rich array of gender-related research issues. These research issues include the interrelations of gender and work with alcohol problems and their resolution.[1]

Compared to other arenas in the overall field of alcohol studies, the attention to women's drinking in relation to work roles and work performance has not been a high priority. Much of what is popularly assumed to be true about employed women's drinking is open to question. To cite two such examples: (1) there is little evidence that on an overall basis, women's work participation is bringing their drinking patterns and drinking problems toward parity with men[2]; and (2) there is little evidence to suggest that the stress of balancing work and nonwork role demands has brought pressures to bear on women that have escalated either their alcohol consumption or their rates of drinking problems.[1,3,4]

This chapter offers an unusual approach to issues surrounding women, work, and alcohol-related problems. The presentation centers on research data about a category of women about whom very little has been reported. These are employed women who have sought help from employee assistance programs (EAPs) for dealing with their own alcohol problems. The research sample includes women who have sought EAP assistance as self-referrals, as well as those whose job behaviors led to a supervisory referral. The overall study sample also includes women whose presenting problems are centered on major symptom areas other than alcohol abuse, as well as those whose diagnosis includes comorbidity of alcohol problems with other problems.

To offer an overview of what follows, we begin with a definition of EAPs. This is followed by a description of our research methods and the means by which this complex data set was collected. We then turn to a description of employed women with alcohol problems who use EAP services. This is followed by comparisons of employed men and women with alcohol problems who use EAP services. We then examine characteristics of women with probable alcohol problems who were not assessed as such by EAP personnel. This is followed by comparisons of those employed women with and without multiple problems who used EAP services, and we conclude with several observations about the implications of these findings.

2. EAPs

EAPs are worksite-based programs designed to assist workplace personnel in identifying and resolving problems involving alcohol or drug abuse, and family, stress, emotional, marital, financial, legal, and other personal concerns that adversely affect an employee's well-being or job performance.[5-7] A variety of services labeled as EAPs are in existence, some of which offer only "bare bones" assistance to employees.[8] The Employee Assistance Professionals Association (EAPA) has developed standards, however, that include a core definition and core functions for EAPs that are addressed only by providing comprehensive services. EAPA guidelines state that alcohol and other drug problems will be addressed effectively if an EAP includes expert consultation and training in identifying and facilitating the resolution of behavioral health and job performance problems; confidential, appropriate, and timely assessment services; referrals for appropriate diagnosis, treatment, and other assistance; links between the workplace and community resources that provide those services; follow-up services; and education on preventing alcohol and other drug problems.

EAPs provide the workplace with a systematic means for dealing with a variety of employee problems. This is valuable because, as Roman[9] pointed out, employee problems often are multiple and interrelated. To be effective, EAPs should be integrated into the performance and benefits management functions of human resource management.

EAPs are usually based on a written policy statement. They provide a means for supervisors, managers, and union shop stewards to obtain guidance in dealing with subordinates or co-workers who need assistance. The guidance is supplied either by an internal EAP coordinator, who is employed by the same organization as the target employees, or by a staff member of an external agency that is retained through a contractual mechanism. Some external agency representatives spend time at the worksites for which they provide services, and some internal program coordinators are located offsite. The structures and sizes of work organizations tend to influence the structures of EAPs as they relate to personnel, corporate medical programs (when they exist), and employee benefit plans.[10]

The EAP model has been well received by employers. In 1991, U.S. national survey data collected from a representative sample of full time employees revealed that, in the United States, 45% of full-time employees who were not self-employed had access to an EAP provided by their employers.[5] Virtually all large workplaces (> 500 workers) provide some form of an EAP, and the majority of medium-sized workplaces (250–500 workers) also provide EAPs. EAP coverage was least likely in small work sites (< 250 workers).[11,12]

On average, approximately 5% of employees working in an organization offering an EAP use the EAP in a 12-month period. While this may appear to be low usage, consideration of cumulative impact over several years indicates the extent of penetration generated by such a usage rate. Approximately 1.5% of employees annually use an EAP because of alcohol- or other drug-related problems in a single year.[13]

EAPs do not replace existing benefits packages. EAPs and third-party coverage for treatment of alcohol-related problems are synergistic, rather than competitive, services.[14] In many instances, management consults with the

EAP to structure the availability of health insurance benefits. New managed-care plans may be supplements to EAPs, and the EAP is sometimes formally integrated into alternative efforts to contain the costs of treating behavioral health problems. In some instances managed-care plans have eliminated an EAP, focusing only on the benefits management function to the detriment of other EAP functions. Alcohol and other drug treatment through EAP referral and integrated EAP/managed-care programs have been shown to be more efficient and effective when compared to the rather scattershot efforts of employees to select providers and use insurance benefits on their own.[8,15]

With regard to health care reform and managed care, third-party coverage is necessary for individuals with stigmatized problems such as alcohol abuse or mental illness to access treatment, but its availability is not sufficient to assure that efforts to access such care will occur. EAPs provide motivation for seeking help and access to helping mechanisms. In addition EAPs are able to use the workplace as a mechanism for referral when other systems, such as the family, do not take action or effectively intervene. EAPs are comprehensive referral mechanisms, allowing social and cultural aspects of employee problems to enter into the referral arrangements, as well as offering the potential for prevention and early intervention.

3. Research Methodology

With support from the National Institute on Alcohol Abuse and Alcoholism, data were collected on 6400 employees from 84 worksites who used the services of EAPs.[5] The natures of the EAP worksites varied based on the type of industry, the number of employees, and the geographical location. Some were corporate headquarters and some were multiple sites of a single corporation. The EAP intake data were collected between early 1990 and mid-1992. Because these data were derived from a large number of EAP clients and administrators for research purposes, they did not present some of the drawbacks of aggregate data based on EAP records that might be available from sites with EAPs. For example, the data we collected make possible multivariate analyses of individuals as well as analysis of clients from different EAPs using a single protocol for data collection. Data were also restricted to clients who made initial contact with their organization's EAP. Dependents of employees were not included in the data set.

We used two data collection instruments. The EAP administrators completed a questionnaire concerning demographic information about each client, referral categories, client treatment history, clinical assessment, treatment regimen, and prognosis. The EAP clients filled out a questionnaire about their job functions and performance, satisfaction with relationships, and the roles of people who were influential in referral or utilization of the EAP. This questionnaire included the CAGE assessment instrument.[16] This queries whether the individual had ever (1) felt it necessary to cut down on drinking, (2) felt annoyed by criticism of the drinking, (3) felt guilty about the drinking, or (4) had a drink as an eye-opener. CAGE responses were a screen for a more comprehensive measure. Clients who scored 1 or more on the CAGE or where there was some concern by the EAP that alcohol may be involved in the presenting problem were administered an Alcohol Dependence Scale (ADS).[17] Each client also completed a short form of the Beck Depression Inventory.[18]

We attempted to gain follow-up information for clients between 18 and 24 months after the initial EAP intake to assess whether the client was still employed, fired, quit, laid off, or retired. Keeping in mind that the sample included a majority of cases with relatively nonserious problems, employment status at follow-up was only attempted for clients (1) with an alcohol or other drug assessment; (2) with ADS scores of 1 or more, even if they were not assessed as having an alcohol-related problem; (3) who were referred to any inpatient treatment; or (4) who scored in the severely depressed category of the BDI. Almost one third ($n = 1990$) of the EAP clients met one or more of the follow-up criteria. We were successful at ascertaining employment status for 81% of those for whom we requested such information.

4. Description of Employed Women with Alcohol Problems Who Use EAP Services

The basic descriptive characteristics of employed women who use EAP services may suggest the effectiveness of EAPs' techniques of intervention. However, it is important to point out two features of this data collection that should guide its generalization and comparison with other findings.

First, we are dealing only with employed women, and with women who are employed by the companies and organizations included in our study. Thus we cannot generalize to all women nor to all working women. Nearly all of the women included in the study have succeeded in establishing an employment relationship. Nearly all of the women have passed through probationary status at their respective workplaces, and thus have full access to employment benefits. This differentiates this sample, in general, from newly employed women and unemployed women (typically defined as seeking work), women who are not employed outside the home, women who move quickly from one brief employment opportunity to another, and from those who work for employers that do not provide EAP services.

These data also do not generalize to women who are employed only part-time, since it is quite rare for part-timers to have routine access to EAP services. This links to the fact that part-timers' employment often does not carry the health insurance benefits necessary to implement EAP referral recommendations. Further, the companies where we collected data were not likely to have the part-time service work occupations that have come to represent large numbers of women workers.

Finally, while more than half of American employers offer EAP services to their employees,[19] the workplaces included in this study are not a random cross section of workplaces, but instead tend to be larger, more likely to offer a broader range of benefits, and less likely to be in the service sector.[11,12] While it is only a rough inference, we would suggest that from employees' point of view, workplaces with EAPs tend to be among the "better" places to work, because EAPs are present in worksites with other progressive personnel management practices.[20]

A second set of significant distinctions centers on the fact that we collected data only about persons who utilized EAP services. We have no knowledge of the characteristics of those women with alcohol problems in these workplaces who did not access the EAP. These alcohol-troubled women included those who went without help as well as those who used some source of services without utilizing the EAP. Thus our findings should not be considered within the context of epidemiological estimates. The data may be interpreted, however, in light of epidemiological estimates of alcohol-related problems among employed women working for organizations that are likely to offer EAPs, a substantial and highly significant segment of the American workforce.

We do not regard this as a limitation or shortcoming of the study, for indeed we have collected data about the dynamics of accessing assistance among persons with problems. This is a much neglected research area that recently has been cited as critical for further understanding if program planning is to facilitate better outreach.[21] Indeed, an attempt to estimate representativeness by gathering prevalence estimates in the sites where these data were collected would have likely confounded the research design. Our access to data was through the EAP coordinators. Due to their professional ethics, these individuals would have insisted that any prevalence-oriented data collection directed at the total employee population, whether by interview or questionnaire, would have to include information about how persons with self-reported problems could access EAP services. We would have thus created a new avenue to EAP usage, which would have affected the characteristics of our study sample.

We now turn to a description of the 238 women in the data set who were assessed by the EAP staff as having a primary or secondary problem with alcohol (see column 1 of Table I). They were relatively young, with an average age of 36.6, and 79% of them were white. Their lack of connection with nuclear families is especially notable, with only 29% of them married, 41% divorced or separated, and 27% never married. They have an average of 1.06 children, with 37% of them having school-age children and 11% having preschool-age children. Most have some college education (1 = high school, 2 = some college, 3 = college graduate), and on average earned between $20,000 and $30,000 per year (4 = $20,000–$30,000, 5 = $30,000–$40,000).

They were generally established employees in their workplaces, having an average of 9 years at their present place of employment. All levels of employment were represented: 18% were professional or technical employees, 4% were executives or upper-level management, 47% were clerical or sales workers, 26% were blue-collar workers, and 5% were first-line supervisors. This distribution may be viewed as consistent with epidemiological evidence: sales workers, managers and administrators, as well as professional and technical workers are included in the highest percentages of consumers of alcoholic beverages compared with other occupational categories.[22]

Many of the women had problems in relation to their work and in their lives generally. Since most respondents in surveys will rate themselves highly (excellent) on the quality of their own job performance, it is notable that on average these women rated their performances as between "average" and "above average." Fully 57% of them felt that their personal problems had a negative effect on their job performance. While 48% responded that they had an attendance problem, only 32% indicated they had received warnings about their attendance. Seventeen percent indicated that they had received warnings from their supervisor about their job performance. On average these 238 women were absent from work 3.3 days and late 1.6 days in the previous month. These data bear on Weisner's[23] finding that women who were new entrants to alcoholism treatment were more likely than men to have concealed drinking problems and delayed seeking assistance until signs of impairment were apparent to others. Receiving warnings about work-related problems may have provided the evidence needed for these women to admit that they were unsuccessfully concealing their drinking.

Without respect to behaviors that might be related to their alcohol problems, 4% had on-the-job accidents during the prior 12 months, and 13% reported off-the-job accidents during that period. Twenty-one percent indicated that they were having legal problems at the time of their referral to the EAP.

In terms of the EAP administrator's classification of the referral of these women, 34% were reported as self-referrals, 21% were formal supervisory referrals, 13% were indicated to be referred by their supervisor through informal channels, and 16% were classified as peer or co-worker referrals. Sixteen percent were classified in an omnibus "other" category, which included family, spouse, friends, and medical and legal system referrals. Weisner[24] found that family members and friends are important referral routes for workers who were new entrants into treatment programs, but only when serious family- and job-related problems and episodes of serious drinking occurred.

The instrument also queried as to the sources that the client felt were influential in bringing about their referral to the EAP. Generally, this would indicate the extent to which their problem behaviors were discussed with persons in these categories. Here, 35% indicated their supervisors influenced their referral decision, 27% indicated influence from a co-worker who had used the EAP, 16% indicated influence from a friend, 11% were influenced by a co-worker who had not used the EAP, and 10% (22% of those who were married) were influenced to some extent by their spouses. In a separate portion of the questionnaire, the women were asked whether their supervisor actually suggested that they use the EAP, for which 29% responded "yes".

In addition, the women were asked to report the most important influence. Supervisors were regarded as most influential for 22%, and the self was most influential for another 22%. Co-workers were most influential for 15% of the women, friends were most influential for 7%, and spouses were most influential for 9% of the married and separated women with alcohol-related problems. One quarter of the women reported someone outside these categories (i.e., doctors, other family members, etc.) had the most influence on their utilization of the EAP.

Social relationships are thought to be importantly related to the chances of success in treatment for alcoholic women.[25] Thus the extent to which employed women are satisfied with various types of relationships in their lives may be important to their receptivity to help and to the outcomes of any recommended treatment regimen. The women in this sample tended to be satisfied with their social relationships. On scales of 1 to 4, with a 1 indicating that the EAP clients were very satisfied and a 4 indicating that they were very dissatisfied, the women scored on average: 1.8 for their current relationships with co-workers, 1.6 with friends, 2.0 with supervisors, 2.7 with spouses, and 1.9 with children. Notable is the lowest relative satisfaction with their relationships with their spouses.

In terms of measures of alcohol problems, these women on average scored 2.2 out of a maximum of 4 on the CAGE, and an average of 9.4 on the Alcohol Dependence Scale (low level of alcohol dependence indicative of psychological rather than physical dependence). They had an average score of 11 on the short form of the Beck Depression Inventory. When BDI scores are categorized, the women scored in between the mild and moderate categories (2 = mild, 3 = moderate). In general, this appears to indicate "early-stage" alcohol problems as the most common characterization of this group of women, with some overlap with depressive symptomatology. This contrasts with findings that suggest that women postpone seeking treatment until they have reached notably problematic levels.[23] Clearly EAP caseloads are composed of women with alcohol problems that are at a much earlier stage than women entrants into treatment.

EAP referrals with alcohol problems enter with other presenting problems as is typical of such women in treatment and epidemiological studies.[26,27] EAP administrators indicated that 51% of these women with alcohol problems also had psychological problems, 29% had other family problems, 21% had other drug problems, 5% had legal problems, and 15% had financial problems. Forty-seven percent of the married or separated women had marital problems. On average, these women had three problem categories (including alcohol-related problems) at EAP intake. This is somewhat consistent with a study[28] of EAP worksites where problem-drinking women employees were diagnosed with family and personality problems, sometimes in combination with alcohol problem assessments and sometimes in place of them.

Sex role stereotyping that projects a negative image of women who drink and potentially stigmatizes those who develop alcohol-related problems[29] may also influence the ways in which women who seek assistance are received by clinicians. Vannicelli[30] found that treatment center staff were inclined to treat women as children and assign a poorer prognosis for recovery compared with men diagnosed as impaired to a similar degree. Likewise, EAP staff are potentially affected by stereotypes in their assessment of clients with alcohol-related problems.

EAP administrators assessed the overall severity of the clients' problems, as well as offering prognoses for recovery and for resuming adequate job performance. These women were given severity ratings on average of 3.8, where a 5 was very severe. The prognosis for recovery ratings were 2.4, on average, where a 2 was good and a 3 was fair. The prognosis for improved job performance was 2.3 for those women who had job performance problems.

The referral decisions reported by the EAP administrator for the sample of employed women were: referral to inpatient treatment, 14%; referral to an outpatient treatment, 43%; referral to a 12-step program only, 18%; a combination of self-help group attendance and EAP counseling, 8%; and EAP counseling only, 5%. The remaining 12% of these clients received no alcohol-specific referral in most of these instances because the alcohol problems were secondary to another presenting problem.

These data stand at strong odds with contentions that EAPs are over users of inpatient treatment or that most alcohol cases are referred by EAPs to inpatient care. Further, the data indicate the preventive potential of EAPs. Also, in terms of "no-cost" treatment, these data indicate that such referrals (EAP, 12-step program) accounted for 31% of the referrals of clients with alcohol problems.

While there are positive features to these patterns of "managed care" within the EAP, there are other possible explanations for these referral decisions. The EAP administrators indicated that for 22% of these employed women, the client's insurance coverage prevented their making the most appropriate referral. Fully 46% of these women clients had health care coverage through an HMO, which often limit EAP involvement.

At follow-up, which occurred between 18 and 24 months after EAP intake, 69% of the women with EAP-assessed alcohol problems were still employed by the organization that was their employer at intake. Fifteen percent had been fired, 9% had quit, and 7% had been laid off. It is interesting to note that in an analysis not shown, more severe levels of alcohol problems were not predictive of being unemployed at follow-up. Surprisingly, those women with more severe problems were more likely to be still employed at follow-up. The retention rate for employment at follow-up is strong testimony for the effectiveness of the EAP, demonstrating its economic value to employees and their families, to employers, and to the larger society which commonly must bear the burden of unemployment.[31]

5. Comparisons of Men and Women with Alcohol Problems Who Use EAP Services

Having offered some foundation of the nature of this sample of employed women who have used the EAP, we now turn to some comparisons that may further describe some of the dynamics of the process of referral, treatment and job retention.

This study offered an unusual opportunity to collect both "objective" assessment information as well as establish the assessments that were made by EAP counselors. The data indicate that these criteria did not generate completely overlapping groups. Using the score of 9 or more on the ADS as a cutoff to indicate the valid presence of an alcohol problem,[32] we found that half (50.8%) of the men who were assessed as having an alcohol problem by the EAP counselor met this criterion. However, for women, only 42% of those assessed by the EAP met the criterion of an ADS score of 9 or more. In most instances, the EAP assessed an alcohol problem as present even when the ADS scores were less than 9. However, 9 out of the 100 women (9%) who scored 9 or more on the ADS and 30 out of 392 men (8.2%) who scored 9 or more on the ADS were not assessed by the EAP as having an alcohol-related problem. Thus, in general, EAP assessments tend to be more likely to find alcohol problems among women that among men, given similar levels of "objective" symptoms.

In this and the following sections we consider the variations between these two bases for assessment of alcohol problems in several ways. We first compare the women with the men who received an alcohol problem assessment from the EAP and look at these findings relative to the differences between these men and women when only high ADS (9 or more) scores were considered.

The comparisons between the women ($n = 238$) and men ($n = 771$) who were assessed by the EAP staff as having a primary or secondary problem with alcohol and between those women ($n = 100$) and men ($n = 392$) with ADS scores of 9 or more are indicated in Table I. Data based on EAP assessments and the significance of gender differences appear in the first three columns and the comparisons based on ADS scores appear in the last three columns.

There are a number of statistically significant differences indicated by t-tests. Most of these are consistent whether EAP assessment or ADS scores were used as the criterion for the presence of an alcohol problem. However, there were more statistically significant gender differences between the comparisons based on EAP assessment than those based on ADS scores, partially because of the larger number of cases in the EAP-assessed groups.

Table I. Mean Comparisons for Women and Men with Alcohol-Related Problems

	EAP assessed			ADS = 9 +		
	Women	Men	Significance	Women	Men	Significance
Individual characteristics						
Age (years)	36.56	38.08	**	35.61	37.57	**
Race (1 = white)	0.79	0.79		0.81	0.81	
Education (2 = some col; 3 = BS)	2.70	2.67	**	2.58	2.60	**
Marital status (1 = married)	0.29	0.50	**	0.34	0.49	**
Preschool children (1 = yes)	0.11	0.17	**	0.11	0.16	
School-age children (1 = yes)	0.37	0.45	**	0.26	0.44	**
Income (4 = $20–30K; 5 = $30–40K)	4.07	4.96	**	4.03	4.85	**
Work characteristics						
Tenure (years)	9.21	11.25	**	9.61	11.07	*
Professional (1 = yes)	0.18	0.15		0.15	0.15	
Executive (1 = yes)	0.04	0.07	**	0.04	0.06	
Clerical (1 = yes)	0.47	0.09	**	0.51	0.08	**
Blue collar (1 = yes)	0.26	0.60	**	0.25	0.64	**
Supervisor (1 = yes)	0.05	0.08	*	0.05	0.06	
Job eval—Self (1 = hi; 5 = lo)	2.29	2.15	**	2.25	2.24	
Job eval—Supr (1 = hi; 5 = lo)	2.57	2.33	**	2.46	2.35	
Supervisor praise (1 = yes)	0.67	0.71		0.71	0.72	
Neg effect on job (1 = yes)	0.57	0.47	**	0.56	0.51	
On-job accident (1 = yes)	0.04	0.08	**	0.03	0.09	*
Off-job accident (1 = yes)	0.13	0.12		0.13	0.10	
Legal problem (1 = yes)	0.21	0.29	**	0.16	0.30	**
Attendance problem (1 = yes)	0.48	0.37	**	0.46	0.43	
Warnings: performance (1 = yes)	0.17	0.13		0.12	0.13	
Warnings: attendance (1 = yes)	0.32	0.25	*	0.29	0.28	
Days missed (count)	3.26	2.57	*	3.69	2.67	*
Days late (count)	1.59	1.05	**	1.56	1.13	

(continued)

Table I. (*Continued*)

	EAP assessed			ADS = 9 +		
	Women	Men	Significance	Women	Men	Significance
Work characteristics (*continued*)						
Offsite work (1 = freq; 5 = never)	3.51	3.01	**	3.50	3.03	**
Physical work (1 = freq; 5 = never)	3.32	2.55	**	3.23	2.55	**
Autonomy (1 = freq; 5 = never)	1.64	1.59		1.62	1.60	
Overtime (1 = freq; 5 = never)	2.16	1.84	**	2.13	1.88	**
EAP reported referral route						
Self (1 = yes)	0.34	0.32		0.35	0.38	
Informal supervisor (1 = yes)	0.13	0.14		0.11	0.13	
Formal supervisor (1 = yes)	0.21	0.22		0.15	0.17	
Peer (1 = yes)	0.16	0.09	**	0.18	0.10	**
Client reported influentials						
Co-worker (1 = yes)	0.11	0.10		0.10	0.10	
Co-worker w/ prior EAP (1 = yes)	0.27	0.19	**	0.28	0.22	
Friend (1 = yes)	0.16	0.17		0.22	0.20	
Supervisor (1 = yes)	0.35	0.37		0.34	0.33	
Spouse (1 = yes)	0.22	0.44	**	0.35	0.51	**
Supervisor suggested EAP (1 = yes)	0.29	0.30		0.27	0.27	
Most influential referral						
Co-worker (1 = yes)	0.15	0.09	**	0.13	0.11	
Friend (1 = yes)	0.07	0.05		0.11	0.06	
Supervisor (1 = yes)	0.22	0.21		0.19	0.16	
Spouse (1 = yes)	0.09	0.27	**	0.21	0.34	
Self (1 = yes)	0.22	0.18		0.18	0.19	
Relationship satisfaction (1 = very satisfied; 4 = very dissatisfied)						
Co-workers	1.78	1.64	**	1.90	1.65	**
Friends	1.63	1.67		1.78	1.80	
Supervisor	1.98	1.78	**	1.92	1.76	
Spouse	2.66	2.09	**	2.60	2.10	**
Child(ren)	1.90	1.63	**	1.78	1.66	**

	238	771		100	392	
Symptoms						
CAGE	2.16	2.49	**	2.71	3.12	**
BDI	11.05	8.30	**	12.58	11.09	**
BDI category (2 = mild; 3 = mod)	2.68	2.29	**	2.88	2.62	**
ADS	9.41	10.63	*	15.15	16.64	**
EAP Assessment						
Marital problem (1 = yes)	0.47	0.41		0.43	0.39	
Family problem (1 = yes)	0.29	0.14	**	0.25	0.13	**
Psychological problem (1 = yes)	0.51	0.23	**	0.49	0.17	**
Legal problem (1 = yes)	0.05	0.11	**	0.05	0.11	*
Financial problem (1 = yes)	0.15	0.13		0.09	0.15	*
Drug problem (1 = yes)	0.21	0.22		0.22	0.25	
Number of problems (1 = yes)	2.97	2.31	**	2.75	2.23	**
Prognosis						
Severity (1 = low; 5 = very severe)	3.79	3.72		3.88	3.96	
Recovery (1 = excellent; 4 = poor)	2.40	2.37		2.36	2.27	
Job performance (1 = excellent; 4 = poor)	2.30	2.13	**	2.08	2.01	
Treatment Recommendation						
Inpatient only (1 = yes)	0.14	0.30	**	0.19	0.40	**
Outpatient only (1 = yes)	0.43	0.46		0.52	0.45	
EAP only (1 = yes)	0.05	0.04		0.01	0.02	
Self-help only (1 = yes)	0.18	0.11	**	0.10	0.10	
EAP–self-help only (1 = yes)	0.08	0.03	**	0.10	0.02	**
No alcohol treatment (1 = yes)	0.12	0.07	**	0.08	0.01	**
Payment						
Inadequate insurance (1 = yes)	0.22	0.14	**	0.26	0.17	**
HMO (1 = yes)	0.46	0.35	**	0.40	0.35	
Follow-up employment status						
Still employed (1 = yes)	0.69	0.74		0.74	0.71	
Fired (1 = yes)	0.15	0.13		0.14	0.13	
Quit (1 = yes)	0.09	0.04	**	0.09	0.06	
Laid off (1 = yes)	0.07	0.09		0.04	0.09	
N	238	771		100	392	

** = p < 0.05,   * = p < 0.10

Female referrals were significantly younger and significantly less likely to be married or to have had children than their male counterparts. The employed women with alcohol problems had significantly lower incomes and shorter tenures in their workplaces. As might be expected, they were less likely to engage in physical work and to work off the premises of their workplace. These women were significantly less likely to have supervisory responsibilities and were significantly less likely than the men with alcohol-related problems to represent either executive/managerial or blue-collar levels. Not surprisingly, women were much more likely to be in the clerical ranks. Of particular interest, however, is that despite these expected gender differences relative to differential gender representation in occupational groupings in organizations, men and women assessed by the EAP as having alcohol problems are substantially represented among the ranks of professionals, managers, or first-line supervisory positions. Despite speculation to the contrary,[33] EAPs do not limit their alcohol-problem client bases to lower status employees.

When these clients were asked to evaluate their job performance, women rated their performance significantly lower than did men. Women also reported that they believed their supervisors would rate their job performance at levels significantly lower than the preceived supervisory ratings reported by men. In the same vein, women were significantly more likely than men to report that their problem had an adverse effect on their job performance. These differences were only significant for the EAP-assessed men and women. There was, however, no difference between men and women in the extent to which they reported supervisory praise for work that is well done for either comparison. For both comparisons, men were significantly more likely to report that they engaged in overtime work, even though both groups indicated relatively high frequency of working overtime. Working overtime could be a stressor or a response to impairment, requiring extra time to complete one's work.

A number of items focused on behaviors that may have been associated with problem drinking. Women were significantly less likely to have experienced an on-the-job accident during the previous 12 months, but there were no differences between the genders in reports of off-the-job accidents. Women who were assessed as having alcohol problems and those with ADS scores more than 9 were significantly more likely than men to be absent from work during the past month and to report lateness to work during the past 30 days. The difference between days late to work was only significant in the EAP assessed comparison.

In terms of routes to the EAP, both the client and the respective EAP administrator were asked to describe the means by which the individual reached the EAP. In terms of the administrators' classifications, there were no differences between the genders in rates of formal supervisory referral, informal supervisory referral, or self-referral. This was consistent with the reports of the clients. There were no differences between the genders in the extent to which they reported that their supervisors had specifically suggested that they come to the EAP for assistance. Further, when asked who was influential in their decision to come to the EAP, there were no differences between the genders in the extent to which their supervisors were seen as influential or the extent to which they indicated that their supervisors had been the most influential parties bringing about their referral.

There were, however, important differences between the genders in other patterns and influences on referral. EAP administrators' reports indicated that women who were assessed to have alcohol-related problems were significantly more likely to come to the EAP as a peer (co-worker) referral than men, supporting other findings of the importance of peers in referring more women workers to EAPs than men.[28] Regarding the clients' own reports, there are no differences between the genders in the extent to which they reported influences from friends in their decision to come to the EAP. In differentiating co-workers who had and had not used the EAP themselves, women were significantly more likely to have been influenced in their referral decision by co-workers who had used the EAP, but there were no gender differences in the reported influence of co-workers who had not used the EAP. Finally, there was a significant and substantial difference between the genders in reported influence of spouses, with the wives of men with alcohol problems more likely to be influential than the husbands of women with alcohol problems.

In attempting to gain more insight into the referral process, we queried the clients as to their reported satisfaction with their relationships with persons in different social categories at the time of their referral. Generally, women who were assessed by the EAP to have alcohol problems reported less satisfactory relationships than comparable men, with significantly lower reported relational satisfaction with supervisors, co-workers, spouses, and children. There was no difference between the genders in reported relational satisfaction with friends. The differences between men and women in satisfaction with relationships with children and supervisors were statistically significant only for the EAP-assessed comparison and not for the ADS-based comparison.

We also examined other presenting problems that were reported by the EAP coordinator. For married and separated clients, there were no differences between men and women in the extent of reported marital problems. Women who were diagnosed with alcohol problems were, however, substantially and significantly more likely to be appraised as having family problems and were more than twice as likely to be assessed with psychological problems. This is consistent with findings that show that alcoholic women referred to EAPs are more likely than men to be diagnosed with personality and family problems.[28] Men were twice as likely as women to report legal problems, but there were no differences between the genders in reported financial problems or drug problems at the time of assessment. For both comparisons, women had, on average, more presenting problems.

Assessment instruments indicated that the men had significantly higher

CAGE scores, whereas the women had significantly higher scores on the Beck's Depression Inventory. Interestingly, the differences were minimal between men and women in their scores on the ADS. Further, there was no difference between the genders in the assessed severity of their alcohol problems, as reported by the EAP administrators, which might suggest that EAP administrators' in diagnoses are not as influenced by negative stereotypes of women problem drinkers as Vannicelli[30] suggested. In multivariate analyses (not shown) the differences between men and women are not due solely to differences in the severity of their alcohol problems.

In terms of EAP administrators' prognoses for individuals' improvement, there were no differences between men and women in the extent to which recovery from their alcohol problem was projected. Administrators did, however, offer a significantly better prognosis for women clients with job performance difficulties to eventually resume an adequate level of job performance.

There were marked differences between the genders in terms of where they were referred for treatment of their alcohol problems. While 14% of the women assessed with alcohol problems were referred to inpatient alcoholism treatment programs, this occurred for 30% of the men (19% vs. 40% of women and men with ADS criteria). Interestingly, there were no gender differences in the referral to outpatient alcoholism treatment. Women were significantly more likely to be referred to self-help groups as their only referral and were significantly more likely than men to be treated through a combination of EAP counseling and self-help group attendance. Women were also more likely to receive no specific referral for treatment of their alcohol problems, reflecting the higher proportion of women for whom the alcohol problem diagnosis was provided in EAP assessment as secondary to another presenting problem, most frequently psychological and/or marital/family problems.

Women were significantly more likely than men to be reported by the EAP administrator to be inadequately covered by insurance in terms of facilitating the most appropriate referral. Further, women who were assessed with alcohol problems were significantly more likely to be covered for health care by an HMO. While the trend for the ADS comparison indicated that women were more likely to be covered by an HMO than men, the difference was not significant.

Nevertheless, there were no significant differences between the genders in the extent to which they were still employed at follow-up. In terms of those no longer employed, there were no differences between the genders in the rates of firings, layoffs, or retirements, but women who had been assessed by the EAP as having alcohol problems were significantly more likely than men to have quit.

6. Comparisons within and between Occupational Categories

There are significant differences between women and men in the types of occupations they perform as well as significant differences in occupational category between women and men who are assessed as having alcohol-related problems. Thus, we compare women and men assessed with alcohol problems according to the other variables of interest, holding constant whether they occupy blue-collar occupations, clerical/sales occupations, or high-status occupations (professional, technical, executive, or managerial). The comparisons allow us to examine differences between women and men in typically mens' jobs (blue-collar), between women and men in typically womens' jobs (clerical), and between high-status women and men.

We then compare differences among women with alcohol-assessed problems in the three different occupational groupings to assess whether differences exist in hierarchical status as well as between the sexes. These comparisons allow us to examine differences between women in typically mens' jobs with women in typically womens' jobs, as well as those in higher-status positions.[22]

There are substantial differences between men and women in each of the three occupational comparisons (Table II). However, there are more significant differences between men and women in blue-collar positions than there are between men and women in clerical positions, with the fewest differences evident between men and women in high-status positions.

Men in blue-collar positions and in high-status positions are more likely to be married than the women in these occupations, but there are no significant differences among the women in marital status. Blue-collar women are less likely than the blue-collar men to have preschool-age children, but the women in the three groups do not differ from each other. The women in high-status positions are less likely to have school-age children than their male counterparts. Blue-collar women are significantly more likely than either of the two other groups of women to have school-age children. The clerical women with alcohol problems are older than the clerical men, but the high-status women are older than the clerical women. While there are no gender differences on race or education level within occupational category, the women differ among the occupational groups. White employed women with alcohol problems are more likely to be represented in high-status occupations than nonwhite alcohol-assessed women and least likely to be in blue-collar positions. The blue-collar women have the lowest average education level and the high-status women have the highest level, as expected. Blue-collar women assessed with alcohol problems earn less than blue-collar men and high-status women earn less than high-status men. While there is no difference, on average, between clerical and blue-collar women, high-status women earn more than either of the other groups of women with alcohol problems.

In terms of work characteristics, we find no differences in tenure between the groups or genders. While blue-collar women report that their supervisors evaluate their job performances lower than is reported by blue-collar males, blue-collar women also report lower ratings than higher-status women. Clerical women with alcohol problems are less likely to report that their supervisors praise them for work well done than for clerical men and also less than

Table II. Comparison of Women and Men within Occupational Status and Comparison of Women by Occupational Status of EAP Assessed Alcohol Problems

	Blue collar			Clerical/sales			High-status occupations		
	Women	Men	Significance	Women	Men	Significance	Women	Men	Significance
Individual Characteristics									
Age (years)	35.88	37.48		35.84	33.53	**b	38.43	40.55	b
Race (1 = white)	0.62	0.72	ac	0.79	0.77	ab	0.92	0.93	bc
Education (2 = some col; 3 = BS)	2.25	2.24	ac	2.53	2.62	b	3.42	3.51	bc
Marital status (1 = married)	0.34	0.49	**	0.24	0.32		0.34	0.55	**
Preschool children (1 = yes)	0.10	0.19	*	0.14	0.14		0.08	0.13	
School-age children (1 = yes)	0.52	0.51	ac	0.37	0.25	*a	0.25	0.40	**c
Income (4 = $20–30K; 5 = $30–40K)	3.65	4.61	**c	3.86	4.00	b	4.89	5.91	**bc
Work Characteristics									
Tenure (years)	10.25	11.31		9.26	7.72		8.17	12.16	
Job eval—Self (1 = hi; 5 = lo)	2.32	2.13		2.23	2.16		2.35	2.17	
Job eval—Supr (1 = hi; 5 = lo)	2.73	2.29	**c	2.60	2.44		2.36	2.35	c
Supervisor praise (1 = yes)	0.64	0.68		0.62	0.77	**b	0.79	0.75	b
Neg effect on job (1 = yes)	0.60	0.46	**	0.59	0.49		0.50	0.48	
On-job accident (1 = yes)	0.06	0.12		0.05	0.04		0.02	0.03	
Off-job accident (1 = yes)	0.13	0.12		0.14	0.09		0.11	0.13	
Legal problem (1 = yes)	0.25	0.33		0.23	0.29		0.15	0.23	
Attendance problem (1 = yes)	0.68	0.43	**ac	0.50	0.43	ab	0.23	0.24	bc
Warnings: performance (1 = yes)	0.15	0.14		0.18	0.09	*	0.20	0.13	
Warnings: attendance (1 = yes)	0.51	0.32	**ac	0.31	0.28	ab	0.13	0.13	bc
Day missed (count)	3.69	2.81	**	3.42	3.26		2.56	1.92	
Days late (count)	1.64	0.65	**	1.62	1.09		1.47	1.78	
Offsite work (1 = freq; 5 = never)	3.70	3.22	**c	3.68	3.46	**b	3.01	2.49	**bc
Physical work (1 = freq; 5 = never)	2.71	2.10	**ac	3.66	3.19	**ab	3.31	3.19	bc
Autonomy (1 = freq; 5 = never)	1.89	1.74	c	1.71	1.81	b	1.29	1.24	bc
Overtime (1 = freq; 5 = never)	2.03	1.85	*a	2.35	2.10	*ab	1.95	1.74	*b

EAP reported referral route									
Self (1 = yes)	0.27	0.32	c	0.26	0.26	b	0.52	0.36	**bc
Informal supervisor (1 = yes)	0.06	0.14	a	0.18	0.19	a	0.09	0.11	c
Formal supervisor (1 = yes)	0.37	0.20	**ac	0.14	0.22	a	0.18	0.25	b
Peer (1 = yes)	0.13	0.08		0.23	0.08	**b	0.09	0.10	
Client reported influentials									
Co-worker (1 = yes)	0.16	0.12	c	0.12	0.09		0.03	0.07	c
Co-worker w/prior EAP (1 = yes)	0.23	0.21		0.32	0.18	**	0.22	0.14	
Friend (1 = yes)	0.10	0.16		0.18	0.22		0.19	0.18	
Supervisor (1 = yes)	0.38	0.37		0.34	0.40		0.32	0.37	
Spouse (1 = yes)	0.20	0.41	**	0.20	0.46	**	0.30	0.47	
Supervisor suggested EAP (1 = yes)	0.34	0.30		0.30	0.32		0.25	0.31	
Most influential referral									
Co-worker (1 = yes)	0.10	0.10	a	0.21	0.06	**ab	0.09	0.10	b
Friend (1 = yes)	0.02	0.04	c	0.07	0.03		0.12	0.06	*c
Supervisor (1 = yes)	0.23	0.20		0.23	0.25		0.20	0.23	
Spouse (1 = yes)	0.08	0.25	*	0.08	0.39	**	0.13	0.29	*
Self (1 = yes)	0.24	0.19		0.18	0.22		0.26	0.16	**
Relationship satisfaction (1 = very satisfied; 4 = very dissatisfied)									
Co-workers	1.92	1.57	**	1.80	1.83		1.62	1.71	
Friends	1.73	1.63		1.59	1.77		1.62	1.72	
Supervisor	1.97	1.74	*	2.07	1.74	**	1.85	1.85	bc
Spouse	2.77	2.03	**c	2.92	1.89	**b	2.13	2.25	
Child(ren)	2.00	1.61	**	1.80	1.44	*	1.93	1.71	
Symptoms									
CAGE	2.08	2.54	**	2.30	2.32		1.98	2.44	**
BDI	11.30	8.10	**c	12.80	9.35	**b	7.64	8.38	bc
BDI category (2 = mild; 3 = mod)	2.70	2.26	**c	2.92	2.41	**b	2.21	2.33	bc
ADS	9.30	11.38		10.62	10.37	b	7.47	9.28	b
EAP Assessment									
Marital problem (1 = yes)	0.54	0.42		0.50	0.27	**	0.36	0.41	
Family problem (1 = yes)	0.31	0.13	**	0.26	0.14	**	0.31	0.18	**

(continued)

Table II. (*Continued*)

	Blue collar			Clerical/sales			High-status occupations		
	Women	Men	Significance	Women	Men	Significance	Women	Men	Significance
EAP Assessment (*continued*)									
Psychological problem (1 = yes)	0.53	0.17	**	0.56	0.35	**	0.42	0.31	*
Legal problem (1 = yes)	0.13	0.12	ac	0.02	0.11	**a	0.05	0.08	c
Financial problem (1 = yes)	0.26	0.16	*ac	0.09	0.11	a	0.14	0.06	**c
Drug problem (1 = yes)	0.29	0.26	c	0.20	0.22		0.14	0.14	c
Number of problems (1 = yes)	3.31	2.30	**a	2.79	2.33	**a	2.94	2.33	**
Prognosis									
Severity (1 = low; 5 = very severe)	3.79	3.82		3.75	3.53		3.84	3.60	*
Recovery (1 = excellent; 4 = poor)	2.56	2.49	c	2.44	2.38	b	2.19	2.13	bc
Job performance (1 = exc; 4 = poor)	2.37	2.17		2.31	2.31		2.16	1.99	
Treatment Recommendation									
Inpatient only (1 = yes)	0.19	0.36	**	0.14	0.25	**	0.10	0.21	**
Outpatient only (1 = yes)	0.35	0.43		0.43	0.39		0.48	0.53	
EAP only (1 = yes)	0.05	0.03		0.05	0.06		0.08	0.04	
Self-help only (1 = yes)	0.24	0.11	**c	0.19	0.15		0.11	0.10	c
EAP-self help only (1 = yes)	0.05	0.03		0.08	0.04		0.11	0.02	
No alcohol treatment (1 = yes)	0.12	0.04	**	0.11	0.11		0.13	0.09	
Payment									
Inadequate insurance (1 = yes)	0.23	0.15		0.25	0.14	*	0.16	0.14	
HMO (1 = yes)	0.57	0.32	**c	0.50	0.40	b	0.30	0.39	bc
Follow-up employment status									
Still employed (1 = yes)	0.65	0.73		0.70	0.68		0.71	0.76	
Fired (1 = yes)	0.17	0.15		0.17	0.11		0.10	0.10	
Quit (1 = yes)	0.02	0.04	c	0.08	0.05	b	0.16	0.04	**bc
Laid off (1 = yes)	0.15	0.07	**a	0.06	0.16	**ab	0.03	0.10	b
N	62	460		111	72		65	240	

** = p < 0.05;   * = p < 0.10;   a = col. 1 & 3 significantly different at p < 0.10;   b = col. 3 & 5;   c = col. 1 & 5

high-status women. Blue-collar women report more negative effects of their personal problems on their job performance than blue-collar men, but these women do not differ from the reports of the women in the other occupational categories. There are no significant differences in accidents or involvement with legal problems among any of the comparison groups. With regard to attendance, blue-collar women report having more problems and having received more warnings than blue-collar men, with the problems and warnings being greatest among the blue-collar women, followed by clerical women, and the least among the high-status women. These differences are reported even though there are not differences in actual days missed. There is more actual lateness among the blue-collar women compared with the blue-collar men, however.

Even looking within occupational categories, we find differences between men and women assessed with alcohol problems with regard to job characteristics. The men in each of the three categories report working offsite to a greater extent than the women, with the high-status women working offsite more than either blue-collar or clerical women. As expected, the men in each of the occupational categories report engaging more frequently in physical work, with significant differences among the women in each of the groups. As expected, the high-status women also report more autonomy than either of the other two groups of women with alcohol-related problems. Men report working more overtime than the women in each of the three occupational groups, with high-status women reporting more overtime work than blue-collar or clerical women, and blue-collar women reporting more overtime work than their clerical counterparts.

We now turn to referral routes to EAP utilization. Blue-collar women (nontraditional occupation) are significantly more likely to be recorded as formal supervisory referral by the EAP (37%) compared with blue-collar men (20%). Blue-collar women are also more likely to be involved in a formal supervisory referral than clerical or high-status women. Co-workers are more likely to be involved in the referral of clerical women (23%) compared with clerical men (nontraditional occupation) (only 8%), and clerical women are recorded as coming to the EAP via this route significantly more than high-status women. Self-referral is recorded as the referral route for high-status women more than for high-status men, and the rate of self-referral for high-status women is twice as much as that recorded for blue-collar and clerical women. Among the influentials reported by the clients to have affected their decision to use the EAP, spouse referrals among those who are married differ for men and women, with men reporting greater influence than women in each of the three groups. These influences do not differ among women across the groups.

In terms of satisfaction with relationships, there are no differences among the high-status men and women with alcohol problems. Blue-collar women are more dissatisfied with their relationships than blue-collar men, and significantly so for relations with co-workers, supervisors, spouses, and children. Clerical women are more dissatisfied with supervisors, spouses, and children than clerical men, but there are no differences in relations with co-workers or friends. Each of the three groups of women are significantly different from each other in terms of their satisfaction with spouses, with the high-status women indicating most dissatisfaction and clerical women showing the least dissatisfaction.

Blue-collar men exhibit higher average CAGE scores than blue-collar women, which is similar to the pattern between high-status men and women with alcohol problems. The men and women do not differ in average ADS scores, however. The women do not differ from each other on their CAGE scores according to their occupational group, but high-status women exhibit lower average ADS scores, indicating earlier intervention for this group of women.

Women with alcohol problems have a broader range of presenting symptoms than men with alcohol problems regardless of occupational category, and blue-collar women have more problems than clerical women. Clerical women are more likely to have marital problems recorded at EAP intake than male clericals, and the women do not differ by occupational category for marital or for other family problems. However, men are less likely to have family problems at intake than the women. Psychological problems are more likely for women with alcohol problems in each of the occupational groups, but not among women in the different occupational groups. Legal problems are greater for clerical men than clerical women, but blue-coller women have significantly more of these problems than women in the other two occupational groups. Financial problems are greater for women than men in the blue-collar and high-status groups, and the blue-collar women have more financial problems than either of the other two groups. Drug problems do not differ between men and women in each of the categories, but blue-collar women are more likely than high-status women to have an illicit drug problem recorded at intake.

Despite the lower ADS and depression scores of the high-status women, the severity of their problems are rated higher than high-status men with alcohol-related problems. While the women do not differ among occupational categories in terms of EAP severity rating, blue-collar women are rated lowest on their prognosis for recovery, and this rating is significantly lower than that given for clerical or high-status women, with high-status women having significantly higher prognostic ratings by the EAP for recovery than clerical women with alcohol problems.

Inpatient treatment recommendations vary by gender for each of the three groups, with women in each group only half as likely to be referred to inpatient treatment. Self-help only is significantly more likely for blue-collar women than blue-collar men, with blue-collar women more than twice as likely as high-status women to be in this referral category. Women are more likely to have inadequate insurance across all three categories, but the difference from the men with alcohol problems is only significant for clerical workers. HMO coverage is significantly more likely for blue-collar women than blue-collar men. HMO coverage is less likely for high-status women than for either blue-collar or clerical women, but the blue-collar and clerical women do not differ in their rate of HMO coverage.

The lack of differences between the genders in sustaining employment at follow-up or in having been fired at follow-up holds across the three occupational groups. There are no significant differences across the three groups of women for those two outcomes. High-status women with alcohol problems are, however, four times more likely to quit their jobs than high-status men, are significantly more likely to quit than women in clerical jobs, and are eight times more likely to quit than women in blue-collar jobs. The difference in voluntary turnover suggests that subtle pressures may be brought on women with alcohol-related problems based on their occupational classification.

It also appears that layoffs do not occur randomly. Blue-collar women are more likely than blue-collar men and clerical women are less likely than clerical men to be laid off at follow-up, suggesting that people in jobs typical of the opposite gender are more likely to bear the burden of layoff. Further, women in blue-collar jobs are more likely to be laid off at follow-up than women in either of the other two job categories, and clerical workers are more likely to be laid off than higher-status women with alcohol problems. Thus, among those who are not still employed at follow-up, it seems that managerial decisions are associated with job status as well as gender.

7. Characteristics of Women with Probable Alcohol Problems Who Were Not Assessed as Such by EAP Personnel

The data revealed 69 women with ADS scores of between 5 and 8, 38 of whom were not assessed by the EAP counselor as having an alcohol problem. When the ADS scores of those who were assessed with alcohol problems was examined, the EAP counselors' diagnoses of alcohol problems appeared to be much more inclusive of lower levels of ADS scores. Looking at what might be seen as the converse of that generalization, we subsequently compared those employed women with ADS scores between 5 and 8 for whom the EAP assessment included no mention of a primary or secondary alcohol problem. In other words, these 38 women comprised a particularly interesting group because they "passed" the scrutiny of EAP assessment despite having levels of alcohol problems that some researchers regard as clear indicators of the presence of an alcohol problem. This may be a reflection of the reluctance of some practitioners to ask the right kinds of questions or to acknowledge signs of potential drinking problems in some types of clients or patients.[34]

Before looking at this group, we should consider the important conceptual differences between those persons who are identified as having an alcohol problem via their ADS score versus those who are diagnosed as such by an EAP counselor. Arguments can be made for the particular validity of each measure.

The ADS score is supposedly an "objective" screen and is specifically focused on the dynamic features of problematic drinking behavior. It captures aspects of drinking that might be missed or overlooked in a clinical interview. Further, by its directness, it requires a particular focus on drinking that might be avoided in the clinical interview. Otherwise, its self-administered feature does not allow for the person's other characteristics to act as markers, filters, or deflections from a diagnostic decision that a person has an alcohol problem. In other words, the scores are generated without knowledge of the person's appearance, social class, or interactional presentation of self. Further, it is a standardized measure that circumvents the influences of bias or inadequate training on the part of the diagnostician. Finally, it has been validated across a variety of groups and settings as an indicator of the presence of alcohol problems.

A "real" assessment of the presence of alcohol problems by a professional diagnostician offers some interesting comparative advantages. While use of the ADS of similar instruments has multiple strengths, it is indeed the case that the one-on-one interview is the normative standard for assessment and diagnosis of behavioral problems. While it is conceivable to fully standardize and automate these processes, there seems to be much reluctance to do so, albeit that reluctance is not necessarily based on clinical evidence. This norm does, however, point strongly to the perceived advantages within the professional community of utilizing a form of "multiple triangulation" in assessment, allowing for a range of objective, self-report, and perceived data about the client to be used as the base for a differential diagnosis.

The in-person diagnostic interview allows the interviewer to use any one of a battery of strategies to deal with aspects of denial of an alcohol problem that may be attempted by the client. Whereas the ADS is limited to specific questions, the interviewer has the opportunity to perhaps lead into these questions in oblique ways that sidestep aspects of denial. One example of this may be persistence or rephrasing of questions when the client "skips" a response, as he or she may easily do on a paper-and-pencil instrument. By the same token, the interviewer is not limited to these specific questions, and he or she can personalize behavioral characteristics as the client's responses unfold. Any standardized instrument must presume standardized perceptions of situated meanings, and an interview can allow for adjustments or interpretations that simply cannot emerge from a quantified response.

It may seem obvious to suggest that maximum validity is achieved by "doing both." This is indeed true, and it would be foolish to recommend anything other than the most complete data collection in arriving at an assessment decision. While our concerns here are directed toward the practitioner, our conceptual distinctions are especially oriented toward research questions. It is clear that there are strong arguments for using an objective, standardized indicator as the primary method of defining cases in research. The special advantage here is replication of data across different populations. Our discussion here should stress, however, that there are very important realities represented by cases that are established as alcohol problems in an actual assessment, recognizing the possibility that there were great variations in how these assessments were conducted. It is this real-world decision that is the basis for a string of subsequent actions that will affect the individual's welfare as well as the possibility of recovery from whatever the real underlying problems happen to be.

We compared the employed women with ADS scores of between 5 and 8 who did not receive an EAP assessment of an alcohol problem with those of scores between 5 and 8 who did recieve such an assessment. There were 31 women in the second group. The reason for taking this "controlled" approach was to ensure that the differences in ADS scores did not account for other differences that might be found. Because of the small numbers in these t-test comparisons, we discuss differences that were found up to the significance level of 0.10.

The women who were not assessed with alcohol problems were significantly less likely to have children, but were similar in age and tenure to those women who received alcohol assessments. They were significantly more likely to have jobs that required them to work off the workplace's premises, a difference that may reflect a lower visibility of their job performance or perhaps engagement in more work-related situations where they learn to cover up the effects of alcohol (i.e., sales). In a similar vein, the women who were not assessed with alcohol problems were significantly more likely to be in executive or managerial positions and significantly less likely to be in clerical positions than women who were EAP assessed as having alcohol-related problems.

A suggestion that their workplace behavior was less visible in terms of identification for women in the ADS 5–8 range who were not assessed as having alcohol-related problems is found in their significantly higher perception of their supervisors' assessments of their job performance. Similarly, they were substantively and significantly more likely to report that their supervisors praised their work. Finally, perhaps reflecting their higher job statuses, they were significantly less likely to report engagement in overtime work.

There were no differences between these two groups in the reported problems that they had in conjunction with their jobs, with the exception that those who were not assessed with alcohol problems reported significantly less absenteeism from work during the 30 days prior to the referral.

There were no significant differences between the groups in terms of the categories of persons who had influenced their decision to come to the EAP or the persons who were most influential. There were no differences in the EAP administrators' classifications of their routes of referral. In addition, there were no differences in their reported levels of satisfaction with their relationships with significant others.

In terms of diagnostic measures, those women who were not assessed as having alcohol problems had significantly lower CAGE scores (1.7 vs. 2.3). In terms of the assessment of their other presenting problems, there were no differences between the groups. There was a trend, on average, for non-assessed women to have higher BDI scores, but the differences were not significant and indicated moderate category levels on the BDI.

Finally, there were no differences between the groups in the extent to which they were still employed at follow-up. Thus, these data did not shed a great deal of light on the features of women who "passed" through the screen of an EAP assessment despite their objective scores indicating the presence of a low-level alcohol problem. There were a few clues to the presence of better relationships with supervisors, higher hierarchical levels (executive and managerial), and lower on-the-job visibility, but they were not compelling explanatory patterns. Thus, for example, evidence of opportunities for "cover-up" should have been shown in lower rates of supervisory referral or supervisory and co-worker involvement in referral.

8. Comparisons of Women with and without Multiple Problems

Comorbidity of alcohol problems with other problems is significant among women who come to the EAP with alcohol problems, as other studies[28] and the foregoing data have indicated. To obtain some insights into the characteristics of women with different configurations of symptoms bearing on comorbidity, we constructed three groups for comparisons across the variables for which data were collected. The comorbidity of interest was a very common pattern, namely, the joint presence of alcohol problems and depression. We constructed the groups on the basis of scores generated through self-administered ADS and BDI assessment instruments.

It was not possible to find an adequate number of women with ADS scores of 9 or above and essentially zero ratings on the BDI. Thus, our "alcohol problem only" group was composed of 28 women with a score of 9 or more on the ADS and categorization in one of the bottom two categories of the four BDI catergories, indicative of mild or less depressive symptomatology. The comorbid group was composed of 88 women with ADS scores of 9 or more and placement in one of the two top categories of the BDI scores, indicative of at least moderate symptomatology. The "depressed only" group was composed of 71 women with ADS scores of 0 and placement in one of the top two categories of BDI scores.

Across these three groups, the comorbid women had significantly lower education than the depressed women. The comorbid women were significantly less likely to have children than the depressed women. There were no differences across the groups in terms of age, race, or marital status.

The comorbid women had significantly lower income from their jobs than did the alcohol problem women and the depressed women. There were no differences across the groups in terms of job tenure. There were no differences in terms of occupancy of professional and technical jobs, but the comorbid women were significantly less likely than the depressed women to occupy executive or managerial positions and significantly more likely than the depressed women to occupy clerical or sales positions.

There were no differences in self-reported job performance or reported perceptions of their supervisors' evaluation of their performance. There were also no differences in the extent to which they had received warnings about poor job performance. However, significantly more comorbid women than depressed women reported that their supervisors praised their work. Nevertheless, more comorbid women than either depressed women or alcohol problem women indicated that their personal problems had had an adverse effect on their job performance. Significantly fewer of the women with alcohol only problems indicated negative effects on job performance than the depressed only group.

In terms of other behaviors that may be associated with these women's problems, the comorbid group had more on-the-job accidents during the past 12 months than the depressed only group, but there were no differences in off the job accidents. The comorbid women had both significantly more days absent during the last 30 days than the depressed women and more days late during the past 30 days than either the alcohol problem women or the depressed women. The comorbid women were also considerably more likely than both the depressed women to report that they had distinctive attendance problems at work and were significantly more likely than both the alcohol problem women and the depressed women to have received warnings about their absenteeism.

A number of differences were found relative to the factors affecting entry of women in the three groups into the EAP. Compared with the depressed women, significantly more of the comorbid women entered through a formal supervisory referral. However, compared with the depressed women, significantly more alcohol problem women entered through such a formal referral. Both the comorbid women and the alcohol problem women were significantly less likely than the depressed women to enter the EAP through a self-referral. A distinctively high proportion, 55%, of the depressed women entered the EAP through this self-referral route compared with 36% of the alcohol problem women and 3% of the comorbid women. There were no differences across the groups in terms of rates of informal supervisory referral or peer (co-worker) referral.

In terms of self-reported influences on referral, the alcohol problem women were less likely than the other two groups to report influence from friends and significantly more likely than the other two groups to report influences from supervisors. Fifty percent of the alcohol problem women reported supervisory influence compared with 28% of the comorbid women and 21% of the depressed women. There were no differences across the three groups in reported influence on referral from co-workers or from spouses.

In terms of the social categories of persons reported as most influential in the decision to go to the EAP, the comorbid women were significantly more likely than the alcohol problem women to report that friends were most influential. Alcohol problem women were significantly more likely than depressed women to report that their supervisors were most influential. There were no differences across the three groups in perceiving greatest influence from co-workers, spouses, or self. Interestingly, compared with the alcohol problem women, significantly more of the comorbid women and depressed women reported that someone had actively discouraged them from using the EAP. Of the depressed women, fully 14% indicated that this had occurred.

In examining the reported satisfaction with relationships with different categories of significant others at the time of the referral to the EAP, a number of notable differences were found. There were no differences across the groups in relational satisfaction with children. The comorbid women were significantly less satisfied with their spousal relationships than either the alcohol problem women or the depressed women. The depressed women were significantly less satisfied with these relationships than the alcohol problem women. The comorbid women were less satisfied with their relationships with their friends than either the alcohol problem women or the depressed women. The comorbid women were significantly less satisfied with their co-worker relationships than the alcohol problem women. Both the comorbid women and the depressed women were significantly less satisfied with their relationships with their supervisors than the alcohol problem women.

The data also indicated other problems that were present and diagnosed at the time of the EAP assessment. There were no differences across the three groups in presenting marital problems, measured only for those who were married or separated. The comorbid women had significantly more family problems than the alcohol problem women. The depressed women had significantly more family problems than both the comorbid women and the alcohol problem women. The alcohol problem women had significantly fewer legal and financial problems than both the comorbid women and the depressed women.

The EAP administrator was asked to provide a rating of the overall severity of the problems being experienced by each client. Here the comorbid women as a group were rated as the most severely troubled, with this being significantly greater than the severity rating for the depressed women. This may be related in turn to the treatment referrals that were made following the assessment.

Twenty-one percent of the comorbid women were referred to inpatient treatment, which was significantly greater than the 14% of the alcohol problem women referred to inpatient treatment, which was, in turn, significantly greater than the 2% of the depressed women who were referred to inpatient care. Sixty-four percent of the alcohol problem women were referred to outpatient treatment, which was significantly greater than the 46% of the comorbid women referred to outpatient, which was, in turn, significantly greater than the 28% of the depressed women who were referred to outpatient care. Twenty percent of the depressed women were referred to self-help groups only, which is significantly greater than the 4% of the alcohol problem women who received such a referral. The 13% of the comorbid women who received such a referral is also significantly greater than the 4% of the alcohol problem women. There were no differences in the proportions of the three groups whose treatment involved a combination of self-help groups and counseling from the EAP. A small proportion (7%) of the depressed women received EAP counseling as their only treatment, which was significantly greater than the 1% of the comorbid women and none of the alcohol problem women who were managed in this way.

In terms of insurance coverage, significantly more of the comorbid women (46%) were covered through HMOs than the alcohol problem women (29%) or the depressed women (22%). The comorbid women were significantly more likely than either the alcohol problem women or the depressed women to have insurance coverage that was not adequate for the EAP counselor to make the most appropriate referral. This was obtained for only 10% of the depressed women compared with 14% of the alcohol problem women and fully 30% of the comorbid women.

In terms of projected outcome noted by the EAP counselor at the time of the assessment, the comorbid women were rated significantly lower than both the alcohol problem women and the depressed women on the prospects for recovery and on the prospects for their eventually resuming an adequate level of job performance.

9. Concluding Observations

These data offer a series of important observations about employed women with alcohol problems who seek services from employee assistance programs. The most important of these is that EAPs are effective in sustaining the employment of most working women with alcohol problems who seek EAP services. Further, the data indicate that EAPs' widely stated (but often doubted) goal of early intervention with alcohol-troubled persons is especially realized among women with alcohol problems. These two conclusions demonstrate the distinctive value of EAPs in dealing with alcohol problems and point toward EAPs' economic benefits for both employees and employers. The important roles of EAPs in pretreatment identification and intervention will not be diminished by any conceivable change in public policies affecting the delivery of alcoholism treatment services.

There are several other more specific conclusions. First, it is clear that women with alcohol problems do not enter EAPs through routes that are strikingly different from those that are followed by men. Second, many of the differences that are revealed are clearly associated with the job statuses occupied by women. Third, employed women with alcohol problems are markedly detached from nuclear families, with substantially low rates of current marriage. Fourth, even when women with alcohol problems are married, their husbands are much less likely to play a role in the referral process than is the case for the wives of employed men with alcohol problems.[35] Finally, these descriptive data offer no indication that women are the target of any form of discrimination in the process of EAP utilization. It is clear, however, that they are considerably more likely to have less adequate insurance coverage than their male counterparts, leading to treatment choices that may be less than ideal.

There is no doubt that there are an important number of differences among these employed women clients across their status levels in the organization. Blue-collar workers seem especially "different" on a variety of measures. Of interest here is that for women, blue-collar work is both lower status and nontraditional for women, bringing two intertwined dynamics into play. In general, upper-status employees seem to have a number of "breaks" in the referral process. Here a germane consideration is the comparable status level between the employee referred to the EAP and the EAP counselor. Greater social distance from lower-level employees, perhaps coupled with gender differences, may lead to reactions by supervisors and subsequently by EAP counselors that might be viewed as less constructive than when this social distance is lessened among referrals from upper-organizational levels.

In examining the differences between women with significant ADS scores who were and were not assessed by the EAP as having alcohol problems, we were able to find little that would suggest patterns of on-the-job "cover-up" peculiar to female employees. If anything, these data suggest that consistent with other findings here status level in the organization is of considerable importance in affecting dynamics of referral activities.

These are virtually the first published data to consider comorbidity within a sample of employed women utilizing EAPs. These data indicate marked differences between employed women with comorbid alcohol problems and depression compared with depressed women without alcohol problems and women with alcohol problems with low levels of depressive symptoms. The comorbid women employees are markedly "worse off" on a variety of job-related, clinical, and treatment indices, underlining the importance that future research be specifically directed toward this group.

ACKNOWLEDGMENT. The research reported herein was supported by Grant No. R01-AA-07250 from the National Institute on Alcohol Abuse and Alcoholism. During preparation of this manuscript, the first two authors were partially supported by Grant No. R01-DA-07417 from the National Institute on Drug Abuse, and the third author was supported by Research Training Grant T32-AA-07473=06 from the National Institute on Alcohol Abuse and Alcoholism.

References

1. Blum TC, Roman PM: Women and work, in Wilsnack RW, Wilsnack SC (eds): *Gender and Alcohol*. New Brunswick, NJ, Publications Division of the Center of Alcohol Studies, Rutgers University, 1995 (forthcoming).

2. Roman PM: *Women and Alcohol Use: A Review of the Research Literature*. Rockville, MD, Alcohol, Drug Abuse and Mental Health Administration, 1988.
3. Shore E: Drinking patterns and problems among women in paid employment. *Alcohol Health Res World* 16(2):160–164, 1992.
4. Wilsnack RW, Wilsnack SC: Women, work and alcohol: Failures of simple theories. *Alcoholism Clin Exp Res* 16:172–179, 1992.
5. Blum TC, Roman PM: A description of clients using Employee Assistance Programs. *Alcohol Health Res World* 16(2):120–128, 1992.
6. Roman PM: Alcoholism and its management in the workplace: Overview, in Galanter M (ed): *Recent Developments in Alcoholism*. New York, Plenum Press, 1988, vol 6, pp 105–111.
7. Roman PM, Blum TC: Dealing with alcohol problems in the workplace, in Galanter M (ed): *Recent Developments in Alcoholism*. New York, Plenum Press, 1993, vol 11, pp 473–491.
8. Committee on Drugs in The Workplace: *Under the Influence*. Washington, National Academy of Sciences Press, 1993.
9. Roman PM: Barriers to the use of constructive confrontation with employed alcoholics. *J Drug Issues* 12:369–382, 1982.
10. Blum TC, Fields DL, Milne SH, Spell CS: The interrelations of drug testing with other human resource management practices and organizational characteristics, in Macdonald S, Roman P (eds): *Drug Testing in the Workplace*. New York, Plenum Press, 1994, pp 279–302.
11. Blum TC, Roman PM, Martin JK: A research note on EAP prevalence, components and utilization. *J Empl Assist Res* 1:209–229, 1992.
12. Bennett N, Blum TC, Roman PM: Presence of drug screening and employee assistance programs: Exclusive and inclusive human resource management practices. *J Organ Behav* 15:549–560, 1994.
13. Blum TC, Roman PM: Employee assistance and human resources management, in Rowland K, Ferris G (eds): *Research in Personnel and Human Resources Management*. Greenwich, CT, JAI Press, 1989, vol 7, pp 258–312.
14. Fennell ML: Synergy, influence and information in the adoption of administrative innovations. *Acad Manage J* 27:113–129, 1984.
15. Mahoney J, Smith D: Mcdonnell Douglas Corporation's EAP produces. *ALMACAN* 19:18–26, 1989.
16. Ewing JS: Detecting alcoholism: the CAGE Questionnaire. *J Am Med Assoc* 252(14):1905–1907, 1984.
17. Horn JL, Skinner HA, Wanberg K, Foster FM: *Alcohol Use Questionnaire (ADS)*. Toronto, Addiction Research Foundation, 1984.
18. Beck AT, Beck RW: Screening depressed patients in family practice: A rapid technique. *Postgrad Med* 52:81–85, 1972.
19. Roman PM, Blum TC: Drug prevention strategies in the workplace, in Coombs RH, Ziedonis D (eds): *Handbook of Drug Abuse Prevention*. Englewood Cliffs, NJ, Prentice Hall, 1995 (forthcoming).
20. Blum TC, Roman PM, Patrick L: Synergism in work site adoption of employee assistance programs and health promotion activities. *J Occup Med* 32:461–467, 1990.
21. Kessler RC, McGonagle, KA, Zhao S, et al: Lifetime and 12-month prevalence of DSM-III-R psychiatric disorder in the United States. *Arch Gen Psychiatry* 51:8–19, 1994.
22. Parker DA, Harford TC: Epidemiology of alcohol consumption and dependence across occupations in the United States. *Alcohol Health Res World* 16:(2):97–105, 1992.
23. Weisner C: The role of alcohol-related problematic events in treatment entry. *Drug Alcohol Depend* 26:93–102, 1990.
24. Weisner C: The alcohol treatment-seeking process from a problems perspective: Responses to events. *Br J Addict* 85:561–569, 1990.
25. Macdonald JG: Predictors of treatment outcome for alcoholic women. *Int J Addict* 22(3):235–248, 1987.
26. Brady KT, Grice DE, Dustan L, Randall C: Gender differences in substance use disorders. *Am J Psychiatry* 150(11):1707–1711, 1993.

27. Helzer J: Psychiatric diagnosis and substance abuse in the general population: The ECA data, in Harris LS (ed): *Problems of Drug Independence*. Rockville, MD, NIDA, 1988, chap 2.
28. Levy MF, Reichman W, Herrington S, Young D: Alcoholic women in industry: Some empirical data. *Int J Group Tensions* 10(1-4):120–129, 1989.
29. Gomberg ESL: Alcoholic women in treatment: The question of stigma and age. *Alcohol Alcohol* 23(6):507–514, 1988.
30. Vannicelli M: Barriers to treatment of alcoholic women. *Subst Alcohol Actions/Misuse* 5:29–37, 1984.
31. Institute of Medicine: *Broadening the Base of Treatment for Alcohol Problems*. Washington, DC, National Academy of Sciences Press, 1990.
32. Ross HE, Gavin DR, Skinner H: Diagnostic validity of the MAST and the Alcohol Dependence Scale in the assessment of DSM-III alcohol disorders. *J Stud Alcohol* 51(6):506–513, 1990.
33. Weiss RM: *Managerial Ideology and the Social Control of Deviance in Organizations*. Westport, CT, Praeger, 1988.
34. Woodall HE: Alcoholics remaining anonymous: Resident diagnosis of alcoholism in a family practice center. *J Fam Pract* 26(3):293–296, 1988.
35. Googins B, Casey JC: Enhancing motivation for treatment: Broadening the constructive confrontation model. *J Empl Assist Res* 1(1):96–111, 1993.

II

Physiology

Richard A. Deitrich, Section Editor

Overview

Richard A. Deitrich

This section, devoted to gender differences in alcohol effects and alcoholism, begins with an examination of some of the genetic, physiological, and biochemical gender-specific effects that might account for some of the differences in the consequences of excessive ethanol intake in women as contrasted to the same or higher intake in men.

The review on alcohol pharmacokinetics by Dr. Thomasson is a valuable contribution in that it pulls together the various studies and looks at the results critically. There is a nice summary of the various studies in table form. The influence of the different genotypes of both alcohol and aldehyde dehydrogenase is reviewed as is the somewhat disputed area of gastric alcohol dehydrogenase and first-pass metabolism.

Dr. Hill has provided a comprehensive review of the mental and physical health consequences of alcohol use in women. She discusses such controversial areas as increased risk for breast cancer and AIDS as being influenced by excessive alcohol intake. One aspect of increased risk for cancer would also be the use of cigarettes by alcohol-abusing women. These two have a markedly synergistic effect on lung cancer, and one wonders if similar increased risk might exist for other types of cancer.

Dr. Gavaler has studied the alcohol effects on hormone levels in post-menopausal women and in those with alcohol-induced cirrhosis. While much of the effort has concentrated on premenopausal women, this chapter demonstrates that there are marked effects of alcohol on hormone levels in the postmenopausal state as well.

Supported in part by grant #AA-00093 from the National Institute on Alcohol Abuse and Alcoholism.

Richard A. Deitrich • Department of Pharmacology, Alcohol Research Center, University of Colorado Health Sciences Center, Denver, Colorado 80262.

Recent Developments in Alcoholism, Volume 12: Women and Alcoholism, edited by Marc Galanter. Plenum Press, New York, 1995

The remaining chapters in this section deal with the evidence of gender differences from animal studies. Dr. Lancaster has provided a bridging review that brings together the studies on animals as they relate to human gender differences.

Dr. McClearn describes the basic genetic differences between the sexes, since it is from these differences that all effects flow. He reviews the X and Y gene structure and the consequences of males having only a single copy of many of the genes on the X chromosome. The less familiar area of the influence of sex on autosomal, or nonsex genes, is discussed, as are concepts of sex-limitation and sex-influence.

Jones and Whitfield review the sex differences that can be studied in genetically defined rodents. They review the use of such animals in delineating the various effects of ethanol. Thus, while a single animal model of human alcoholism is difficult to obtain, it is possible to separate the myriad effects of ethanol in genetically defined animals and study these effects one at a time. Thus, alcohol self-administration, hypnotic sensitivity, hypothermic sensitivity, and locomotion are discussed. In addition there are genetic models for dependence on alcohol. Since it is abundantly clear that there is a genetic influence in the actions of ethanol on these behaviors and further that human alcoholism is caused by the effect of ethanol on behavior (secondary to basic effects of the chemistry of the brain and body), we are forced to conclude that there is a solid foundation for genetic risk factors in humans of both genders. Unfortunately, it is also clear that these effects on behavior are due to more than a single gene in each case. Thus, the task of identifying the genes responsible for either gender-specific effects in animals or humans or for the overall risk of alcoholism in humans is indeed a difficult one.

The crucial area of "reinforcing" properties of ethanol and the relationship with the dopamine system in the brain is covered by Drs. Blanchard and Glick. This is particularly important to the understanding of the similarities of action of various drugs, including nicotine, opiates, cocaine, and alcohol.

Drs. Brot, Koob and Britton have addressed the anxiolytic effects of steroid hormones and the interrelationships with ethanol, especially in the actions on the GABA receptor. This is an area that has been especially active in recent years with the discovery that some steroid compounds are anesthetic agents and further that they interact with GABA receptors.

As a careful reading of this section will show, there is a great deal to be learned about gender differences. It is repeatedly pointed out that while women generally drink less and have lower rates of alcoholism, they are at greater risk for many of the damaging effects of ethanol for the amount of alcohol that they do consume. It is also pointed out that, in general, female animals drink more, not less, than males. All of this is complicated by the large differences between the estrous cycle in animals and the menstrual cycle in women.

After reading the various chapters in this section as well as in the rest of this volume, one recalls Professor Higgins' lament in *My Fair Lady*, "Why can't a woman . . . be more like a man?" It is clear, however, as far as alcohol is concerned, that this will never be the case. So we must put forth greater effort to understand those differences, learn from them, and eventually decrease the damage caused by alcohol with better prevention and treatment methods for both genders.

Gender Differences in Alcohol Metabolism

Physiological Responses to Ethanol

Holly R. Thomasson

Abstract. A gender difference in alcohol pharmacokinetics has been suggested to explain why women are more vulnerable to ethanol's toxic effects. The results of animal experiments suggest that females exhibit higher alcohol metabolic rates than males as a result of hormonal differences. Experimental results examining gender differences in human alcohol metabolism have been inconsistent; the diversity of experimental protocols and variety of pharmacokinetic parameters reported have made comparisons of these studies very difficult. Variability in alcohol metabolic rate between individuals of the same sex is often significant, preventing an assessment of gender differences in some studies. This chapter attempts to summarize the findings of studies from the last decade that examined the role of gender and sex hormone differences on ethanol metabolism in men and women. The role of body composition, genetic factors, gastric and hepatic alcohol dehydrogenase, and gastric absorption in creating gender differences in alcohol metabolism is discussed. Suggestions are offered that may result in better cross-study comparisons and more consistent experimental results.

1. Introduction

Several independent studies have shown that women develop alcoholic cirrhosis and alcoholic hepatitis at younger ages and at lower accumulated alcohol intakes than men.[1–5] The factors that cause women to be more vulnerable to alcoholic liver disease continue to elude us. Adult female rats and mice have faster alcohol metabolic rates than male animals.[6,7] Since immature and

Holly R. Thomasson • Eli Lilly and Company, Lilly Laboratory for Clinical Research, Wishard Memorial Hospital, Indianapolis, Indiana 46202.

Recent Developments in Alcoholism, Volume 12: Women and Alcoholism, edited by Marc Galanter. Plenum Press, New York, 1995

older female animals[8,9] do not have faster ethanol elimination rates than males, the effect is believed to be hormonal. These results suggest that differences in ethanol pharmacokinetics between males and females may be a reasonable physiological explanation for the gender difference in ethanol toxicity. Faster ethanol oxidation in women may expose liver tissue to higher levels of acetaldehyde, a highly reactive molecule that forms adducts with cell surface and blood proteins[10,11] and is believed to contribute to the development of cirrhosis. Indirect evidence of this hypothesis can be obtained by comparing the ethanol pharmacokinetics between healthy men and women and between individuals under the influence of different levels of sex hormones.

2. Variability in Human Alcohol Metabolism: General Considerations

Ethanol pharmacokinetics have been extensively studied in humans.[12–17] A high degree of interindividual variation in alcohol metabolic rates, usually two- to threefold, has been described.[18–21] The intrasubject variation, usually of smaller magnitude than intersubject variation, is also important when interpreting multiple assessments of pharmacokinetic measures in subjects under different conditions.[22–24] When this degree of variability is found between groups of individuals of the same sex, it is often difficult to identify gender as the only cause of rate differences between groups of men and women. It seems wise to examine the repeatability of ethanol metabolic parameters before declarations about gender differences are made from study data.

The high intraindividual variability on ethanol metabolism reported by several groups[21,24] contrasts with the report of Kopun and Propping[18] where the intrasubject coefficient of variation for β_{60}, the slope of the descending blood alcohol concentration (BAC)–time curve, of twins tested 2 months apart was under 10%. Passananti et al.[25] also measured β_{60}s in eight men on four occasions 1 week apart and reported an average of 8% coefficient of variation of intrasubject β_{60}. Their study design included men of similar age given oral ethanol in the fasted state and also controlled for other potentially important environmental factors such as medication, tobacco use, and the quantity of ethanol consumed in the recent past. A smaller study involving two men and five women showed a 95% test–retest reproducibility of the intrasubject β_{60}s.[26] These three studies suggest that the reproducibility of β_{60} measurements in well-controlled studies is high enough that gender differences can be distinguished from intrasubject variation, as long as the variation due to gender differences is greater than 10%.

Environmental and genetic heterogeneity accounts for much of the interindividual variation in ethanol metabolism. Some environmental factors are part of the study protocol and therefore under the control of the investigator.

Some of these include the presence or absence of food in the stomach,[27–29] the food composition of the meal,[30,31] the concentration of the ethanol or the beverage form given,[32,33] and the route and rate of administration.[34] All of these influence ethanol absorption and, thus, ethanol pharmacokinetics. If studies are performed following a meal, the food composition can change the rate of ethanol metabolism as well.[27,30,31] Circadian rhythm is believed by some to alter ethanol metabolic rates[35] and others suggest the variation is not meaningful for ethanol metabolic rate.[36] The subject's age,[8] recent ethanol drinking,[18,37] smoking history,[18] and the history or presence of liver disease[38] or other illness[25] may all influence ethanol pharmacokinetics. Chronic heavy drinking increased the rate of ethanol metabolism in men[38] and women[39] and in animal models of alcoholism[40]; however, in other studies the findings are not as clear.[41,42]

The results of studies measuring ethanol elimination rates of identical and fraternal twins ascribed about 50% or more of the observed variation to genetic factors.[18,21,24] The alcohol dehydrogenase (ADH) and aldehyde dehydrogenase (ALDH) gene loci are likely to be genetic determinants of ethanol metabolic differences in humans.[43] Together, ADH and ALDH catalyze the first and second steps of ethanol metabolism. ADH controls the rate-limiting step. Genetic polymorphism exits at two of the ADH loci, ADH2 and ADH3. There are striking differences in V_{max} among the low K_m ADH isozymes encoded by ADH2 and ADH3,[43,44] suggesting that individuals with different ADH genotypes should display different ethanol metabolism profiles.[45]

The ADH2 loci has three alleles, ADH2*1, ADH2*2, and ADH2*3.[43,44] Each allele encodes a subunit protein that forms homo- and heterodimer isozymes of ADH2. ADH2*1 encodes the β_1 ADH subunit, found in 95% of Caucasians and a majority of African-Americans but rarely in Asians.[43,46] ADH2*2 encodes the β_2 subunit, found in 70–95% of Asian peoples, rarely in Caucasians, and not at all in African-Americans.[43,46] ADH2*3 encodes the β_3 subunit, identified only in a minority (15%) of African-Americans.[43] The V_{max} of both β_2 and β_3 are 300–400 min^{-1}, but β_3-containing isozymes have a K_m near 34 mM (150 mg/dl) which implies their contribution to ethanol metabolism is not significant until very high blood ethanol levels are reached.[45]

The ADH3 locus has two alleles, γ_1 and γ_2, which also associate as homo- and heterodimer isozymes. ADH3*1 encodes the γ_1 subunit, found in high frequency in African-Americans and Asians. ADH3*2 encodes the γ_2 subunit, found in equal frequency with γ_1 in Caucasians but rarely in African-Americans and Asians. The K_ms of the γ_1 and γ_2 homodimer isozymes are very similar; however, the V_{max} of γ_1 homodimer isozyme is about twice that of γ_2 homodimer isozyme.[43,45]

The ALDH2 locus also has two alleles: ALDH2*1, encoding an active isozyme subunit, and ALDH2*2, encoding an inactive isozyme subunit. The ALDH2*2 allele is dominant; therefore, homo- and heterozygotes of ALDH2*2 have a deficiency of the low K_m ALDH2 activity.[44,47] Persons with ALDH2 deficiency experience elevated acetaldehyde levels in the blood and unpleasant symptoms characterized primarily by a facial flush reaction after modest amounts of alcoholic beverage consumption.[47,48]

Since ethnic groups vary considerably in the frequencies of the *ALDH2, ADH2,* and *ADH3* alleles,[46] the ethanol metabolism of subjects from these groups may show significant differences. A study of Caucasians, who exhibited polymorphism at *ADH3* but not at the *ADH2* or *ALDH2* loci, did not have differences in mean ethanol elimination rates.[49] The influence of *ADH2*-encoded isozyme subunits, β_1, β_2, and β_3, may be larger, however, since the differences in V_{max} among them are more than tenfold larger than the differences in V_{max} described between γ–ADH homodimer isozymes.[44,50] In African-Americans, those subjects with β_3-containing ADHs had significantly faster ethanol metabolic rates.[51,52] The role of the *ADH2*2*-encoded, high catalytic activity isozyme, β_2, is still being studied; initial data suggest that subjects who have β_2 homodimer ADH have higher ethanol metabolic rates than subjects with β_1-containing ADH isozymes.[47,53]

The Asian population, which has a high frequency of *ADH2*2* alleles, also has a high frequency of the *ALDH2*2* allele. ALDH2 deficiency, due to the presence of *ALDH2*2*, is associated with reduced ethanol metabolic rates.[47,53]

In summary, whenever opposite sex twins/siblings or men and women with identical *ADH* or *ALDH* genotypes are subjects in ethanol metabolic studies, there is a much better chance of identifying gender differences unencumbered by some of the known genetic variation.

3. Comparison Studies of Metabolic Rate in Men and Women

In the last decade, most human ethanol metabolic studies involved only male subjects, but a small number compared rates in men and women. Table I is a summary of 12 studies. The ethanol dose used, the route of administration, the number of subjects, and a measure of ethanol metabolism are reported for each study. To assist the reader in comparing these reports, the β_{60} for men and for women is shown in mg/dl/hr from each report even if other pharmacokinetic measures were compared. If β_{60} was not available and could not be estimated, an elimination rate corrected for differences in body weight or volume of ethanol distribution (V_d), usually designated the elimination rate (ER), was shown in mg/kg body weight/hr. Only one group did not report β_{60} or ER; the area under the blood ethanol concentration versus time curve (AUC) was the variable used.[54] These results were derived from the control group values when the study also involved testing of alcoholics, subjects on drugs, or subjects given daily ethanol as in the study of metabolic tolerance by Holtzman *et al.*[41] Goist and Sutker[54] reported testing subjects using ethanol doses corrected for body weight on one occasion and doses corrected for body

Table I. Reported Ethanol Pharmacokinetic Measures for Men and Women

Reference	Dose	Subjects (N)		Results[a]
Thomasson et al.[55] (ADH2*1/*1)	Anthropometric equations used to reach $C_0 = 0.08$[b] 0.6 g/kg (δ) 0.5 g/kg ($\female$) oral	Men Women	(45) (45)	β_{60}[c] 11.5 ± 2 mg/dl/hr[d] 14.1 ± 3 mg/dl/hr
Smith et al.[39]	0.8 g/kg oral	Men Women	(11) (9)	β_{60} 13.5 mg/dl/hr[d] 16.0 mg/dl/hr
Mishra et al.[56] (siblings)	0.6 g/kg intravenous	Men Women	(9) (9)	β_{60} 13.5 ± 1.6 mg/kg/hr[d] 20.5 ± 2.3 mg/kg/hr
Sutker et al.[58,e]	0.50 g/kg (low) 0.76 g/kg (high) oral	Men Women	(10) (8)	β_{60} 15.0 ± mg/dl/hr[d] (low) 11.3 ± mg/dl/hr[d] (high) 15.2 ± mg/dl/hr (low) 14.2 ± mg/dl/hr (high)
Cole-Harding and Wilson[62]	0.8 g/kg + to reach peak BAC 0.1 g/dl oral	Men Women	(75) (59)	β_{60} 17.2 ± 0.40 mg/dl/hr[d] 20.8 ± 0.55 mg/dl/hr
Goist et al.[54]	1.2 ml/liter TBW[f] 0.63 g/kg oral	Men Women	(12) (12)	AUC[g] 10.4 ± 1.44 mg ·5 min/ml 10.0 ± 1.91 mg ·5 min/ml
Martin et al.[24] (twins)	0.75 g/kg oral	Men Women	(194) (208)	β_{60} 15.5 ± 5.0 mg/dl/hr 15.9 ± 5.1 mg/dl/hr
Holtzman et al.[41]	45 g/day, 0.64 g/kg oral	Men Women	(7) (5)	β_{60} 16.5 ± 1.4 mg/dl/hr[d] 20.9 ± 1.3 mg/dl/hr
Arthur et al.[57]	0.5 g/kg intravenous	Men Women	(10) (10)	β_{60} 13.6 ± 5.3 mg/dl/hr 14.8 ± 3.6 mg/dl/hr
Sutker et al.[59,h]	0.5 g/kg oral	Men Women	(9) (7)	ER[i] 102.6 ± 16 mg/kg/hr 111.8 ± 11 mg/kg/hr
Marshall et al.[60]	0.5 g/kg/oral	Men Women	(10) (9)	ER 97 ± 5 mg/kg/hr 87 ± 4 mg/kg/hr

(continued)

Table I. (*Continued*)

Reference	Dose	Subjects (N)		Results[a]
Jones and Jones[61]	0.5 g/kg oral			β_{60}
		Men	(10)	18.3 ± 3.0 mg/dl/hr
		Women	(20)	20.0 ± 1.7 mg/dl/hr

[a]The mean $\pm$ SE is given, where available, except Martin *et al.*, Arthur *et al.*, and Thomasson *et al.* where mean $\pm$ SD is given. All used blood alcohol concentration data.
[b]C_0, the theoretical blood alcohol concentration at time zero in g/dl.
[c]β_{60}, the slope of the pseudolinear portion of the blood alcohol vs. time curve using linear regression analysis.
[d]$p < 0.05$; refers to the comparison of men vs. women.
[e]An average β_{60} from three test sessions is reported here. Results were corrected for the differce in total body water. SE was not reported.
[f]TBW, total body water based on anthropometric calculations.
[g]AUC, the area under the blood alcohol concentration vs. time curve.
[h]ERs corrected for difference in total body water.
[i]ER, the ethanol elimination rate (see text).

water at another time. For reasons that will be discussed, the results of the latter are shown in Table I. Nine of the 12 studies used small numbers of subjects. The diversity of doses, protocols, and method of calculating results precludes combining the results from all the studies to calculate a β_{60} for men and women.

Methods of determining ethanol concentrations included the use of the ADH method or, more recently, gas chromatography. Ethanol was measured in venous or capillary blood samples in all but one study where plasma was obtained.[41] Since plasma is a fraction of whole blood and about 93% water, ethanol concentrations in plasma will be higher than those obtained from whole blood if the results of each are not properly corrected for water content. Uncorrected BAC data from plasma samples shifts the BAC–time curve toward higher ethanol concentrations compared to uncorrected whole blood data, but should not change the slope of the pseudolinear curve which represents β_{60}. However, many studies did not choose to analyze β_{60}. Uncorrected plasma-derived data for AUC and ER estimates, which are frequently derived from the y-intercept C_0 and the y-intercept MIN_0 of the pseudolinear descending BAC–time curve, would be higher than the same estimates from uncorrected whole blood data.

Table I shows the actual doses used in each study converted to grams of absolute ethanol per kilogram body weight. Two studies used ethanol doses adjusted for total body water (TBW), using anthropometric equations. Therefore, the g/kg doses shown for these two reports are an approximation.[54,55] The dose range, 0.5 to 0.76 g/kg, is surprisingly small for these diverse studies.

Two of the protocols used intravenous ethanol[56,57] while the remainder gave oral doses over various lengths of time using several ethanol dilutions. In several studies, ethanol was given to fasted subjects[41,54,56–60] while in others a light breakfast was given followed by ethanol 1 or 2 hours later.[55,61] The use of different routes of administration, the fed or fasted state, and different dilutions of alcohol created differences in absorption time and subsequently in peak BAC levels. These differences prevent satisfactory cross-study analysis.

Approximately half of the published reports (5 of 11) concluded that women had faster ethanol metabolic rates than men when β_{60} was compared.[39,41,56,58,62] Six studies, including one that involved hundreds of twins, concluded there were no significant gender differences in ethanol metabolism.[24,54,57,59–61] In several of the studies where β_{60} or AUC was different between men and women, the gender differences disappeared when the rates were corrected for body water, V_d, or body weight.[59–61] The explanation for apparent gender differences in rate "uncorrected" for body weight or TBW has been attributed to gender differences in body composition. Women have proportionately more body fat and less body water than men of the same body weights. Since ethanol is dispersed in body water, body weight-adjusted doses of ethanol distribute in the smaller V_ds of women and cause a higher peak BAC.[54,58,60,63] Subjects with higher peak BACs and/or higher theoretical zero-time BACs (C_0s) may have higher β_{60}s by virtue of receiving a greater ethanol dose. This has been noted in animal studies but is still controversial in humans.[58] In any case, most studies in Table I showed significantly higher C_0s for women, a difference that placed women higher on the BAC–time curve and potentially confounded β_{60} comparisons with those of men.[24,54_56,60,61]

The solution to the problem of equivalent ethanol dosing of subjects with differences in body composition, TBW, and V_d is unresolved. Cole-Harding and Wilson[62] chose to give an initial oral ethanol dose adjusted by body weight and followed it with "topping off" doses to bring the BAC up to a desired level before allowing the descending BAC curve to begin. Other groups adjusted the ethanol dose for the subjects' V_d or estimated TBW rather than adjusting for body weight.[54,55] Goist et al.[54] gave body weight-adjusted and TBW-adjusted doses to the same subjects on different occasions. A comparison of the BAC–time data showed women still had higher peak BACs than the men; however, the TBW-adjusted doses came closer to producing equivalent peak BACs and C_0s in men and women. Thomasson et al.[55] reported a gender difference in C_0 in spite of the use of TBW-adjusted ethanol doses; C_0 was 82 ± 6 mg/dl for men and 79 ± 5 mg/dl for women ($p < 0.01$). In that study, TBW estimates were made from anthropomorphic calculations derived by Watson et al.[63] The use of these equations for African-American subjects has not been tested before; therefore, this may be the source of the undesirable gender difference in C_0. Nonetheless, the comparison of mean β_{60}s between men and women had a much smaller p value (Table I, $p < 0.001$) than the mean C_0s, suggesting that women may actually have faster ethanol metabolic rates than men. The body weight-adjusted dose used by Smith et *al.*[39] did not result in higher C_0s in the women, perhaps due to slower ethanol absorption in those women. Gender differences in ethanol absorption is discussed in a later section. Smith *et al.*[39] also reported a higher mean β_{60} in women than men.

It is apparent from the variety of pharmacokinetic parameters used in these studies that there is still considerable debate over which parameter most accurately reflects human ethanol metabolism and is best for cross-gender comparisons. The classical approach to ethanol elimination kinetics was to view it as a zero-order process.[64] Further study has shown that BACs are not linear over time and ethanol elimination rates are not independent of ethanol concentration.[13,58] Other models, including those that employ Michaelis-Menten kinetics, more accurately describe ethanol pharmacokinetics.[13,16,39,65–67] After the administration of ethanol, an absorption and distribution phase is followed by a pseudolinear phase of apparent zero-order characteristics when moderate doses of ethanol are given. Between the BACs of 5 to 15 mM (25 to 65 mg/dl) most hepatic ADH isozymes are saturated; therefore, the elimination rate is nearly constant.[44,45] Below 5 mM the BAC falls in a distinctly nonlinear fashion as the concentration of ethanol in the body falls below the K_m of the hepatic ADHs.

Wilson and Erwin[68] argued in favor of comparing mean β_{60}s of different ethnic groups, rather than AUC or ER, because β_{60} is an expression of ethanol metabolic rate that is not influenced by differences in V_d resultant from differences in obesity or leanness. This advice could be applied to gender comparisons of ethanol metabolism, since disparate body composition is one of the major differences that precludes equivalent dosing. No body weight correction of β_{60} should be made, especially when the protocol uses TBW-adjusted ethanol doses; the dose adjustment alone should suffice.

In addition to the use of a sufficiently large dose of ethanol, the accurate calculation of β_{60} requires that the absorption of the ethanol be fairly rapid so that BAC–time points during absorption are not included in the pseudolinear portion. Using data points from the absorption phase results in falsely high C_0 and β_{60} values.[68]

Since accurate β_{60} calculations and cross-gender comparisons depend on equivalent ethanol absorption in both genders, the influence of sex hormones on gastric motility or of gender on gastric ethanol metabolism may create inequities in β_{60}. Ethanol is readily absorbed from the duodenum; however, there is evidence that a portion of the ethanol dose is also absorbed through the wall of the stomach.[28] The fraction of an oral dose absorbed in the stomach is largely dependent on the mucosal exposure time and possibly mucosal metabolism, which in turn depends on the gastric emptying rate and gender. Women may have less gastric metabolism of oral ethanol compared with men (see Section 6). This would explain the higher peak BACs and AUCs of women compared with men.[59,60] Faster duodenal absorption of ethanol in women because of faster gastric emptying of ethanol might also explain higher BACs in women. Gender differences in gastric emptying of solids and liquids have been reported[69,70]; however, the researchers concluded that premenopausal women usually had slower, not faster, gastric emptying of solids and in some cases liquids than men. Unfortunately, these studies did not examine the gastric emptying of ethanol. There are also reports of menstrual cycle-related changes in gastric emptying rate of liquids, though not ethanol in particular.[71] These differences may contribute to gender differences in peak BAC, AUC, and metabolic rate in some studies, especially those where the timing of the ethanol study was designed to control for the phase of the subjects' menstrual cycle or where oral contraceptive use was not controlled.

Studies using twins or genotyped subjects can reduce genetic variability and allow better evaluation of gender differences. Martin et al.[24] studied 206 twin pairs, including 39 opposite sex pairs. Unfortunately, the report only shows that the within-pair variance in the β_{60} values was smaller than the between-pair variance for these male–female dizygotic twin pairs. There was no comparison of the mean β_{60}s for the men and women of this twin subset; however, this was not the focus of the study. Mishra et al.[56] reported significantly higher peak BACs, ERs, and β_{60}s for the women of nine sibling pairs. There was no corresponding gender difference in plasma acetate concentration. It is possible that women had faster utilization of acetate as well as faster ethanol metabolism than the men.

The examination of gender differences in ethanol metabolism in subjects for whom the *ADH2, ADH3,* and *ALDH2* genotypes are known are still being completed. African-Americans and Caucasians, all of whom had the *ADH2*1/*1* genotype, participated in a study of ethanol metabolism measurement where the women had significantly higher mean β_{60} values and higher mean ERs compared with the men (Table I).[55] A separate analysis looked at the gender differences in mean β_{60}s within ethnic groups. Fifty African-American men and women, 25 of each sex, and 20 Caucasians, 10 of each sex, were involved. The gender differences of these subgroups showed similar results; women had higher β_{60}s compared with men. The women participating in these studies were taking oral contraceptives, and their ethanol metabolism was studied 1–4 days following the end of their menstrual flow, a time when estrogen and progesterone levels are low. Testing women at this point in their cycle should minimize the effect of these sex hormones on ethanol metabolic rate, if the level of sex hormones indeed makes a difference.

4. The Role of Sex Hormones in Ethanol Metabolism

Another way to explore gender differences in ethanol metabolism, especially those related to sex hormones, is by measuring ethanol pharmacokinetics during different phases of the menstrual cycle. Animal studies have shown higher ethanol metabolic rates in adult females compared with males or immature or older females.[6,7] This suggests that the presence of higher levels of progesterone or estrogen in mature females enhances the rate of ethanol metabolism.[6–9] However, exogenous estrogen did not change ethanol metabolic rates in rats[9,72] even when the hepatic ADH activity was increased.[72,73]

The early studies of Jones and Jones[74] suggested that women had faster ethanol absorption, higher peak BACs, and longer MIN_0s or total time of intoxication during the premenstrual phase when estrogen and progesterone levels were lowest. Following this report, others found no difference in ethanol metabolic rate during different stages of the menstrual cycle[75–78] or significantly faster rates associated with higher estrogen and progesterone phases of the cycle.[58,60,62,79–81] Only two investigators measured the hormone levels of the participants, and one of these eliminated several anovulatory subjects from the analysis.[60,81] In spite of similar attempts to document and account for the influence of the level of the sex hormones on testing of ethanol metabolism, their conclusions appear to disagree. Marshall et al.[60] reported that there were no cyclical differences in peak BAC, AUC, ER, β_{60}, or V_d when subjects were tested in the early follicular, ovulatory, and midluteal phases. Sutker et al.[81] measured the same parameters during the same phases and found an increase in β_{60}, ER, and AUC during the high progesterone and estrogen midluteal phase compared with the other two cycle phases and no differences in peak BAC or absorption throughout the cycle. The importance of female sex hormones during ethanol metabolism remains unsettled.

Women taking oral contraceptives (OC) should have more predictable hormone levels during the menstrual cycle. When the women on OC were analyzed separately from those cycling naturally, significantly lower peak BACs and β_{60}s were found.[74,78,80] Other investigators have reported no difference in ethanol metabolism associated with OC use.[62,75,82] Two of these studies also reported there were no important differences in ethanol metabolism during the different phases of the menstrual cycle in women cycling naturally.[62,75] This may mean that earlier studies were measuring differences in β_{60} that resulted from the higher peak BACs of those on OCs, which is in itself significant. Cole-Harding and Wilson[62] note that differences in the amount of synthetic hormone in OCs has declined dramatically between the 1980s and the earlier studies, a factor that may account for the difference in study results.

The sex hormone fluctuations of women may not be as important as testosterone levels in men on the rate of ethanol metabolism. Castration of male rats resulted in increased hepatic ADH activity, an effect that was reversed by the administration of exogenous testosterone.[9] In a unique study, nine prostate cancer patients underwent ethanol metabolic rate testing before and after orchiectomy for prostate cancer.[83] After an approximately tenfold drop in testosterone levels following surgery, the β_{60}s and ERs of these men were reduced significantly without a change in the peak BAC or V_d. They speculated that the change in β_{60} was the result of increased hepatic ADH activity, as was the case in the rat studies.[84] This theory remains untested in humans since liver biopsy would be necessary for evidence of changes in hepatic ADH.

5. Gender Differences in Hepatic ADHs and Cytochrome P450

Differences in hormone levels appear to control the level of expression of hepatic ADH genes in animals. Androgens, estrogen, thyroid hormones, and growth hormone have been implicated as having a role in the expression of rat ADHs.[73,85–87] The mass of the ADH enzyme in rat liver is directly proportional to ADH activity, which correlates well with ethanol elimination rate.[87] These findings suggest that future experiments to measure the rates of ethanol elimination of men and women (β_{60}) should correct for differences in liver mass as grams of ethanol per minute per gram of liver tissue rather than per kg body weight. If estimates of liver mass are accurate and gender differences are found in the corrected β_{60}s, this would provide indirect evidence of gender differences in ADH mass in humans, a factor that could significantly alter individual responses to ethanol.

Gender differences in the amount or activity of hepatic ADH in humans are suspected but unproved. A study of the total liver ADH activity from autopsy specimens suggested men had higher levels of activity than women[85]; however, enzyme degradation and the effect illness may have had on hepatocyte function could have compromised the reliability of these results. Currently, the absence of a noninvasive means to estimate hepatic ADH activity in healthy men and women prevents the investigation of hepatic ADH activity under different circumstances.

During social drinking the class I ADHs are the major hepatic ethanol-metabolizing catalysts; however, the microsomal enzyme, cytochrome P450IIE1 also contributes to ethanol metabolism. Its greatest contribution occurs during moderately high blood alcohol concentrations due to its relatively high K_m for ethanol (10 mM or 50 mg/dl) and following chronic ethanol ingestion. A known polymorphism in the human P450IIE1 5'-flanking region sequence is associated with a difference in transcription rates.[88] It is not known if differences in the sex hormones affect the regulation or induction of cytochrome P450IIE1.[89] Such differences could explain the greater hepatic toxicity of ethanol in women. No such gender differences are known, and, in fact, little is known about regulation of the human P450IIE1 gene or the biological significance of the polymorphism described.

6. Gender Differences in the Gastric Metabolism of Ethanol

Women may have decreased ethanol metabolism in the stomach as a reasonable explanation for their higher peak BACs, even with TBW-adjusted ethanol doses.[90,91] The significance of gastric mucosal metabolism and the gender differences ascribed to this phenomenon are controversial. By comparing the difference in bioavailability (AUC) of identical oral and intravenous (or intraduodenal) ethanol doses, Frezza et al.[90] found that men, but not women, experience a prehepatic "first-pass" metabolism of ethanol. These differences in AUC were noted only with low doses of ethanol (< 0.30 g/kg) given after a full meal; fasted subjects did not demonstrate the phenomenon.[92] It is difficult, if not impossible, to distinguish the difference between hepatic first-pass and gastric metabolism of ethanol in humans.[86] Therefore, another interpretation of the Frezza *et al.* study is that women have less hepatic ADH mass (or activity) and thus less hepatic first-pass metabolism of ethanol than men. Furthermore, ethanol bioavailability is highly dependent on the rate of administration.[34] The rate of the intravenous administration may have been faster than the rate at which ethanol was absorbed during oral administration.[93,94] If this were the case, the differences in AUC measured between men and women may have represented differences in the rate of absorption of the ethanol, not its metabolism.

The discovery that women under the age of 50 have lower gastric ADH activity compared with men[95,96] seemed to support the gender difference in gastric metabolism of ethanol. Multiple ADH activity bands have been identified in gastric mucosal samples following starch gel electrophoresis and isoelectric focusing.[97,98] Several of these bands represent the previously identified γ-ADH and χ-ADH; however, several ADH activity bands are unique to the stomach mucosa. One of these, now designated σ-ADH, is a high activity form of ADH with a V_{max} of 1500 min^{-1} (pH 7.5).[99] The σ-ADH was responsible for at least 75% of the gastric mucosal ethanol-oxidizing activity.[99] This enzyme is unlike the low activity stomach-specific ADH identified earlier.[100] The relationship of these two gastric ADHs to each other is not known. It is also unclear how a decrease in the overall gastric ADH activity in women occurs; σ-ADH activity bands were seen in all biopsy samples from women even as overall mucosal ADH activity was diminished.[95,98] The quantity and precise location of σ-ADH in the stomach mucosa are also unknown. Current estimates of the ethanol-metabolizing capacity of σ-ADH and stomach mucosa suggest that the contribution of the stomach may be no more than 1–10% that of the liver in ethanol metabolism.[34,99]

7. Summary and Recommendations for Future Work

The increased susceptibility of women to alcoholic cirrhosis and hepatitis has been attributed to their smaller volume of distribution for ethanol, decreased first-pass metabolism or more rapid absorption, and more rapid metabolism of ethanol. The gender differences observed in ethanol metabolic rate (β_{60}) were often eliminated when the rate was corrected for gender differences in V_d or body weight. Since women have a significantly smaller V_d for ethanol, doses adjusted by body weight routinely result in higher peak BACs in the women, inadequately compensating for the gender difference in body composition. This way of dosing should probably be abandoned in favor of doses based on knowledge or calculation of the subject's total body water. Examination of β_{60} from studies using TBW-adjusted doses should not include a "correction" for body weight or V_d. Several studies using this approach have reported significantly faster ethanol metabolism in women compared with men, suggesting a gender difference really exists. However, questions remain concerning the role of gastric motility, gastric metabolism, and genetics confounding the rate estimates of these oral ethanol studies. Comparisons of the metabolic rate using siblings or twins and studies of subjects of known *ALDH2, ADH2,* and *ADH3* genotype, where significant polymorphism exists, may have the advantage of reducing genetic variability in ethanol metabolism and reveal gender differences more clearly. Other sources of variability in ethanol metabolism should be minimized, including the study of women in the same phase of their menstrual cycle or using only those on oral contraceptives. The administration of intravenous ethanol to fasted subjects completely avoids the gender differences that may exist due to gastric metabolism, absorption, or the emptying rate of the ethanol and should allow more careful determination of hepatic alcohol oxidation rates.

References

1. Spain DM: Portal cirrhosis of the liver: A review of two hundred necropsies with references to sex differences. *Am J Pathol* 15:215–218, 1945.
2. Morgan MY, Sherlock S: Sex-related differences among 100 patients with alcoholic liver disease. *Br Med J* 1:939–941, 1977.
3. Wilkinson P, Santamaria JN, Randin JG: Epidemiology of alcoholic cirrhosis. *Aust Ann Med* 18:222–226, 1969.
4. Saunders JB, Walters JRF Davies P, *et al:* A 20-year prospective study of cirrhosis. *BR Med J* 282:263–266, 1981.
5. Gavaler JS: Sex-Related Differences in ethanol-induced liver disease: Artifactual or real? *Alcohol Clin Exp Res* 6:186–196, 1982.
6. Eriksson CJP, Malmstrom KK: Sex differences in consumption and elimination of ethanol in albino rats. *Ann Med Exp Fenn* 45:398–392, 1967.
7. Wilson JR, Erwin VG, DeFries JC, *et al:* Ethanol dependence in mice: Direct and correlated responses to ten generations of selective breeding. *Behav Genet* 14:226–232, 1984.
8. Collins AC, Yeager TN, Lebsack ME, Panter SS: Variations in alcohol metabolism: Influence of sex and age. *Pharmacol Biochem Behav* 3:973–978, 1975.
9. Rachamin G, MacDonald JA, Wahid S, *et al:* Modulation of alcohol dehydrogenase and ethanol metabolism by sex hormones in the spontaneously hypertensive rat. *Biochem J* 186:483–490, 1980.
10. Sorrell MF, Tuma DJ: Hypothesis: Alcoholic liver injury and covalent binding of acetaldehyde. *Alcohol Clin Exp Res* 9:306–309, 1985.
11. Lin RC, Lumeng L: Alcohol and hepatic protein modification in liver pathology and alcohol, in Watson RR (ed): Liver Pathology and Alcohol, Totowa, NJ, Humana Press, 1991, pp 221–240.
12. Wilkinson PK: Pharmacokinetics of ethanol: A review. *Alcohol Clin Exp Res* 4:6–21, 1980.
13. Holford NHG: Clinical pharmacokinetics of ethanol. *Clin Pharmacokinet* 13:273–292, 1987.
14. Wilkinson PK: Pharmacokinetics of ethanol: A review. *Alcohol Clin Exp Res* 4:6–21, 1980.
15. Lundquist F, Wolthers H: The kinetics of alcohol elimination in man. *Acta Pharmacol Toxicol* 14:265–286, 1958.
16. Von Wartburg J-P: Pharmacokinetics of alcohol, in Crow KE, Batt RD (eds): *Human Metabolism of Alcohol.* Boca Raton, FL, CRC Press, 1989, vol 11, pp 9–22.
17. Kalant H: Absorption, diffusion, distribution and elimination of ethanol: Effects on biolog-

ical membranes, in Kissin B, Begleiter H (eds): *The Biology of Alcoholism.* New York, Plenum Press, 1971, vol 1, p 1046.

18. Kopun M, Propping P: The kinetics of ethanol absorption and elimination in twins an supplementary repetitive experiments in singleton subjects. *Eur J Clin Pharmacol* 11:337–344, 1977.

19. Wagner JG: Intrasubject variation in elimination half-lives of drugs which are appreciably metabolized. *J Pharmacokinet Biopharm* 1:165–173, 1973.

20. Jones AW: Interindividual variations in the disposition and metabolism of ethanol in healthy men. *Alcohol* 1:385, 1984.

21. Vessell ES, Page JG, Passananti GT: Genetic and environmental factors affecting ethanol metabolism in man. *Clin Pharmacol Ther* 12:192–201, 1971.

22. Wagner JG, Wilkinson PK, Ganes DA: Parameters V_m and K_m for elimination of alcohol in young male subjects following low doses of alcohol. *Alcohol Alcohol* 24:555–564, 1989.

23. Wagner JG: Intrasubject variation in elimination half-lives of drugs which are appreciably metabolized. *J Pharmacokinet Biopharm* 1:165–173, 1973.

24. Martin NG, Perl J, Oakeshott JG, et al: A twin study of ethanol metabolism. *Behav Genet* 15:93–109, 1985.

25. Passanati GT, Wolff CA, Vesell ES: Reproducibility of individual rates of ethanol metabolism in fasting subjects. *Clin Pharmacol Ther* 47:389–396, 1990.

26. Thomasson HR, Christian J, Reed T, Li T-K: Reproducibility of human alcohol metabolic rate testing. *Alcohol Clin Exp Res* 14:345, 1990.

27. Sedman AJ, Wilkinson PK, Sakmar E, et al: Food effects on absorption and metabolism of alcohol. *J Stud Alcohol* 37:1197–1214, 1976.

28. Cortot A, Jobin G, Ducrot F, et al: Gastric emptying and gastrointestinal absorption of alcohol ingested with a meal. *Digest Dis Sci* 31:343–348, 1986.

29. Lin, Y-J, Weidler DJ, Garg DC, Wagner JG: Effects of solid food on blood levels of alcohol in man. *Res Commun Chem Pathol Pharmacol* 13:713, 1976.

30. Keegan A, Batey R: Dietary carbohydrate accelerates ethanol elimination, but does not alter hepatic alcohol dehydrogenase. *Alcohol Clin Exp Res* 17:431–433, 1993.

31. Rogers J, Smith J, Starmer GA, Whitfield JB: Differing effects of carbohydrate, fat and protein on the rate of ethanol metabolism. *Alcohol Alcohol* 22:345–353, 1987.

32. Roine RP, Gentry T, Lim RT, et al: Effect of concentration of ingested ethanol on blood alcohol levels. *Alcohol Clin Exp Res* 15:734–738, 1991.

33. Pfeiffer A, Hogl B, Kaess H: Effect of ethanol and commonly ingested alcoholic beverages on gastric emptying and gastrointestinal transit. *Clin Invest* 70:487–491, 1992.

34. Smith T, DeMaster EG, Furne JK, et al: First-pass metabolism of ethanol is negligible in the rat. *J Clin Invest* 89:1801–1806, 1992.

35. Sturtevant RP, Sturtevant FM: Circadian rhythms in rates of ethanol metabolism, in Crow KE, Batt RD (eds): *Human Metabolism of Alcohol.* Boca Raton, FL, CRC Press, vol 1, pp 23–39, 1989.

36. Yap M, Mascord DJ, Starmer GA, Whitfield JB: Studies on the chronopharmacology of ethanol. *Alcohol Alcohol* 28:17–24, 1993.

37. Kater RMH, Carulli N, Iber FL: Differences in the rate of ethanol metabolism in recently drinking and nondrinking subjects. *Am J Clin Nutr* 22:1608–1617, 1969.

38. Mezey E, Tobon F: Rates of ethanol clearance and activities of the ethanol-oxidizing enzymes in chronic alcoholic patients. *Gastroenterology* 61:707–715, 1971.

39. Smith GD, Shaw LJ, Maini RJ, et al: Mathematical modelling of ethanol metabolism in normal subjects and chronic alcohol misusers. *Alcohol Alcohol* 28:25–32, 1993.

40. Salaspuro PM, Lieber CS: Non-uniformity of blood ethanol elimination: Its exaggeration after chronic consumption. *Ann Clin Res* 10:294–297, 1978.

41. Holtzman JL, Gebhard RL, Eckfeldt JH, et al: The effects of several weeks of ethanol consumption on ethanol kinetics in normal men and women. *Clin Pharmacol Ther* 38:157–161, 1985.

42. Pieper WA, Skeen MJ: Changes in rate of ethanol elimination associated with chronic admin-

istration of ethanol to chimpanzees and Rhesus monkeys. *Drug Metab Dispos* 1:634–641, 1973.

43. Crabb DW: The liver, in Galanter M (ed): *Recent Developments in Alcoholism*. New York, Plenum Press, 1993, vol 11, pp 207–230.

44. Bosron WF, Li T-K: Genetic polymorphism of human liver alcohol and aldehyde dehydrogenases, and their relationship to alcohol metabolism and alcoholism. *Hepatology* 6:502–510, 1986.

45. Bosron WF, Crabb DW, Li T-K: Relationship between kinetics of liver alcohol dehydrogenase and alcohol metabolism. *Pharmacol Biochem Behav* 18(Suppl 1):223–227, 1983.

46. Goedde HW, Agarwal DP, Fritze G, *et al*: Distribution of *ADH2* and *ALDH2* genotypes in different populations. *Hum Genet* 88:344–346, 1992.

47. Thomasson HR, Crabb DW, Edenberg HJ, Li T-K: Alcohol and aldehyde dehydrogenase and alcoholism. *Behav Genet* 23:131–136, 1993.

48. Mizoi Y, Ijiri I, Tatsuno Y, *et al*: Relationship between facial flushing and blood acetaldehyde levels after alcohol intake. *Pharmacol Biochem Behav* 10:303–311, 1979.

49. Couzigou P, Fleury B, Groppi A, *et al*: Role of alcohol dehydrogenase polymorphism in ethanol metabolism and alcohol-related diseases. *Adv Exp Med Biol* 284:263–70, 1991.

50. Burnell JC, Bosron WF: Genetic polymorphism of human liver alcohol dehydrogenase and kinetic properties of the isoenzymes, in Crow KE, Batt RD (eds): *Human Metabolism of Alcohol*. Boca Raton, FL, CRC Press, 1989, vol 2, pp 65–75.

51. Thomasson HR, Beard JD, Li T-K: Faster ethanol metabolic rate demonstrated in subjects with *ADH2*3* alleles. *Alcohol Clin Exp Res* 17:495, 1993.

52. May DG, Thomasson HR, Martier S, *et al*: Ethanol metabolism in women: Relative importance of ADH genotype and intake. *Alcohol Clin Exp Res* 16:605, 1992.

53. Mizoi Y, Kogame M, Fukunaga T, *et al*: Polymorphism of aldehyde dehydrogenase and ethanol elimination. *Alcohol* 2:393–396, 1985.

54. Goist KC Jr, Sutker PB: Acute alcohol intoxication and body composition in women and men. *Pharmacol Biochem Behav* 22:811–814, 1985.

55. Thomasson HR, Beard JD, Li T-K: Gender differences in ethanol metabolism. *Alcoholism: Clin Exp Res* 18:921, 1994.

56. Mishra L, Sharma S, Potter JJ, Mezey E: More rapid elimination of alcohol in women as compared to their male siblings. *Alcohol Clin Exp Res* 13:752–754, 1989.

57. Arthur MJP, Lee A, Wright R: Sex differences in the metabolism of ethanol and acetaldehyde in normal subjects. *Clin Sci* 67:397–401, 1984.

58. Sutker PB, Goist KC Jr, Allain AN, Bugg F: Acute alcohol intoxication: Sex comparisons on pharmacokinetic and mood measures. *Alcohol Clin Exp Res* 11:507–512, 1987.

59. Sutker PB, Tabakoff B, Goist KC Jr, Randall CL: Acute alcohol intoxication, mood states and alcohol metabolism in women and men. *Pharmacol Biochem Behav* 18(Suppl 1):349–354, 1983.

60. Marshall AW, Kingstone D, Boss M, Morgan MY: Ethanol elimination in males and females: Relationship to menstrual cycle and body composition. *Hepatology* 3:701–706, 1983.

61. Jones MB, Jones MK: Alcohol effects in women during the menstrual cycle. *Ann NY Acad Sci* 273:577–587, 1976.

62. Cole-Harding S, Wilson JR: Ethanol metabolism in men and women. *J Stud Alcohol* 48:380–387, 1987.

63. Watson PE, Watson ID, Batt RD: Total body water volumes for adult males and females estimated form simple anthropometric measurements. *Am J Clin Nutr* 33:27–39, 1980.

64. Widmark EMP: Verteilung und Umwandlung des Ethyl Alkohols in Organismus des Hundes. *Biochem Z* 267:128–134, 1933.

65. Rango RE, Kreeft JH, Sitar DS: Ethanol "dose-dependent" elimination: Michaelis-Menten vs. classical kinetic analysis. *Br J Clin Pharmacol* 12:667–673, 1981.

66. Wilkinson PK, Sedman AJ, Sakmar E, *et al*: Blood ethanol concentrations during and following constant-rate intravenous infusion of alcohol. *Clin Pharm Ther* 19:213–223, 1975.

67. Watson PE, Watson ID, Batt RD: Prediction of blood alcohol concentrations in human subjects: Updating the Widmark equation. *J Stud Alcohol* 42:547–556, 1981.

68. Wilson JR, Erwin VG: Rate of alcohol metabolism: Do not "correct" the β_{60} estimates for comparisons among ethnic groups. *J Stud Alcohol* 44:1093–1096, 1983.
69. Hutson WR, Roehrkasse RL, Wald A: Influence of gender and menopause on gastric emptying and motility. *Gastroenterology* 96:11–17, 1989.
70. Datz FL, Christian PE, Moore JA: Gender-related differences in gastric emptying. *J Nucl Med* 28:1204–1207, 1987.
71. Wald A, Van Theil DH, Hoechstetter L, *et al:* Gastrointestinal transit: The effect of the menstrual cycle. *Clin Pharmacol Ther* 17:578–584, 1975.
72. Mezey E, Potter JJ, Tsitouras PD: Liver alcohol dehydrogenase activity in the female rat: Effects of ovariectomy and estradiol administration. *Life Sci* 29:1171–1176, 1981.
73. Torres A, Kling OR, Zeiner AR: Effects of elevated female sex steroids on enzyme induction in rats. *Alcohol Clin Exp Res* 9:187, 1985.
74. Jones MB, Jones MK: Women and alcohol: Intoxication, metabolism, and the menstrual cycle, in Greenblatt M, Schuckit MA (eds): *Alcoholism Problems in Women and Children.* New York, Grune and Stratton, 1976, pp 103–136.
75. Hay WM, Nathan PE, Heermans HW, Frankenstein W: Menstrual cycle, tolerance and blood alcohol level discrimination ability. *Addict Behav* 9:67–77, 1984.
76. Brick J, Nathan, PE, Westrick E, *et al:* The effect of menstrual cycle on blood alcohol levels and behavior. *J Stud Alcohol* 47:472–477, 1986.
77. Mello NK: Some behavioral and biological aspects of alcohol problems in women, in Kalant OJ (ed): *Alcohol and Drug Problems in Women.* New York, Plenum Press, 1980, vol 5, pp 263–298.
78. Jones BM, Jones MK: Ethanol metabolism in women taking oral contraceptives. *Alcohol Clin Exp Res* 8:24–28, 1984.
79. Zeiner AR, Kegg PS: Menstrual cycle and oral contraceptive effects on alcohol pharmacokinetics in Caucasian females. *Alcohol Clin Exp Res* 4:233, 1980.
80. Zeiner AR, Kegg PS: Menstrual cycle and oral contraceptive effects on alcohol pharmacokinetics in Caucasian females, in Galanter M (ed): *Currents in Alcoholism.* New York, Grune and Stratton, 1981, vol 8, pp 47–56.
81. Sutker PB, Goist KC Jr, King AR: Acute alcohol intoxication in women: Relationship to dose and menstrual cycle. *Alcohol Clin Exp Res* 11:74–79, 1987.
82. Jeavons CM, Zeiner AR: Effects of elevated female sex steroids on ethanol metabolism and acetaldehyde metabolism in humans. *Alcohol Clin Exp Res* 8:352–358, 1984.
83. Mezey E, Oesterling JE, Potter JJ: Influence of male hormones on rates of ethanol elimination in man. *Hepatology* 8:742–744, 1988.
84. Mezey E, Potter, JJ: Effect of dihydrotestosterone on rat liver alcohol dehydrogenase activity. *Hepatology* 2:359–365, 1982.
85. Azevedo E, Smith M, Hopkinson DA, Harris H: A study of possible factors influencing the variation in liver alcohol dehydrogenase activity in individuals of the "usual" ADH phenotype. *Ann Hum Genet* 38:31–37, 1974.
86. Mezey E, Sharma S, Rennie L, Potter JJ: Sex differences in gastric alcohol dehydrogenase activity in Sprague-Dawley rats. *Gastroenterology* 103:1804–1810, 1992.
87. Crabb DW, Bosron WF, Li T-K: Ethanol metabolism. *Pharmacol Ther* 34:59–73, 1987.
88. Hayashi S-I, Watanabe J, Kawajiri K: Genetic polymorphisms in the 5'-flanking region change transcriptional regulation of the human cytochrome P450IIE1 gene. *J Biochem* 110:559–565, 1991.
89. Gonzalez FJ, Liu SY, Yano M: Regulation of cytochrome P450 genes:molecular mechanisms. *Pharmacogenetics* 3:51–57, 1993.
90. Frezza M, Padova C, Pozzato G, *et al:* High blood alcohol levels in women: The role of decreased gastric alcohol dehydrogenase activity and first pass metabolism. *N Engl J Med* 322:95–99, 1990.
91. Caballeria J, Frezza M, Hernandez-Munoz C, *et al:* Gastric origin of the first-pass metabolism of ethanol in humans: Effect of gastrectomy. *Gastroenterology* 97:1205–1209, 1989.
92. DiPadova C, Worner TM, Julkunen RJK, Lieber CS: Effect of fasting and chronic alcohol consumption of the first-pass metabolism of ethanol. *Gastroenterology* 92:1169–1173, 1987.

93. Thomasson HR, Nowak TV, Kalbfleisch J, Li T-K: Bioavailability of ethanol by oral and intraduodenal administration. *Clinical Research* 42:241A, 1994.
94. Lucey MR, Demo-Dananberg L, Young J, *et al:* The interplay of age, sex, and gastric function on ethanol metabolism. *Gastroenterology* 104:A945, 1993.
95. Seitz HK, Egerer G, Simanowski UA, *et al:* Human gastric alcohol dehydrogenase activity: Effect of age, sex and alcoholism. *Gut* 34:1433–1437, 1993.
96. Baraona E, Yokoyama A, Ishii H, *et al:* Lack of alcohol dehydrogenase isoenzyme activities in the stomach of Japanese subjects. *Life Sci* 49:1929–1934, 1991.
97. Lumeng L, Lehman GA, Mathis JG, Blitz GP: The relationship of the molecular forms of alcohol dehydrogenase in human gastric mucosa to those in liver. *Hepatology* 1:528, 1981.
98. Thomasson HR, Cutler C, Stone CL, *et al:* Multiple forms of gastric alcohol dehydrogenase consistently identified in gastric biopsies. *Gastroenterology* 104:1007A, 1993c.
99. Stone CL, Thomasson HR, Bosron WF, Li T-K: Purification and partial amino acid sequence of a high-activity human stomach alcohol dehydrogenase. *Alcohol Clin Exp Res* 17:911–918, 1993.
100. Moreno A, Pares X: Purification and characterization of a new alcohol dehydrogenase from human stomach. *J Biol Chem* 266:1128–1133, 1991.

Mental and Physical Health Consequences of Alcohol Use in Women

Shirley Y. Hill

Abstract. Chronic consumption of alcohol in levels typically consumed by alcoholic women clearly produces adverse health consequences, including a shorter life expectancy. The health consequences of alcohol use appear to depend on the characteristics of the person consuming the alcohol (genetic vulnerability to particular diseases, the particular point in the life span when the majority of the alcohol is consumed, and the pattern of consumption typical for that individual). For adolescence and young adulthood, emphasis is placed on increased rates of accidental and suicidal mortality. For middle age, breast cancer risk and risk for developing osteoporosis is discussed. Finally, use of alcohol alone and in combination with psychoactive drugs presents special problems for older women. Other specific adverse effects of alcohol are reviewed with respect to gender differences in cardiovascular, hepatological, and neuropathological outcome, as well as with respect to HIV/AIDS. Psychiatric comorbidity and domestic violence are also discussed with respect to gender differences.

1. Introduction: Prevalence of Use and Abuse in Females

Alcohol is the most widely used drug in the United States as it is in most societies. An estimated 47 million girls and women over the age of 12 reported using alcohol in the month preceding the most recent National Institute of Drug Abuse (NIDA) sponsored household survey.[1] Only a minority of women who drink will ever become alcoholic. If few women become alcoholic, why should we consider alcohol use a major health concern? The answer is

Shirley Y. Hill • Alcoholism and Genetics Research Program, Department of Psychiatry, University of Pittsburgh School of Medicine, Pittsburgh, Pennsylvania 15213.

Recent Developments in Alcoholism, Volume 12: Women and Alcoholism, edited by Marc Galanter. Plenum Press, New York, 1995

that many women suffer some problems associated with drinking even though they may not be alcoholic. Increased risk of ill health has been associated with relatively low levels of alcohol use (e.g., liver disorders in women). Therefore, a review of the health consequences of alcohol use must cover not only risks found in alcoholic or alcohol-dependent women but all use of alcohol at any level and at any point in the life span.

The last decade has provided a unique opportunity to assess changing patterns of alcohol consumption in women. Prior to the initiation of community surveys in the 1980s, estimates of the rates of alcoholism and alcohol abuse among women were made on the basis of treated cases alone. With the advent of community surveys, age- and sex-specific rates of particular psychiatric illnesses including alcoholism became available. Also, data became available on patterns of use among women by age group as a result of national surveys.

Wilsnack *et al.*[2] in collaboration with the National Opinion Research Center (NORC) conducted a national survey of women's drinking practices, noting rates of heavy drinking by age group among women. They found the highest levels of heavy drinking reported was for women between the ages of 35 and 49 (9%), with those aged 21 to 34 showing slightly lower rates (6%). At approximately the same time that this NORC survey was being conducted, the Epidemiological Catchment Area (ECA) program was engaged in a national survey of specific psychiatric disorders including alcoholism in the community. The ECA project used trained interviewers to assess the number and variety of symptoms reported by the respondents and compared these with established DSM III criteria. This study[3] reported rates of alcohol abuse/dependence by sex and age, allowing comparison with the Wilsnack data gathered at approximately the same time (1980–1982). The ECA data indicated that only 1.8% of women in the 25–44 age group are alcoholic.

Thus, while few women meet criteria for alcohol dependence, there is substantial use of alcohol in young adult women that may persist into middle adulthood or beyond. This provides the potential for numerous health consequences to occur, at each stage of the life cycle. For example, during young adulthood non–problem-drinking behavior can have serious health consequences for unborn offspring. Review of the literature concerning prenatal consequences of alcohol use is beyond the scope of this chapter. However, there are a number of excellent reviews of this topic for the interested reader.[4,5] As a woman matures and moves into middle adulthood new risks become more salient: heart disease, breast cancer, and osteoporosis. While we do not know precisely the effects of alcohol use on health among women social drinkers, we do know the effects of excessive use on morbidity and mortality.

2. Adverse Health Consequences in Alcoholic Women

There are a number of adverse health consequences associated with use of alcohol among persons drinking at levels significantly high enough to cause interpersonal, legal, and social problems and who, therefore, would be considered alcoholic or alcohol dependent. For example, comparison of mortality ratios for alcoholics compared with nonalcoholics indicates that alcoholics have increased mortality ranging from 2.0 to 7.0 depending on which study is consulted (see Hill,[6] for review). When mortality ratios for men and women are compared, it is clear that women fare less well than men.[6] Smith *et al.*[7] completed an 11-year follow-up on 100 alcoholic women with a mean age of 44 years, finding over one third deceased. These authors conclude that the average alcoholic woman in their series had her life span shortened by over 15 years as a result of drinking. While the health consequences of excessive use of alcohol are clear, establishing safe levels among nonalcoholic women is a challenge. Risk for organ damage is most likely the result of not only the amount of alcohol a woman consumes, but also in what pattern it is consumed (e.g., continuously or episodically), the age of the woman, and her genetic makeup with its particular vulnerabilities for specific diseases (e.g., heart disease or breast cancer). Recognizing that assessment of health risk in association with alcohol use is complex, this chapter will begin by covering the alcohol-related health problems of women by stages in the life span.

3. Alcohol-Related Health Consequences by Life Stage

3.1. Use of Alcohol and Other Drugs among Adolescents and Young Adults

Substance use among adolescents has risen dramatically in the last two decades.[8] The 1990 national school-based Youth Risk Behavior Survey,[9] which periodically measures the prevalence of particular health behaviors among youth (grades 9–12) in the United States, has noted that a third of all students reported having consumed five or more drinks on one occasion in the past month. Alcohol use on college campuses continues to be heavy,[10,11] with 56% of college freshman reporting drinking five or more drinks at one time in the past month.[10] Thus, alcohol use appears to be a quite common occurrence among high school and college-age students and is not typical of just the more deviant groups as it was in previous generations. Therefore, the impact on mental and physical health is substantial.

Among the greatest health risks to adolescents and young adults who abuse alcohol, sometimes in combination with other drugs, are those involving violent death (accidents, suicide, and homicide). In the United States, suicide is the third leading cause of death for 15- to 24-year-olds. It has been known for some time now that both fatal and nonfatal suicide attempts are associated with acute and chronic use of alcohol, with alcoholics showing rates of completed suicide 6–20 times higher than that of the general population.[12] In the general population, women have higher rates of attempted suicide than men, though they are less likely to complete suicide.[13,14] However, for alcoholic women, the rate of completed suicide appears to exceed those for alcoholic men (see Hill,[6] for review). This suggests that females with serious alcohol or drug problems are not reticent about using methods of suicide with clear lethality. As a result, adolescent girls and young adult women who abuse alcohol, alone or in combination with other psychoactive drugs, may be at especially high risk for suicide.

Among adolescents who attempt suicide, those who use illicit drugs outnumber controls by 8:1 to 10:1.[15] Others have reported a threefold increase in risk for suicide among adolescent substance abusers in outpatient treatment for substance abuse compared with age and sex matched non–drug-using controls.[16] These authors note that out of a total of 89 self-reported suicide attempters, significantly more were female than male.

Moreover, there is accumulating evidence that psychoactive substance abuse among adolescents is related to greater frequency and repetitiveness of suicide attempts and more medically lethal attempts, both of which reflect greater seriousness of intention and greater suicidal ideation among youth who abuse drugs.[17] Others have noted the greater likelihood of suicide by firearms among adolescents who are alcohol-intoxicated at the time of the attempt.[18] Additionally, adolescents who have both depressive and substance use disorders have a greater likelihood of suicidal behavior.[17]

In summary, alcohol and other drug use affects the health of adolescents and young adults most conspicuously by elevating rates of suicide attempts and completed suicides. Clinical depression also plays a role, amplifying the impact of substance use and abuse. Because females of all ages appear to be at greater risk for affective disorders, alcohol use and abuse among adolescent females is particularly worrisome. Additionally, other reckless behavior (driving under the influence of drugs, unprotected sexual activity) may be more likely for the individual who is depressed, impulsive, or otherwise feels life is not worth living.

3.2. Alcohol Use in Middle-Aged Women

Use of alcohol alone or in combination with other drugs poses a new set of problems and possibly even some benefits to middle-aged women. Illicit drug use appears to decline markedly among middle-aged women.[1] However, several studies have noted that women in comparison to men are the major recipients of psychoactive drug prescriptions in the United States.[19,20] Thus, while women, particularly middle-aged and older women, on the whole are not major consumers of illicit drugs, they do have access to a variety of psychoactive drugs that may be used alone or in combination with alcohol.

3.2.1. Breast Cancer. There is increasing evidence that moderate levels of alcohol use may have deleterious effects on women's health. For example, one in ten women in the United States will develop breast cancer. While the peak time for cancers to occur is after the age of 55, the time required for one cell to go awry until it is manifest by radiological means (a mass of 1 cm) can be as long as 5–10 years.[21] Thus, alcohol exposure during the middle years could have significant impact on women's health if indeed a link between alcohol intake and breast cancer can be established. Retrospective and prospective studies have yielded conflicting results. Lowenfels and Zevola[22] reviewed the existing literature for the time period 1974–1987, concluding that only three of nine cross-sectional studies[23–25] gave evidence for a correlational association. However, the positive studies do give substantial evidence for an association.

Rosenberg and colleagues[25] report a relative risk for women who drank any alcohol compared with those not drinking to be 1.9, utilizing a large case-control study of 1152 women with breast cancer and a control group of women with nonmalignant disorders. Harvey et al.[23] noted that women who had one or fewer drinks daily did not experience any increased risk compared with nondrinkers, whereas significant increased risk was noted among those women who drank one to two drinks daily [1 drink odds ratio (OR = 1.3) or 2 drinks (OR = 1.7)].

Finally, the third cross-sectional study of note was one performed in Milan, Italy[24] which found similar results. Compared to the relative risks for women who had never drunk alcohol, the relative risks for those reporting one to three drinks and those reporting more than three drinks daily were 1.24 and 1.93, respectively. Three prospective studies[26–28] have also shown increased relative risks for developing breast cancer among women who drink. The value of the prospective approach in which a large population of women are followed before any of them are diagnosed with breast cancer is that the results are not dependent on retrospective recall of alcohol use as they are in cross-sectional designs.

A meta-analysis of data from 21 published studies evaluated the possible relationship between the quantity of alcohol consumed and risk for breast cancer.[29] Pooling data from all sources, dose–response curves were calculated. Results based solely on the cross-sectional, case-control study designs revealed a relative risk of 1.4 when women who drank two drinks per day were compared with nondrinkers. For the prospective studies that followed women before they developed breast cancer, the average relative risk was 1.7. Thus, this meta-analysis appears to support a link between alcohol consumption and risk of breast cancer at intakes of 24 g/d (1 oz absolute ethanol or 2 drinks per day).

In summary, though a majority of studies using the cross-sectional approach found no relationship between alcohol use and breast cancer, the three prospective studies that found positive results appear quite impressive. A dose–response relationship was established, and confounding variables were taken into account in the statistical analyses of obtained data. Moreover, all of the prospective studies showed significant associations. Thus, it may be concluded that one or fewer alcohol drinks daily may not be deleterious, but higher levels may be associated with increased risk. Determining whether or not alcohol consumption promotes breast cancer is an important issue. Breast cancer is a major cause of cancer mortality in most industrialized countries. If the relative risk for developing breast cancer in association with drinking is, in fact, 2.0 for US women[30]—60% of whom drink, 7% of whom develop breast cancer—then an estimated third or more of all breast cancer is due to alcohol consumption alone, according to estimates provided by Webster and colleagues.[31]

3.2.2. Osteoporosis and Bone Fractures. Alcohol and bone mineralization is another topic of extreme importance to the woman in her middle years. The relationship between alcohol intake and bone formation is a complex one. Chronic alcoholism is associated with increased risk of bone fractures, possibly due to the direct effects of ethanol on osteoblast function (see Diamond,[32] for review).

Because of these well-known deleterious effects of chronic alcoholism on bone mineral density (BMD) with its attendant increase in bone fractures, it has come as somewhat of a surprise that moderate alcohol consumption in postmenopausal women correlates positively with central and peripheral BMD. Laitinen et al.[33] studied 351 healthy Finnish women between the ages of 20 and 76 years. The effects of age and several physical and lifestyle factors on BMD were determined. BMD diminished with age, significantly so after menopause. However, when moderate users of alcohol were contrasted with abstainers, the postmenopausal women who had consumed alcohol showed a positive correlation between alcohol intake and BMD. Specifically, the postmenopausal alcohol users had significantly higher BMD in the sites evaluated. The beneficial effect of moderate doses of alcohol on BMD was found only among the postmenopausal women, however.

Finding a positive relationship between moderate alcohol use and greater BMD is intriguing, particularly in view of recent reports by Gavaler and Van Thiel,[34] Teoh et al.[35] and Mello et al.[36] that acute moderate alcohol consumption is associated with increased plasma estradiol levels. The beneficial effects of estrogen in preventing osteoporosis are now well known. The levels of estradiol reported by Gavaler and Van Thiel[34] are in the range normally prescribed for postmenopausal women desiring estrogen replacement therapy.

Finally, it has been known for some time that alcohol use is associated with increased risk of cardiomyopathy,[37] hypertension,[38] and other cardiovascular disorders in men. Only recently have we begun to assess the potential for increased risk of coronary heart disease (CAD) among women. Klatsky et al.[38] have analyzed data from 123,840 individuals with 10,002 deaths due to CAD and have found that use of alcohol in both men and women was associated with lower risk for CAD, through risks for hypertension, hemmorrhagic stroke, and cardiomyopathy were increased for both men and women. Specifically, a protective effect of lighter drinking was found for CAD in that relative risks were less than 1.0 for those who consumed up to six drinks per day. Similarly, the Nurses Health Study[39] found relative risks of CAD less than 1.0 among women who drank up to 25 g/day (approximately 15 drinks per week). However, heavy drinking (six or more drinks per day) is associated with an eightfold increase in cardiomyopathy among women.[38] Thus, drinking does not appear to increase the risk of CAD in women who drink moderately or even heavily, though cardiomyopathy and hypertension are associated with drinking in women as they are in men.

In summary, while moderate to heavy alcohol consumption may present problems for middle-aged women, particularly those who drink and use psychoactive drugs, there is some evidence that low levels of alcohol use may be beneficial to postmenopausal women. This is based on observed increases in estradiol among women who drink an average of five drinks per week. These increases in estradiol may have functional significance to women at risk for osteoporosis as a result of their postmenopausal status. Illicit drug use is of minor importance statistically to the middle-aged woman in that use of drugs of this type appear to be part of a "maturing out" phenomena.

3.3. Alcohol Use during the Later Years

Most surveys have ignored alcohol use among older adults on the premise that the problem is relatively small. Also, both cross-sectional[3] and longitudinal data[40] confirm that there is an "aging out" of heavy drinking in the 60s for both men and women. Also, the ECA data suggest that older men far outnumber older women with respect to alcohol disorders than they do among younger age groups. However, significant drug and alcohol interactions may be more frequent among older adults.

Alcohol use need not be at alcoholic levels to have deleterious effects on the health of the individual; this is particularly true when alcohol is used in combination with other psychoactive drugs. Among the problems resulting from these interactions are mental confusion and an increased likelihood of falls or other accidents. In fact, alcohol in combination with other substances is the most frequent cause of emergency episodes in the Drug Abuse Warning Network system.[41] There is reason to believe that older women may be at greater risk for alcohol–drug interactions than older men. Alcohol problems of women often go undetected by physicians.[42] Moreover, alcohol problems of the elderly are often unrecognized by physicians who may prescribe psychoactive drugs.[43] Even though alcohol dependence is rarer among older women, they do represent a significant portion of women in treatment for alcoholism. For example, Schuckit et al.[44] found 16% of their treated sample of alcoholic women to be over the age of 55, with a mean age of 61 years.

There is evidence that older women are prescribed psychoactive drugs, as well as other drugs, at a rate that is 2.5 times higher than that for older men.[20] In that study, 447 men and women over the age of 60 were interviewed as part of a stratified household survey of older adults. They found 62% of their sample currently using prescription drugs, with cardiovascular medications being the most frequently prescribed medication used (39% of prescriptions). Interestingly, the second most common prescription medications being used were tranquilizers and sedatives (13.6%). Approximately 44% of this sample of individuals over the age of 60 continued to use alcohol, 25% infrequently and 19% frequently. Thus, this study indicates that approximately one in five persons over the age of 60 uses alcohol frequently and one in six are taking prescribed tranquilizers or sedatives. Data from the National Household Survey on Drug Abuse (NHSDA) household survey from 1985 support the notion that women are more likely to report medical use in the past year than are men. While use in women appears to exceed that in men through age 64, there is evidence that a reversal occurs after age 65. The national survey data indicate significantly higher reported use of prescription psychoactive drug use among women aged 45 to 64 than for those over 65. Over the age of 65, men appear to be more likely to report past year medical use of sedatives, tranquilizers, and stimulants.

Summarizing the results of studies comparing use of alcohol and illicit and licit (prescribed) psychoactive medications indicates that women, especially elderly women, may be major consumers of psychoactive medications with only a minority of women experiencing problems related to alcohol or illicit drug use. However, given the potential for adverse drug–alcohol interactions, it is important to determine the extent of misuse in this population of older adults. For example, there is evidence that older white women may use prescribed and over-the-counter medications at a somewhat higher level than minority women; however, there is reason to believe that ethnic minority women may be at greater risk for complications. Kail[45] has noted that older minority women (black, Hispanic, Native American, Asian-American) may have more difficulty communicating with their physicians about proper usage of medications or need for them. Barriers to adequate health care may include differences in language, perceptions of illness, and differing expectations of the doctor and the patient.

4. Liver Pathology

Drinking appears to be more detrimental to women than men with respect to alcohol-related liver disease (see Hill,[6] for review). A number of studies have found gender differences in the incidence of chronic advanced liver disorders (hepatitis and cirrhosis) among alcoholic individuals.[46–50] What is particularly intriguing is why women should be more vulnerable to developing liver disorders than men, particularly in view of their lower levels of consumption. Higher cirrhosis rates among female than male alcoholics in association with lower consumption among women was first reported by Pequignot et al.[51] and Wilkinson et al.[47] and more recently by Loft et al.[50] and Hislop et al.[52]

A number of theories have been advanced regarding women's greater susceptibility, including an autoimmune phenomena.[49] Recently, evidence has been offered suggesting that the first-pass metabolism of alcohol differs in men and women.[53] This may explain the fact that women reach higher blood levels than men after an equivalent oral dose.[54]

While the liver is the principal site for ethanol metabolism, other tissues contribute as well. Animal studies have shown that when alcohol is ingested, a fraction of the load does not enter the systemic circulation but rather is metabolized by gastric mucosa where some alcohol dehydrogenase (ADH) is found. Alcohol dehydrogenase activity measured in endoscopic gastric biopsies revealed gastric ADH in women was 59% less than that in men.[53] These authors conclude that increased bioavailability of alcohol resulting from decreased gastric oxidation may enhance women's vulnerability to biomedical consequences of ethanol use. Greater vulnerability to liver problems in women may be the result of lesser metabolism in the gastrointestinal tract.

5. Neuropathological Effects of Alcohol

In view of the gender differences in liver pathology among alcoholics, coupled with the greater bioavailability of alcohol to the tissues, it would be important to know whether or not women alcoholics suffer a higher incidence of brain pathologies common to alcoholic individuals. A number of indices of brain pathology have been examined in alcoholic men including neuropsychological test performance,[55] brain ventricular size and size of cerebral sulci utilizing CT scans[55] and more recently magnetic resonance imaging (MRI) techniques.[56] Few studies have addressed the issue of neuropathological changes in women alcoholics. However, one MRI study involving ten young alcoholics was negative[57] as was a previous study using CT methodology[58] indicating minimal neuropathology in female alcoholics. However, women alcoholics appear to have dramatic changes in brain electrophysiological characteristics.[59] Specifically, the amplitude of the P300 wave of the event-related potential is diminished in alcoholic women relative to both normal controls and their nonalcoholic sisters. Nevertheless, the world's literature on possible brain changes due to drinking among alcoholic women is extremely small.

6. Psychiatric Comorbidity

Alcohol problems rarely occur in isolation as the only presenting problem. A reasonably accurate estimate of comorbidity in the general population is available from data obtained as part of the Epidemiological Catchment Area (ECA) study.[60] This study was conducted in the United States in the mid-1980s and provided data on comorbidity of alcoholism abuse and other psychiatric disorders by age and sex. The project involved interviews with 20,000 community dwellers and took 10 years to complete between inception and analysis of data.

The ECA data demonstrate that while 44% of male alcoholics have some other psychiatric disorder, among female alcoholics approximately 65% meet criteria by lifetime for some other diagnosis.[61] Because the data collected in the ECA study were cross sectional, it is difficult to know which disorder came first in the life history of the individuals interviewed. In such situations it is difficult to know whether alcohol use exacerbated symptoms of psychiatric disorders that already existed or whether the alcohol use was an attempt on the part of the individual to self-medicate psychiatric conditions. Longitudinal studies are needed to address this question. Using retrospective report of the respondents, Helzer and colleagues[61] noted that overall alcoholism preceded depression in 78% of cases, whereas among women depression preceded alcoholism in 66% of cases.

The lifetime prevalence of major depression is higher among women than men; 10.2% of women and 5.2% of men reported at least one episode lasting two or more weeks with significant symptomatology that interfered with normal occupational and social functions.[62] Therefore, it is not surprising that more female substance abusers have concurrent depressive disorders.

In summary, it is difficult to know what is cause and what is consequence when one attempts to look at the consequences of alcohol abuse/dependence on the mental health problems of women. Also, alcohol-dependent women may simultaneously be dependent on drugs, substances that have their own set of physical and mental health consequences.[63] The ECA data showed prevalence ratios of 8.8 for women alcoholics (prevalence in alcoholics to prevalence in nonalcoholics). Moreover, the significant amount of comorbidity for major depressive disorder seen among alcoholic women (prevalence ratio of 2.7) signals a high risk for suicidal behavior. Also, it is currently unknown to what degree health-promoting behavior and avoidance of potential risk to one's health is altered by depressive disorders. If there is an association between being depressed and taking risks, it could have important implications for decreasing the spread of HIV infections.

7. Domestic Violence

Persons in treatment for substance abuse frequently report family histories of abuse and neglect, a problem that far too often is transmitted from generation to generation.[64] The percentage of batterers who assault their partners while intoxicated has been reported to be as high as 70 to 90%.[65-67] Alcohol appears to be the most widely used substance associated with battery. Roberts[67] reported that 60% of batterers interviewed were under the influence of alcohol at the time of the battering incident for which they were charged. Another 32% were under the influence of drugs other than alcohol, while another 22% of the cases reported use of both alcohol and drugs at the time of the incident. Use of both drugs and alcohol was associated with more severe battering in that study.

The frequency with which some form of physical abuse of women occurs in the United States is quite high. Appleton[65] interviewed all women coming through an emergency department of a general hospital who were conscious and able to be interviewed during a 10-week period. From this sample of 620 completed questionnaires, they found that 35% of women in ongoing relationships reported history of battery. Having a history of battery was significantly related to psychiatric history in either partner and alcohol use. In addition to the interviews conducted in the general sample, 30 acutely battered women who were seen in the same emergency department were also interviewed. The partners of these battered women in 47% of cases battered children as well; in 85% of the cases they drank "more than moderate" amounts of alcohol and in 13% of cases were reported to have used drugs. Thus, there is an increased likelihood of familial violence as a consequence of drinking and drug use among partners of women who batter them. However, there is also some evidence that this abuse may lead to higher rates of substance abuse in women who are victimized.

Clinical studies have reported higher rates of incest and sexual abuse among women found in treatment for alcoholism.[68] The validity of these observations has been further tested by extension to a general population sample.[69] Data obtained from a national survey of women in 1986 in which women were asked to report their level of drinking and possible problems incurred from drinking revealed that twice as many problem drinkers as nonproblem drinkers reported experiencing at least one incident of sexual abuse before the age of 18.[69,70] A similar survey of women living in New Zealand was conducted in which the women were queried about sexual and physical abuse along with their current drinking practices.[71] Significantly more women who reported abuse as adults were problem drinkers. However, this study found no significant difference in the rates of problem drinking among these adult women who had been abused as children.

Others have noted a link between physical and/or sexual abuse and significantly greater use of cocaine, marijuana, and alcohol among teenagers.[72] Bayatpour and colleagues[72] interviewed 352 pregnant teenagers in a prenatal clinic concerning their use of substances before they knew they were pregnant and found that 17% used marijuana and alcohol and 23% used tobacco. Those who had been abused were compared with a nonabused cohort. These investigators found increased use of drugs as well as increased prior suicidality among the teenagers who had been abused.

In summary, alcohol and drug use is associated not only with increased intrafamilial abuse (both physical and sexual), but also appears to perpetuate the cycle of increased drinking into the next generation by increasing the likelihood that the abused female will increase her drinking to abusive levels. However, it is also likely that alcoholism is familial and quite possibly mediated genetically in women as it is in men.[73] Therefore, the likelihood of a woman becoming alcoholic whose parents are alcoholic can be expected to be greatly elevated over the population prevalence. These parents, because of their own alcoholism, will be at greater risk for dysfunctional behavior, including physical and sexual abuse of their children, than persons drawn from the general population. At any rate, whether or not sexual and physical abuse are causative of further problem drinking is open to debate. Clearly, however, it is one consequence of parental alcohol and drug abuse.

8. Human Immunodeficiency Virus and Acquired Immune Disease

Alcohol abuse/dependence may increase the likelihood of the spread of infection because of the direct effects of particular drugs on the immune system (e.g., alcohol has been implicated in this role). Another way in which alcohol abuse might be expected to increase the likelihood of virus spread is through its acute effects on mood. Intoxicated individuals may engage in unsafe sexual behavior. These same individuals might otherwise practice "safe sex" were their judgment not impaired by intoxication.

Currently, there is controversy concerning the role of alcohol and drug use on risky behavior. Stall et al.[74] reported that the frequency of combining drugs and sex are all positively associated with risky sexual behavior for acquiring AIDS. Similarly, McCusker et al.[75] reported that reduction of alcohol use appears to have positive benefits for homosexually active men. Those who stopped using marijuana or reduced their frequency of alcohol use were significantly more likely to stop unsafe sexual practices. These associations would appear to be important in view of the relatively higher use of drugs and alcohol among gay men than heterosexual men drawn from the same geographic areas of San Francisco.[76] However, others have argued that data reporting an association are largely correlational and that when gay and bisexual men are asked to keep a weekly diary of use of drugs and risky behaviors, no relationship is found.[77] Penkower et al.[78] examined 644 homosexual men and found elevated risk for seroconversion in relation to only 3 of 11 factors examined: heavy drinking, moderate to heavy drug use, and younger age. These variables were associated with increased number of sexual partners, anonymous sex, and failure to use condoms.

Based on these observations in gay men, it may be assumed that heavy alcohol use in women might similarly increase the spread of infection. One example of this might be the woman who is a chronic alcohol abuser who develops a depressive disorder (depressed mood for 2 or more weeks, coupled with five or more clinical symptoms, e.g., sleep difficulties, suicidal ideation). The depressive disorder may be induced by chronic use of alcohol, but may not be of sufficient severity for the woman to seek treatment either for the alcohol problem or the mood disorder. Nevertheless, depressed individuals who are not overtly suicidal (no specific plan) may nevertheless view life as without purpose or meaning and be more vulnerable to engaging in risky behaviors with full knowledge of its dire consequences. Nemoto et al.[79]

have addressed this issue among 262 intravenous drug users in methadone clinics in New York City. Among the female intravenous drug users, the HIV-positive subjects reported larger numbers of sex partners than those who were HIV-negative, and those with more partners were more likely to be depressed.

The tragedy of the AIDS epidemic appears to be hitting women and children especially hard. Romano et al.,[80] reporting on a cross-sectional seroepidemiological study of 1567 heterosexual intravenous drug users who had been seen at the AIDS Regional Reference Center in Palermo, Italy between 1985 and 1990, revealed that antibodies to HIV-1 were observed more frequently in females (66.4%) than males (49.0%). They also found that the odds of being infected with HIV-1 increased by 49% for each year of intravenous drug use after adjustment for other variables.

The European Collaborative Study examined a large number of children born to HIV-infected mothers. In all, 1528 women and 356 children under the age of 13 had been reported to the WHO European AIDS surveillance center. These data indicate that half of the women were intravenous drug users of child-bearing age and three quarters of the children had acquired their infection from a mother who had AIDS or was at risk for AIDS.[81] Coupled with this trend is a high level of spread among teenagers due to high levels of sexual activity. Karen Hein,[82] Director of the Adolescent AIDS Program at Montefiore Medical Center, Bronx, New York, recently stated that "the new face of AIDS worldwide is the face of teenaged girls." She noted that the number of 13- to 21-year-olds in the United States who have become infected with HIV has risen by 77% in two years, and half of this rise is due to heterosexual intercourse. This represents about 1% of US teenagers. A report by Catania et al.,[83] based on a national probability survey, revealed that across all social strata between 15 and 31% of subjects nationally and 20 to 41% in cities with high prevalence of AIDS report having experienced at least one HIV risk factor (multiple sexual partners, a risky partner, or transfusion recipient) in the past 5 years.

In summary, further work is needed to identify the role that alcohol use, alone and in combination with other drugs, plays in risky behavior particularly with respect to women and most particularly female youth. New health policies are needed for reaching women who are at high risk for acquiring sexually transmitted infections, including HIV. These may include identifying women and young girls who are psychiatrically impaired by depression, either as a primary disorder or secondary to substance abuse. Identifying women, particularly adolescents and young adults, who are frequent substance users, though not necessarily drug dependent, and who might be more likely to take chances while intoxicated is especially important. The chronic substance abusers who regularly share needles or other drug paraphernalia are also of special concern because of the risk not only to women but to their unborn children.

9. Conclusions

Alcohol is the most widely used drug in the United States among women and girls over the age of 12. Only a minority of women become alcoholic. Nevertheless, there are known risks and some possible benefits of consuming alcohol in quantities well below the level consumed by alcoholic women. In addition to the direct effects of ethanol on the cardiovascular system, liver, brain, and gastrointestinal tract, there are indirect effects of alcohol that may substantially alter one's health. For example, women who drink excessively may be more prone to alcohol-induced depressive disorders, are more likely to associate with others who drink excessively thereby increasing her risk of domestic violence, and are possibly at increased risk for exposure to HIV because of intoxication. Because alcohol use is the "port of entry" for the young woman who later moves into the use of other drugs of abuse, providing educational materials concerning the health consequences of not only excessive alcohol use, but moderate alcohol exposure as well, may be particularly beneficial as a primary prevention technique.

ACKNOWLEDGMENTS. Preparation of this chapter was supported in part by awards from the National Institute on Alcohol Abuse and Alcoholism, AA005909 and AA05808.

References

1. National Institute on Drug Abuse, Division of Epidemiology and Prevention Research: *National Household Survey on Drug Abuse: Population Estimates 1991* (DHHS Publication No. ADM-92-1887). Washington, DC, US Government Printing Office, 1991.
2. Wilsnack RW, Wilsnack SC, Klassen AD: Women's drinking and drinking problems: Patterns from a 1981 national survey. *Am J Public Health* 74:1231–1238, 1984.
3. Robins LN, Helzer J, Weissman MN, *et al*: Lifetime prevalence of specific psychiatric disorders in three sites. *Arch Gen Psychiatry* 41:949–958, 1984.
4. Streissguth AP, Grant TM, Barr HM, *et al*: Cocaine and the use of alcohol and other drugs during pregnancy. *Am J Obstet Gynecol* 164:1239–1243, 1991.
5. Day N: The effect of alcohol use during pregnancy, in Zagon I, Slotkin T (eds): *Maternal Substance Abuse and the Developing Nervous System.* Orlando, FL, Academic Press, 1992, pp 27–44.
6. Hill SY: Vulnerability to the biomedical consequences of alcoholism and alcohol-related problems among women, in Wilsnack S, Beckman L (eds): *Alcohol Problems in Women.* New York, Guilford Press, 1984, pp 121–154.
7. Smith EM, Cloninger CR, Bradford S: Predictors of mortality on alcoholic women: A prospective follow-up study. *Alcohol Clin Exp Res* 7:237–243, 1983.
8. O'Malley PM, Bachman JG, & Johnston LD: Period, age, and cohort effects on substance use among young Americans: A decade of change, 1976–1986. *Am J Public Health* 78:1315–1321, 1988.
9. Kolbe LJ: An epidemiological surveillance system to monitor the prevalence of youth behaviors that most affect health. *Health Educ* 21:44–48, 1990.
10. Werner MJ, Greene JW: Problem drinking among college freshmen. *Adolesc Health* 13:487–492, 1992.

11. West R, Drummond C, Eames K: Alcohol consumption, problem drinking and anti-social behaviour in a sample of college students. *Br J Addict* 85:479–486, 1990.

12. Goodwin DW: Alcohol in suicide and homicide. *Q J Stud Alcohol* 34:144–156, 1973.

13. Gibbs JP: Suicide, in Merton RK, Nisbet RA (eds): *Contemporary Social Problems*, 2nd ed. New York, Harcourt, Brace & World, 1966, pp 281–321.

14. Bratfos O: Attempted suicide. *Acta Psychiatr Scand* 47:38–56, 1971.

15. Kirkpatrick-Smith J, Rich A, Bonner R: *Alcohol Abuse and Suicide Ideation in Adolescents*. Presentation American Association of Suicidology, April 14, 1989, San Diego, CA.

16. Berman AL, Schwartz RH: Suicide attempts among adolescent drug users. *Am J Dis Child* 144:310–314, 1990.

17. Crumley FE: Substance abuse and adolescent suicidal behavior. *J Am Med Assoc* 263:3051–3056, 1990.

18. Brent DA, Perper JA, Allman CJ: Alcohol, firearms, and suicide among youth. Temporal trends in Allegheny County, Pennsylvania, 1960 to 1983. *J Am Med Assoc* 257:3369–3372, 1987.

19. Cooperstock R, Parnell P: Research on psychotropic drug use. *Soc Sci Med* 16:1179–1196, 1982.

20. Guttmann D: Patterns of legal drug use by older Americans. *J Addict Dis* 3:337–356, 1978.

21. DeVita VT, Hellman S, Rosenberg SA (eds): *Cancer: Principles and Practice of Oncology*, 3rd ed. Philadelphia, Lippincott, 1989.

22. Lowenfels AB, Zevola SA: Alcohol and breast cancer: An overview. *Alcohol Clin Exp Res* 13:109–111, 1989.

23. Harvey EB, Schairer C, Brinton LA, *et al:* Alcohol consumption and breast cancer. *J Natl Cancer Inst* 78:657–661, 1987.

24. LaVecchia C, Decarli A, Franceschi S, *et al:* Alcohol consumption and the risk of breast cancer in women. *J Natl Cancer Inst* 75:61–65, 1985.

25. Rosenberg L, Shapiro S, Slone D, *et al:* Breast cancer and alcoholic-beverage consumption. *Lancet* 1:267–270, 1982.

26. Hiatt RA, Bawol RD: Alcoholic beverage consumption and breast cancer incidence. *Am J Epidemiol* 120:676–683, 1984.

27. Schatzkin A, Jones DY, Hoover RN, *et al:* Alcohol consumption and breast cancer in the epidemiologic follow-up of the first national health and nutrition examination survey. *N Engl J Med* 316:1169–1173, 1987.

28. Willett WC, Stampfer MJ, Colditz GA, *et al:* Moderate alcohol consumption and the risk of breast cancer. *N Engl J Med* 316:1174–1180, 1987.

29. Longnecker MP, Berlin JA, Orza MJ, Chalmers TC: A meta-analysis of alcohol consumption in relation to risk of breast cancer. *J Am Med Assoc* 260:652–656, 1988.

30. Rosenberg L, Slone D, Shapiro S, *et al:* Noncontraceptive estrogens and myocardial infarction in young women. *J Am Med Assoc* 244:339–342, 1980.

31. Webster LA, Layde PM, Wingo PA, Ory HW: Alcohol consumption and risk of breast cancer. *Lancet* 2:724–726, 1983.

32. Diamond T, Stiel D, Lunzer M, *et al:* Ethanol reduces bone formation and may cause osteoporosis. *Am J Med* 86:282–288, 1989.

33. Laitinen K, Valimaki M, Keto P: Bone mineral density measured by dual-energy x-ray absorptiometry in healthy Finnish women. *Calcif Tissue Int* 48:224–231, 1991.

34. Gavaler JS, Van Thiel DH: The association between moderate alcoholic beverage consumption and serum estradiol and testosterone levels in normal postmenopausal women: Relationships to the literature. *Alcohol Clin Exp Res* 16:87–92, 1992.

35. Teoh SK, Mendelson JH, Mello NK, Skupny A: Alcohol effects on naltrexone-induced stimulation of pituitary, adrenal, and gonadal hormones during the early follicular phase of the menstrual cycle. *J Clin Endocrinol Metab* 66:1181–1186, 1988.

36. Mello NK, Mendelson JH, Teoh SK: Neuroendocrine consequences of alcohol abuse in women. *Ann N Y Acad Sci* 562:211–240, 1989.

37. Klatsky AL: The relations of alcohol and the cardiovascular system. *Annu Rev Nutr* 2:51–71, 1982.
38. Klatsky AL: Blood pressure and alcohol intake, in Laragh JH, Brenner BM (eds): *Hypertension: Pathophysiology, Diagnosis and Management*. New York, Raven Press, 1990, pp 277–294.
39. Stampfer MJ, Colditz GA, Willett WC, *et al:* A prospective study of moderate alcohol consumption and the risk of coronary disease and stroke in women. *N Engl J Med* 319:267–273, 1988.
40. Fillmore KM: Women's drinking across the adult life course as compared to men's. *Br J Addict* 82:801–811, 1987.
41. National Institute on Drug Abuse: *Data from the Drug Abuse Warning Network (DAWN): Annual Data, 1987* (DHHS Publication No. ADM-88-1584). Rockville, MD, US Department of Health and Human Services, 1987.
42. Smith AR: Alcoholism and gender: Patterns of diagnosis and response. *J Drug Issues* 16:407–420, 1986.
43. Dunham RG: Noticing alcoholism in the elderly and women: A nationwide examination of referral behavior. *J Drug Issues* 16:397–406, 1986.
44. Schuckit MA, Morrissey ER, O'Leary MR: Alcohol problems in elderly men and women. *J Addict Dis* 3:405–416, 1978.
45. Kail BL: Drugs, gender and ethnicity: Is the older minority woman at risk? Introduction to drug use and minority older women. *J Drug Issues* 19:171–189, 1989.
46. Viel B, Donoso S, Salcedo D, Varela A: Alcoholic drinking habit and hepatic damage. *J Chronic Dis* 21:157–166, 1968.
47. Wilkinson P, Santamaria JN, Rankin JG: Epidemiology of alcoholic cirrhosis. *Australas Ann Med* 18:222–226, 1969.
48. Krasner N, Davis M, Portmann B, Williams R: Changing pattern of alcoholic liver disease in Great Britain: Relation to sex and signs of autoimmunity. *Br Med J* 1:1497–1550, 1977.
49. Morgan MY, Sherlock S: Sex-related differences among 100 patients with alcoholic liver disease. *Br Med J* 1:939–941, 1977.
50. Loft S, Olesen KL, Dossing M: Increased susceptibility to liver disease in relation to alcohol consumption in women. *Scand J Gastroenterol* 22:1251–1256, 1987.
51. Pequignot G, Chabert C, Eydoux H, Courcoul MA: Increased risk of liver cirrhosis with intake of alcohol. *Rev Alcohol* 20:191–202, 1974.
52. Hislop WS, Bouchier IAD, Allan JG, *et al:* Alcoholic liver disease in Scotland and northeastern England: Presenting features in 510 patients. *Q J Med* 52:232–243, 1983.
53. Frezza M, di Padova C, Pozzato G, *et al:* High blood alcohol levels in women. The role of decreased gastric alcohol dehydrogenase activity and first-pass metabolism. *N Engl J Med* 322:95–99, 1990.
54. Jones BM, Jones MK: Male and female intoxication levels for three alcohol doses or do women really get higher than men? *Alcohol Tech Rep* 5:11–14, 1976.
55. Hill SY: Comprehensive assessment of brain dysfunction in alcoholic individuals. *Acta Psychiatr Scand* 62(Suppl 286):57–75, 1980.
56. Zipursky RB, Lim KO, Pfefferbaum A: MRI study of brain changes with short-term abstinence from alcohol. *Alcohol Clin Exp Res* 13:664–666, 1989.
57. Kroft CL, Gescuk B, Woods BT, *et al:* Brain ventricular size in female alcoholics: An MRI study. *Alcohol* 8:31–34, 1991.
58. Cala LA, Thickbroom GW, Black JL, *et al:* Brain density and cerebrospinal fluid spaces on the cranial CT scan in normal volunteers. *Am J Neuroradiol* 2:41–47, 1981.
59. Hill SY, Steinhauer SR: Event-related potentials in women at risk for alcoholism. *Alcohol* 10:349–354, 1993.
60. Robins LN, Regier DA (eds): *Psychiatric Disorders in America: The Epidemiological Catchment Area Study*. New York, Free Press, 1991.
61. Helzer JE, Burnam A, McEvoy LT: Alcohol abuse and dependence, in Robins LN, Regier DA (eds): *Psychiatric Disorders in America: The Epidemiological Catchment Area Study*. New York, Free Press, 1991, pp 81–115.

62. Weissman MM, Bruce ML, Leaf PJ, *et al:* Affective disorders, in Robins LN, Regier DA (eds): *Psychiatric Disorders in America: The Epidemiological Catchment Area Study.* New York, Free Press, 1991, pp 53–80.
63. Hill SY: Health implication of substance abuse in women. *World Health Organization.* Presentation given to WHO in Geneva, Switzerland, August 3–5, 1993.
64. Gorney B: Domestic violence and chemical dependency: Dual problems, dual interventions. *Psychoactive Drugs* 21:229–238, 1989.
65. Appleton W: The battered woman syndrome. *Ann Emerg Med* 9:84–91, 1980.
66. Fagan JA, Stewart DK, Hansen KV: Violent men or violent husbands? in Finkelhon D, Gelles RJ, Hotaling GT, Strauss MA (eds): *The Dark Side of Families: Current Family Violence Research.* Beverly Hills, Sage Publications, 1983, pp 49–67.
67. Roberts A: Substance abuse among men who batter their mates: The dangerous mix. *Subst Abuse Treat* 5:83–87, 1988.
68. Rohsenow DJ, Corbett R, Devine D: Molested as children: A hidden contribution to substance abuse? *J Subst Abuse Treat* 5:13–18, 1988.
69. Wilsnack SC, Klassen AD: *Childhood Sexual Abuse and Problem Drinking in a US National Sample of Women.* Paper presented at the Women's Issues Related to Alcohol Abuse and Violence Conference, University of Illinois at Chicago, College of Nursing, September 1992.
70. Wilsnack SC, Klassen AD, Brett ES, Wilsnack RW: Predicting onset and chronicity of women's problem drinking: A five-year longitudinal analysis. *Am J Public Health* 81:305–318, 1991.
71. Romans-Clarkson SE, Walton VA, Herbison GP, Mullen PE: Alcohol-related problems in New Zealand women. *Aust N Z J Psychiatry* 26:175–182, 1992.
72. Bayatpour M, Wells RD, Holford S: Physical and sexual abuse as predictors of substance use and suicide among pregnant teenagers. *J Adolesc Health* 13:128–132, 1992.
73. Hill SY, Smith TR: Evidence for genetic mediation of alcoholism in women. *J Subst Abuse* 3:159–174, 1991.
74. Stall R, McKusick L, Wiley J, *et al:* Alcohol and drug use during sexual activity and compliance with safe sex guidelines for AIDS: The AIDS Behavioral Research Project. *Health Ed Q* 13:359–371, 1986.
75. McCusker J, Westenhouse J, Stoddard AM, *et al:* Use of drugs and alcohol by homosexually active men in relation to sexual practices. *J Acquir Immune Defic Syndr* 3:729–736, 1990.
76. Stall R, Wiley J: A comparison of alcohol and drug use patterns of homosexual and heterosexual men: The San Francisco Men's Health Study. *Drug Alcohol Depend* 22:63–73, 1988.
77. Weatherburn P, Davies PM, Hickson FCI, *et al:* No connection between alcohol use and unsafe sex among gay and bisexual men. *AIDS* 7:115–119, 1993.
78. Penkower L, Dew MA, Kingsley L, *et al:* Behavioral, health and psychosocial factors and risk for HIV infection among sexually active homosexual men: The Multicenter AIDS Cohort Study. *Am J Public Health* 81:194–196, 1991.
79. Nemoto T, Foster K Sr, Brown LS Jr: Effect of psychological factors on risk behavior of human immunodeficiency virus (HIV) infection among intravenous drug users (IVDUs). *Int J Addict* 26:441–456, 1991.
80. Romano N, Vitale F, Alesi DR, *et al.:* The changing pattern of human immunodeficiency virus type 1 infection in intravenous drug users. Results of a six-year seroprevalence study in Palermo, Italy. *Am J Epidemiol* 135:1189–1196, 1992.
81. European Collaborative Study: Mother-to-child transmission of HIV infection. *Lancet* 2:1039–1043, 1988.
82. Hein K: Invisible epidemic now becomes visible as HIV/AIDS pandemic reaches adolescents. *J Am Med Assoc* 270:16, 1993.
83. Catania JA, Coates TJ, Stall R, *et al:* Prevalence of AIDS-related risk factors and condom use in the United States. *Science* 258:1101–1106, 1992.

Alcohol Effects on Hormone Levels in Normal Postmenopausal Women and in Postmenopausal Women with Alcohol-Induced Cirrhosis

Judith S. Gavaler

Abstract. The effects of alcoholic beverage consumption on the hormonal status of postmenopausal women will be reviewed. Focused attention on the effect of social drinking among 244 normal postmenopausal women has revealed that moderate alcohol intake exerts a major influence not only on estradiol, testosterone, and the estimate of aromatization of testosterone to estradiol but also on the estrogen-responsive pituitary hormones in normal postmenopausal women. The hormonal status of 66 postmenopausal women with alcohol-induced cirrhosis is compared with normal alcohol-abstaining control women. As expected, there are significant differences in levels of all hormones; furthermore, hormonal interrelationships are also disrupted. Of major interest are findings that hormone levels in alcoholic cirrhotic postmenopausal women are related to the severity of liver disease. This observation supports a role for cirrhosis per se in the hormonal disruptions noted. Of further interest are findings that hormone levels may have prognostic value in postmenopausal women with alcohol-induced liver disease.

1. Alcohol and Postmenopausal Estrogenization

Until recently, the effect of alcoholic beverage consumption on the hormonal status of postmenopausal women has been largely limited to data obtained in postmenopausal women with alcohol-induced cirrhosis.[1–7] However, in the absence of data obtained in postmenopausal women with postnecrotic cir-

Judith S. Gavaler • Oklahoma Medical Research Foundation, and Oklahoma Transplantation Institute, Baptist Medical Center, Oklahoma City, Oklahoma 73112.

Recent Developments in Alcoholism, Volume 12: Women and Alcoholism, edited by Marc Galanter. Plenum Press, New York, 1995.

rhosis from causes other than alcohol, it has been difficult to delineate the hormonal effects of alcohol abuse from those of cirrhosis per se. Further, although substantial numbers of normal postmenopausal women consume alcoholic beverages, albeit sometimes infrequently and usually in moderation, systematic studies of the hormonal effects of such alcohol consumption are rare.

In postmenopausal women, hormonal research has focused on the identification of factors that influence estrogen levels because higher estrogen levels are associated with a decreased risk of both osteoporosis and coronary heart disease. Until recently, alcoholic beverage consumption has not been evaluated as a factor with the potential to alter postmenopausal estrogen levels.

The possibility that alcohol might influence postmenopausal estrogen levels has strong underpinnings. It is well established that the major source of postmenopausal estrogen is from the conversion of androgens produced by the adrenal glands and ovarian stroma to estrogens via the action of the enzyme aromatase. It is also well known that the activity of aromatase is increased in postmenopausal women. Thus factors that increase aromatization or the production of androgen substrate are likely to be factors that may elevate postmenopausal estrogen levels. Studies in male volunteers and experimental animals have demonstrated that alcohol not only increases the aromatization of androstenedione to estrone and of testosterone to estradiol but also increases the adrenal production of substrate androgens.[8-11] Thus, the probability that alcohol might influence postmenopausal estrogen concentrations is high.

2. Effects of Moderate Alcohol Consumption on Hormone Levels in Normal Postmenopausal Women

2.1. Detection of an Effect of Alcohol on Hormone Levels

The effect of moderate alcoholic beverage consumption on hormone levels has been evaluated in several study samples of normal postmenopausal women.[12-16] The presence of postmenopausal ovaries as a source of androgens and body fat mass as the primary site of aromatization of androgens to estrogens are established determinants of postmenopausal estrogen levels; these factors must therefore be taken into account when analyzing alcohol effects on levels of estrogens and of the pituitary hormones that are influenced by estrogen. Characteristics of four study populations of normal postmenopausal women are summarized in Table I. As may be seen, the study populations are heterogeneous with respect to age, duration of menopause, and the prevalence of ovariectomy and obesity.

The alcohol consumption patterns and the relationship of estradiol levels with alcoholic beverage consumption are shown in Table II. As shown, even

Table I. Characteristics of the Study Samples of Normal Postmenopausal Women

	Pittsburgh ($n = 128$)	Copenhagen ($n = 62$)	Lisbon ($n = 34$)	Madrid ($n = 20$)
Age (years)	57.7 ± 0.4	64.0 ± 1.0	58.2 ± 1.3	57.1 ± 1.4
Menopause duration (years)	8.8 ± 0.5	14.8 ± 1.2	10.9 ± 1.6	8.2 ± 1.6
Ovariectomy	27%	5%	26%	20%
Body mass index				
Acceptable	50%	63%	41%	35%
Overweight	38%	35%	53%	50%
Obese	12%	2%	6%	15%
Use of estrogen				
replacement therapy	0%	0%	0%	0%

in a setting where the effect of the known postmenopausal estrogen determinants of ovariectomy and estimated body fat mass are not controlled, estradiol levels are statistically elevated among alcoholic beverage consumers in three of the four study samples; interestingly, basal estradiol levels among the alcohol abstainers also appear to vary among the four nationality groups. Also shown, the bivariate correlation coefficients of estradiol levels with total weekly drinks, where the abstainers have a value of zero, are statistically significant in three of the four study samples, as well as in the combined study population of 244 normal postmenopausal women. It must be pointed out that this analytic approach demonstrated no detectable effect of moderate alcoholic beverage consumption on testosterone, the estimate of aromatization of testosterone to estradiol (the E_2:T ratio), nor on levels of the pituitary hormones: luteinizing hormone (LH), follicle stimulating hormone (FSH), and prolactin.

Table II. Estradiol and Alcoholic Beverage Consumption Relationships in Normal Postmenopausal Women

	Pittsburgh ($n = 128$)	Copenhagen ($n = 62$)	Lisbon ($n = 34$)	Madrid ($n = 20$)	ALL ($n = 244$)
Alcohol users	79%	95%	31%	75%	76%
Total weekly drinks[a]	5.7 ± 0.6	6.9 ± 0.8	12.4 ± 2.6	5.4 ± 1.3	6.4 ± 0.8
Prevalence of alcohol intake at <2 drinks/day[a]	90%	85%	82%	87%	87%
Correlation coefficient of estradiol with total weekly drinks	$r = 0.31$[b]	$r = 0.47$[b]	$r = 0.45$[b]	$r = 0.15$	$r = 0.36$[b]
Estradiol (pg/ml)					
abstainers	27.5 ± 3.6	35.1 ± 3.4	41.6 ± 2.3	46.7 ± 8.6	35.1 ± 3.5
users	44.3 ± 3.0[b]	68.1 ± 2.5[b]	89.0 ± 26.8[b]	45.4 ± 5.8	54.6 ± 4.4[b]

[a]Among alcohol users.
[b]At least $p < 0.05$.

Table III. Determinants of Hormone Levels[a] in 244 Normal Postmenopausal Women Using Stepwise Multiple Linear Regression

Dependent variable[b]	Estradiol	Testosterone	E_2:T ratio	LH	FSH	Prolactin
Weekly drinks of wine	Yes	No	Yes	Yes	Yes	No
Drink (yes/no)	No	Yes	No	No	No	Yes
Age	No	Yes	Yes	Yes	Yes	No
Menopause duration	No	No	No	Yes	No	No
Ovariectomy (yes/no)	Yes	No	Yes	Yes	Yes	Yes
Weight	Yes	Yes	No	No	No	Yes
Body mass index	No	Yes	No	Yes	Yes	Yes
Nationality	Yes	No	Yes	No	Yes	Yes
Adjusted R^2	0.344	0.254	0.241	0.164	0.211	0.302
Significance	$p < 0.000$	$p < 0.000$	$p < 0.000$	$p < 0.000$	$p < 0.000$	$p < 0.000$

[a]Normalizing logarithmic transformations used in analyses.
[b]Did a specified dependent variable enter the equation with a statistically significant β coefficient?

In contrast, when controlling for relevant independent variables using stepwise multiple linear regression, the influence of moderate alcoholic beverage consumption on postmenopausal steroid and pituitary hormone levels becomes apparent, particularly when the adjusted R^2 values are viewed from the standpoint of the percent of variation explained by the independent variables entering the equation. As may be seen in Table III, either total weekly drinks of wine or the variable distinguishing abstainers from alcohol consumers (DRINK) enter the equations for estradiol, testosterone, the E_2:T ratio, LH, FSH, and prolactin.

2.2. The Context of Moderate Alcoholic Beverage Consumption

Several additional points need to be noted: First, daily alcohol consumption of one drink/day has been defined as moderate/acceptable intake level for women by agencies of the US government.[17] Second, the increases in estradiol occurred in the absence of any change in measures of liver injury or function.[18] Third, the prevalence of alcoholic beverage consumption at levels of less than two drinks/day is 87% in the entire study sample of 244 normal postmenopausal women. Fourth, although the correlation coefficient of 0.36 between estradiol levels and total weekly drinks is statistically significant, it must be noted that actual shape of the regression line is that of a steady increase in estradiol concentrations up to an alcohol intake level of approximately one drink/day, above which estradiol concentrations plateau even with higher alcohol intake.

The congruence of findings related to a defined level of moderate/acceptable alcohol consumption in a large study sample of normal postmenopausal women among whom moderate drinkers predominate, among whom there is no evidence of liver injury, and among whom estradiol increases but then reaches a plateau at the defined level of moderate/acceptable alcohol consumption is remarkable, particularly when viewed within the context of coronary heart disease risk.[19–23] Specifically, the increases in estradiol with moderate alcohol intake provide a direct link for the reproducible findings that the risk of coronary heart disease in postmenopausal women is statistically reduced at consumption levels of one drink/day compared with both excessive drinkers and alcohol abstainers.

These findings in normal postmenopausal women clearly demonstrate that moderate alcoholic beverage consumption exerts a statistically significant effect on hormone levels. These findings also demonstrate that the effect of moderate alcoholic beverage consumption on postmenopausal hormone levels may be sufficiently subtle so as to require not only a statistically adequate sample size but also a multivariate analytic approach to allow detection of the effect. By extension, it is clear that disease states which may be related to postmenopausal estrogenization such as osteoporosis, breast cancer, and uterine cancer should be carefully evaluated from the standpoint of alcoholic beverage consumption.

3. Hormonal Relationships in Postmenopausal Women with Alcohol-Induced Cirrhosis

3.1. The Study Sample

The impetus to examine the possibility that moderate alcoholic beverage consumption might influence estrogen levels in normal postmenopausal women stemmed from several studies in postmenopausal women with alcohol-induced cirrhosis and from a myriad of studies in alcoholic cirrhotic men that reported an association between increased estrogen levels and alcohol abuse sufficient to cause cirrhosis.[1–3,5,6] In addition, a few of the reports in postmenopausal women suggested that prolactin levels were increased while LH and FSH levels were decreased. In general, the reports on postmenopausal women were based on results obtained in small study samples ($n < 21$) without the benefit of multivariate analyses. Thus the opportunity remained to fully evaluate the hormonal status of a large study sample of alcoholic cirrhotic postmenopausal women using a broad range of analytic methods.

The characteristics of a sample of 66 postmenopausal women with alcohol-induced liver disease are summarized in Table IV. As may be seen, there are no statistical differences in age, weight, body mass index (BMI), or the prevalence of ovariectomy between alcoholic cirrhotic women and normal alcohol-abstaining control women. In contrast, as may be seen in Table V, the

Table IV. Characteristics of 66 Postmenopausal Women with
Alcohol-Induced Cirrhosis

	Alcoholic cirrhotic women (n = 66)	Normal alcohol-abstaining controls (n = 27)
Age (years)	56.8 ± 1.2	57.7 ± 1.0
Weight (kg)	67.1 ± 1.8	66.4 ± 3.0
Body mass index	24.8 ± 0.6	25.5 ± 5.7
Ovariectomy	21.2%	29.6%
Estrogen replacement therapy	0%	0%

findings of earlier studies were confirmed and extended by the statistically
significant differences in levels of estradiol, testosterone, the estimate of
aromatization (E_2:T ratio), and all three estrogen-responsive pituitary hormones. Further, the hormonal relationships observed in the normal alcohol-
abstaining control women are either undetectable (e.g., nonsignificant
correlation coefficients between estradiol and LH, FSH, and BMI) or even
reversed (e.g., positive significant correlation of age with LH and FSH) in the
alcoholic cirrhotic women.

3.2. Liver Disease Severity as a Determinant of Hormone Levels

The above hormone data clearly demonstrate that the hormonal status of
postmenopausal women with alcohol-induced cirrhosis is disrupted in a ma-

Table V. Hormone Levels[a] and Relationships in 66 Postmenopausal Women
with Alcohol-Induced Cirrhosis

	Alcoholic cirrhotic women (n = 66)	Normal alcohol-abstaining controls (n = 27)
Estradiol (pg/ml)	62.7 ± 10.4[b]	27.5 ± 3.3
Testosterone (ng/ml)	0.49 ± 0.05[b]	0.74 ± 0.08
E_2:T ratio	172 ± 27[b]	44.5 ± 5.8
LH (μ/ml)	8.0 ± 1.4[b]	24.0 ± 2.8
FSH (μ/ml)	28.0 ± 4.4[b]	63.3 ± 5.5
Prolactin (ng/ml)	16.4 ± 2.2[b]	5.7 ± 0.4
Correlation of estradiol with		
LH	r = +0.07	r = −0.32[b]
FSH	r = +0.08	r = −0.35[b]
BMI	r = −0.07	r = +0.36[b]
Correlation of age with		
LH	r = +0.39[b]	r = −0.51[b]
FSH	r = +0.37[b]	r = −0.37[b]

[a]Normalizing logarithmic transformations used in analysis.
[b]At least $p < 0.05$.

jor manner. What is not clear is the relative contribution to alterations in hormonal status made by alcohol abuse and that made by the presence of cirrhosis. The issue of the role of cirrhosis per se can perhaps be obliquely addressed by evaluating whether or not there are changes in levels of hormones that are associated with varying degrees of liver disease severity.

Markers of the status of liver disease in the sample of postmenopausal women with alcohol-induced cirrhosis are summarized in Table VI. As expected, mean levels of biochemical markers of liver function (e.g., albumin, total bilirubin, and prothrombin time) and liver injury [e.g., gamma glutamyltranspeptidase (GGTP)] are outside the normal range. The prevalence of major complications of cirrhosis related to portal hypertension is greater than 50% in the entire sample. Child's class is based on levels of albumin, total bilirubin, and prolongation of the prothrombin time, and on the degree of both ascites and encephalopathy. Fortunately, the distribution of the women by Child's class demonstrates that the study sample is composed of women at various stages of cirrhosis severity, a prerequisite for sensibly evaluating relationships between cirrhosis severity and levels of hormones.

Based on the direction of differences in postmenopausal hormone levels between normal controls and alcoholic cirrhotic women, if hormone levels are related to cirrhosis severity, then the following could be hypothesized: Levels of LH, FSH, and testosterone might be inversely related, while estradiol, the E2:T ratio, and prolactin might be directly related to severity markers that increase with increasing cirrhosis severity (total bilirubin, prothrombin time, GGTP, and Child's class score) and oppositely correlated with albumin, which diminishes with increased severity. The results of such analyses are summarized in Table VII. There are several points to be emphasized: (1) Levels of each hormone and the E_2:T ratio are all statistically correlated with at least one measure of cirrhosis severity. (2) These significant correlation coefficients are inverse or direct, consistent with the a priori hypothesis. (3) The prevalence of appropriate hormone correlations is higher for the biochemical markers of

Table VI. Liver Disease Status in 66 Postmenopausal Women with Alcohol-Induced Cirrhosis

Marker	Value	Normal range
Albumin (mg/dl)	3.1 ± 0.1	(≥ 3.5)
Prothrombin time (sec)	14.8 ± 0.4	(≤ 11.5)
Total bilirubin (mg/dl)	5.1 ± 1.0	(0.3 − 1.5)
GGTP (μ/ml)	136 ± 21	(< 32)
AST/ALT ratio	2.5 ± 0.3	(< 1)
Ascites	68.7%	
Encephalopathy	53.0%	
Child's class		
A	24.6%	
B	56.1%	
C	19.3%	

Table VII. Correlations Coefficients for Hormone Levels[a] with Markers of Liver Disease Severity in 66 Postmenopausal Women with Alcohol-Induced Cirrhosis

	Estradiol	Testosterone	E_2:T ratio	LH	FSH	Prolactin
Child's Score	ns	ns	ns	-0.260^b	ns	ns
Total bilirubin	ns	-0.295^b	$+0.345^b$	-0.424^b	-0.363^b	ns
Albumin	ns	ns	ns	$+0.260^b$	$+0.273^b$	-0.213^b
Prothrombin time	ns	-0.247^b	ns	-0.534^b	-0.494^b	ns
GGTP	$+0.354^b$	ns	$+0.369^b$	ns	ns	$+0.283^b$

[a]Normalizing logarithmic transformations used in analyses.
[b]At least $p < 0.05$.

function and injury than for the composite variable Child's class. Taken together, these findings suggest that the severity of cirrhosis significantly influences levels of hormones; therefore, it must be concluded that, in addition to alcohol abuse, cirrhosis per se makes a major contribution to the observed disruption of postmenopausal hormone levels and interrelationships.

3.3. Potential Prognostic Value of Hormone Levels

Given the evidence that hormone levels are related to cirrhosis severity, a preliminary report of the prognostic value of hormone levels among postmenopausal women with alcohol-induced cirrhosis is of relevance.[24] Hormone levels were examined in 36 postmenopausal women at the time of evaluation for liver transplantation. The group was dichotomized on the basis of whether or not transplantation was later performed. These two groups were then subdivided: transplant recipients were grouped on the basis of survivorship at time of follow-up, while women who did not receive a transplant were grouped on the basis of death occurring before transplantation could be performed or still being alive at the time of follow-up.

The results of this study are summarized in Table VIII. As may be seen, lower values for estradiol and the E_2:T ratio and higher levels of LH appeared

Table VIII. Predictive Potential of Hormone Levels[a] in Alcoholic Cirrhotic Postmenopausal Women at Time of Evaluation for Liver Transplantation

	No liver transplant		Liver transplant	
	Alive ($n = 13$)	Dead ($n = 11$)	Survivors ($n = 7$)	Nonsurvivors ($n = 5$)
Estradiol	44.1 ± 25.8	89.1 ± 44.9	29.5 ± 8.2^b	87.7 ± 6.9
E_2:T ratio	104 ± 24	163 ± 44	106 ± 37^b	443 ± 172
LH	7.8 ± 2.0	3.5 ± 1.6	6.7 ± 3.4^b	1.6 ± 0.5

[a]Normalizing logarithmic transformations used in analyses.
[b]At least $p < 0.05$ transplant survivors vs. nonsurvivors.

to distinguish statistically those who survived and those who did not survive following liver transplantation. A similar pattern was observed for LH and the E_2:T ratio in postmenopausal women who died before transplantation could be performed and those still alive and waiting for a liver transplant. These data suggest that further work in a study group of adequate sample size using multivariate survival analyses may well yield exceedingly useful information.

4. Summary

Data have now been accumulated which demonstrate that moderate alcoholic beverage consumption significantly influences a broad spectrum of hormones in normal postmenopausal women. Data have now also been accumulated which demonstrate that the combination of alcohol abuse and alcohol-induced cirrhosis plays a major role in the disruption of postmenopausal hormonal status. Particularly interesting are new data which suggest not only that cirrhosis severity has a detectable effect on levels of postmenopausal hormones, but also that levels of certain hormones may have a predictive value related to risk of death.

The results of these studies raise intriguing questions: What is the strength of the effect of alcohol abuse compared with that of cirrhosis in the disruption of postmenopausal hormonal status? Do hormone levels actually predict death in alcoholic cirrhotic postmenopausal women? Do hormone abnormalities reverse following liver transplantation? The more we learn, the more questions arise; the complexity of the emerging questions will provide a challenge in performing the research that remains to be done.

ACKNOWLEDGMENT. This work has been supported by grant R01 AA06772 from the National Institute on Alcohol Abuse and Alcoholism. The author thanks Marilyn Bonham-Leyba for her assistance in the preparation of the manuscript.

References

1. Hugues JN, Perret G, Adessi G, et al: Effects of chronic alcoholism on the pituitary–gonadal function of women during menopausal transition and in the postmenopausal period. Biomedicine 29:279–283, 1978.
2. Hugues JN, Coste T, Perret G, et al: Hypothalamo–pituitary ovarian function in thirty-one women with chronic alcoholism. Clin Endocrinol 12:543–551, 1980.
3. James VHT, Green JRB, Walker JG, et al: The endocrine status of postmenopausal cirrhotic women in Chiandussi M, Langer L, Chopra IJ, Martini L (eds): The Endocrines and the Liver. San Diego, CA, Academic Press, 1982, pp 417–419.
4. Carlstrom K, Eriksson S, Rannevik G: Sex steroids and steroid binding proteins in female alcoholic liver disease. Acta Endocrinol 111:75–79, 1986.
5. Jasonni VM, Bulletti C, Bolelli GF, et al: Estrone sulfate, estrone and estradiol concentrations in normal and cirrhotic postmenopausal women. Steroids 41:569–573, 1983.

6. Gavaler JS, Van Thiel DH: Hormonal status of postmenopausal women with alcohol-induced cirrhosis: Further findings and a review of the literature. *Hepatology* 16:312–319, 1992.

7. Gavaler JS: Effects of alcohol use and abuse on the endocrine status in expanded study samples of postmenopausal women, in Zakhari S (ed): *Alcohol and the Endocrine System* (NIAAA Research Monograph No. 23). NIH Pub. No. 93-3533. Washington, DC: US Government Printing Office, 1993, pp 171–187.

8. Longcope C, Pratt JH, Schneider S, Fineberg E: Estrogen and androgen dynamics in liver disease. *J Endocrinol Invest* 7:629–634, 1984.

9. Gordon GG, Altman K, Southren AL, *et al:* Effect of alcohol (ethanol) administration on sex-hormone metabolism in normal men. *N Engl J Med* 295:793–797, 1976.

10. Gordon GG, Olivo J, Fereidoon F, Southren AL: Conversion of androgens to estrogens in cirrhosis of the liver. *J Clin Endocrinol Metab* 40:1018–1026, 1975.

11. Cobb CF, Van Thiel DH, Gavaler JS, Lester R: Effects of ethanol and acetaldehyde on the rat adrenal. *Metabolism* 30:537–543, 1981.

12. Gavaler JS, Love K: Detection of the relationship between moderate alcoholic beverage consumption and serum levels of estradiol in normal postmenopausal women: Effects of alcohol consumption quantitation methods and sample size adequacy. *J Stud Alcohol* 53:389–394, 1992.

13. Gavaler JS, Love K, Van Thiel DH, *et al:* An international study of the relationship between alcoholic beverage consumption and postmenopausal estradiol levels, in Kalant H, Khanna JM, Israel Y (eds): *Proceedings of the Fifth ISBRA (International Society for Biomedical Research on Alcoholism) Congress.* New York, Pergamon Press, 1991, pp 327–330.

14. Gavaler JS: Alcohol and nutrition in postmenopausal women. *J Am Coll Nutrition* 12:347–356, 1993.

15. Gavaler JS, Van Thiel DH: The association between moderate alcoholic beverage consumption and serum estradiol levels in normal postmenopausal women: Relationship to the literature. *Alcohol Clin Exp Res* 16:87–92, 1992.

16. Gavaler JS, Deal SR, Van Thiel DH, *et al:* Alcohol and estrogen levels in postmenopausal women: The spectrum of effect. *Alcohol Clin Exp Res* 17:786–790, 1993.

17. US Department of Agriculture, US Department of Health and Human Services: *Nutrition and Your Health: Dietary Guidelines for Americans.* Home and Garden Bulletin No. 232. Washington DC, US Government Printing Office, 1990.

18. Gavaler JS: Alcohol effects in postmenopausal women: Alcohol and estrogens, in Mendelson JH, Mello NK (eds): *Medical Diagnosis and Treatment of Alcoholism.* New York, McGraw Hill, 1992, pp 623–638.

19. Klatsky AL, Friedman GD, Siegelaub AB: Alcohol consumption before myocardial infarction: Results from the Kaiser-Permanente epidemiologic study of myocardial infarction. *Ann Int Med* 81:294–301, 1974.

20. Petitti DB, Wingerd J, Pellegrin F, Ramcharan S: Risk of vascular disease in women: Smoking, oral contraceptives, non-contraceptive estrogens and other factors. *J AM Med Assoc* 242:1150–1154, 1979.

21. Ross RK, Paganini-Hill A, Mack TM, *et al:* Menopausal oestrogen therapy and protection from death from ischemic heart disease. *Lancet* 1:858–860, 1981.

22. Cullen K, Stenhouse NS, Wearne KL: Alcohol and mortality in the Busselton Study. *Int J Epidemiol* 11:67–70, 1982.

23. Gordon T, Kannel WB: Drinking habits and cardiovascular disease: The Framingham Study. *Am J Heart* 105:667–673, 1983.

24. Gavaler JS, Van Thiel DH, Deal, SR: Surgical risk in alcoholic cirrhotic postmenopausal women: Prognostic value of levels of hormones. *J Surg Oncol Suppl* 3:52–54, 1993.

Gender Differences in Animal Studies

Implications for the Study of Human Alcoholism

Francine E. Lancaster

Abstract. The reasons for gender differences in alcohol intake, responses to alcohol, and consequences of alcohol abuse in humans and in animals are poorly understood. Animal models for
the study of alcoholism have been focused primarily on the study of male rodents, although
researchers have observed that female rodents drink more alcohol than males and have sex-
related differences in drinking patterns and responses to alcohol. In humans, the difference
between the sexes is the opposite of rodents, with males drinking more than females. These
results suggest differences between the sexes and differences between humans and rodents in
drinking behavior and responses to alcohol which may be based on a complex interaction of
social, genetic, hormonal, neurobiologic, and environmental factors. Four new studies are introduced to identify sex-distinct genetic influences in alcohol-related phenotypes, sex-based differences in behavioral responses to alcohol, sex differences in responses of brain reward systems to
alcohol, and interactions of the anxiolytic effects of alcohol with steroids and the estrous cycle.

1. Gender Differences in Response to Alcohol

Alcohol research involving humans and animals has been dominated by investigations of males. Only recently the problems and mechanisms for alcoholism in female animals have been studied; and recently, interest has increased in including women in study populations. Increasingly, clinical and

Francine E. Lancaster • Department of Biology, Texas Woman's University, Denton, Texas
76204.

Recent Developments in Alcoholism, Volume 12: Women and Alcoholism, edited by Marc Galanter.
Plenum Press, New York, 1995

experimental studies are showing that women have higher blood alcohol levels than men after drinking the same amount of alcohol based on body size[1] and greater vulnerability to damage by alcohol than men.[2] Women, within a shorter period of time and with lower alcohol intake, are more likely to develop alcohol-induced liver disease and brain damage.[3–5] Liver damage and shrinking of the brain from loss of white matter have been detected in women categorized as moderate drinkers.[6] These insidious effects of alcohol intake remained largely undetected until recent improvements in the technology of brain imaging and new interest in including female subjects in study populations.[7]

The reasons for the differences in pattern of drinking and the differential risk for consequences of alcohol intake for males and females are poorly understood.[8] Social factors, which have played a part in concealing problems associated with alcoholism of women, and the research focus on males, have limited the study of women, resulting in a deficit of information regarding drinking practices for women in our society.[9] In the past, when most women did not work outside the home, they were able to conceal problems with alcohol and were enabled by family members to continue drinking.[10] With changes in social roles, women are more likely to experience some of the work-related problems of alcoholism previously experienced predominantly by men.[11] However, hypotheses that alcohol intake by women would converge to meet levels consumed by men when women began working outside the home have not been proved.[12] Although women make up about half the work force, women still drink significantly less than men.[13]

Currently, animal models for the study of alcoholism, alcohol preference, and voluntary alcohol intake are focused primarily on the study of male rodents, although researchers have observed that female rodents will drink more alcohol than males[14,15] and have sex-related differences in drinking patterns and responses to alcohol.[16] In humans, the difference between the sexes is the opposite of rodents, with males drinking more than females.[17] These results suggest differences between the sexes and differences between humans and rodents in drinking behavior and responses to alcohol, which may be based on a complex interaction of social, genetic, hormonal, neurobiologic, and environmental factors.

1.1. Genetics and Environment

Gender differences in heritability of alcoholism suggest that women are more likely to experience type I alcoholism, which is environmentally influenced and associated with adult onset of alcohol abuse in either biological parent.[18] Type II alcoholism, male-limited and having strong genetic transmission from father to son, is not thought to be experienced by females.[19] However, scientific evidence to explain this protection of females from type II alcoholism remains unclear. A preliminary study of incarcerated female alcoholics suggests that some female alcoholics in families with a history of alcoholism strongly resemble males with the highly heritable, male-limited type II alcoholism.[20] Other reports suggest negligible heritance of alcoholism for females and late-onset alcoholism for males,[21] and stress the importance of environmental factors.

An observation common to both human and animal research on alcoholism is that males and females of similar genetic background (siblings or littermates) differ significantly in alcohol intake and responses to alcohol.[22,23] The source of differences between the sexes may be related to the influence of steroid hormones on gene expression, alcohol metabolism, and pharmacokinetics of alcohol in brain reward centers.

1.2. Hormone Secretion, Brain Function, and Behavior

Gender differences in hormonal secretion, brain function, and behavior begin during development, continue throughout life, and are influenced by environmental factors (Fig. 1). Individual life experiences as unique and varied as peer pressure,[24] *in utero* alcohol[25] and drug exposure, experience with alcohol and drug abuse, smoking,[26] employment status, marital status, stress,[27] and history of physical and sexual abuse[28] can have an impact on behavior through complex interactions of the nervous and endocrine systems. Although animal models have reflected differences between the sexes, few studies have attempted to model the potential impact of complex environmental factors experienced by humans on gender differences in drinking behavior and response to alcohol.

2. Gender Differences in the Brain

An area of research that has received little attention is the investigation of gender differences in the brain related to alcohol intake, responses to alcohol, and the consequences of alcohol abuse (see Lancaster,[29] for review). Through the influence of steroid hormone levels during development, certain areas of the brain develop differently in females than in males. In turn, these sexually dimorphic brain areas influence many neuronal reactions of the brain and therefore affect many behaviors throughout life. Other behaviors are modulated differentially in males and females not only through the activity of the sexually dimorphic brain but also through responses of neurons to the fluctuation of steroid hormones throughout life.[30]

2.1. Neurosteroids in the Brain

Neurosteroids can be synthesized *de novo* in glial cells[31,32] in the brain or formed as metabolites from circulating, peripherally synthesized steroids.[33] Steroid hormones are found in different levels in males and females during development and throughout life, depending on biological and environmen-

GENDER DIFFERENCES

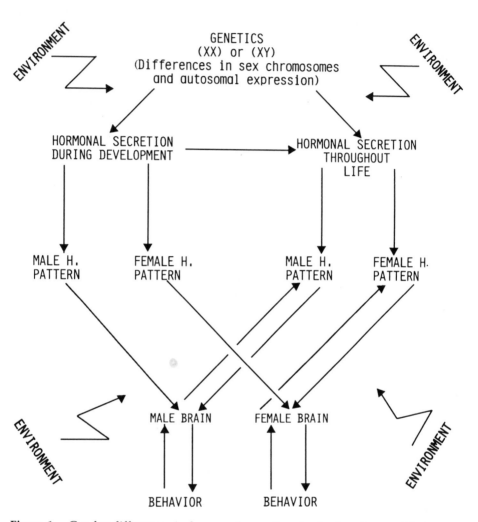

Figure 1. Gender differences in hormonal secretion, brain function, and behavior begin during development, continue throughout life, and are influenced by genetic and environmental factors.

tal factors such as age, estrous or menstrual cycles, stress, and alcohol or drug use.[34] Several neurosteroids act as agonists or antagonists[35] of the γ = aminobutyric acid A ($GABA_A$) receptor, by binding at a unique steroid site.[36] Some neurosteroids enhance N-methyl-D-aspartate (NMDA) currents in neurons,[37] while inhibiting GABA and glycine receptors.[38] Thus, interactions between neurons and glial cells have a role in modulating excitatory and inhibitory activity of the nervous system, and therefore influence behavior through the influence of neurosteroids.[39] Neurochemical and behavioral data suggest that many of the effects of alcohol are mediated through $GABA_A$[40] and NMDA receptors.[41] Thus, neuroactive steroids may influence alcohol-mediated changes in GABA and NMDA activity.

Neurosteroids may be responsible in part for the differences between males and females in the response of the GABA system to alcohol. Recent studies report gender differences in the response of the GABA system to alcohol, showing greater effect of the partial $GABA_A$ receptor inverse agonist Ro 15-4513 in disrupting the influence of alcohol on operant behavior in male mice than in female mice.[42] Further study of the influence of alcohol on neurosteroid production in the brain is needed to determine whether the gender differences observed in alcohol intake[43] and consequences of alcohol abuse are linked to gender differences in circulating steroids, differences in neurosteroid levels, or the influence of alcohol on glial cell production of neurosteroids.

3. New Research Findings

New and exciting studies on gender differences in the brain regarding alcohol intake and responses to alcohol are currently being developed and are reported in this volume. Early results identify sex-distinct genetic influences in alcohol-related phenotypes in mice (Chapter 11), sex-based differences in behavioral responses to alcohol by recombinant inbred strains of mice (Chapter 12), sex differences in responses of brain reward systems to alcohol (Chapter 13), and interactions of the anxiolytic effects of alcohol with steroids and the estrous cycle (Chapter 14).

References

1. Frezza M, di Padova C, Pozzato G, et al: High blood alcohol levels in women. The role of decreased gastric alcohol dehydrogenase activity and first-pass metabolism. N Engl J Med 322:95–99, 1990.
2. Morgan MY, Sherlock S: Sex-related differences among 100 patients with alcoholic liver disease. Br Med J 1:939–941, 1977.
3. Blume SB: Women's health: Issues in mental health, alcoholism, and substance abuse. Pub Health Rep Suppl Jul–Aug:38–42, 1987.
4. Norton R, Dwyer T, MacMahon S: Alcohol consumption and the risk of alcohol related cirrhosis in women. Br Med J 295:80–82, 1987.
5. Lishman WA, Jacobson RR, Acker C: Brain damage in alcoholism: Current concepts. Acta Med Scand Suppl 717:5–17, 1987.
6. Harper C, Kril JJ: Neuropathology of alcoholism. Alcohol Alcohol 25:207–216, 1990.
7. Harper C, Smith NA, Kril JJ: The effects of alcohol on the female brain: A neuropathological study. Alcohol Alcohol 25:445–448, 1990.
8. Farid B, Clarke ME: Characteristics of attenders to community based alcohol treatment centre with special reference to sex difference. Drug Alcohol Depend 30:33–36, 1992.

9. Richman JA, Rospenda KM: Gender roles and alcohol abuse. *J Nerv Ment Dis* 180:619–626, 1992.

10. Roman PM, Blum TC: Life transitions, work, and alcohol: An overview and preliminary data. *Alcohol Clin Exp Res* 16:149–158, 1992.

11. Gomberg ESL: Women and alcohol: Use and abuse. *J Nerv Ment Dis* 181:211–219, 1993.

12. Mercer PW, Khavari KA: Are women drinking more like men? An empirical examination of the convergence hypothesis. *Alcohol Clin Exp Res* 14:461–466, 1990.

13. Wilsnack RW, Wilsnack SC: Women, work, and alcohol: Failure of simple theories. *Alcohol Clin Exp Res* 16:172–179, 1992.

14. Li T-K, Lumeng L: Alcohol preference and voluntary alcohol intakes of inbred rat strains and the National Institutes of Health heterogenous stock of rats. *Alcohol Clin Exp Res* 8:485–486, 1984.

15. Adams N, Shihabi ZK, Blizard DA: Ethanol preference in the Harrington derivation of the Maudsley reactive and nonreactive strains. *Alcohol Clin Exp Res* 15:170–174, 1991.

16. Lancaster FE, Spiegel KS: Sex differences in pattern of drinking. *Alcohol* 9:415–420, 1992.

17. Harford TC, Parker DA, Grant BF, Dawson DA: Alcohol use and dependence among employed men and women in the United States in 1988. *Alcohol Clin Exp Res* 16:146–148, 1992.

18. Goodwin DW: Alcoholism and genetics. *Arch Gen Psychiatry* 42:171–174, 1985.

19. Cloninger CR, Christiansen KO, Reich T, Gottesman II: Implications of sex differences in the prevalences of antisocial personality, alcoholism, and criminality for familial transmission. *Arch Gen Psychiatry* 35:941–951, 1978.

20. Lex BW, Scholar W, Bower T, Mendelson JH: Putative type II alcoholism characteristics in female third DUI offenders in Massachusetts: A pilot study. *Alcohol* 8:283–287, 1991.

21. Pickens RW, Svikis DS, McGue M, *et al:* Heterogeneity in the inheritance of alcoholism. A study of male and female twins. *Arch Gen Psychiatry* 48:19–28, 1991.

22. Mishra L, Sharma S, Potter JJ, Mezey E: More rapid elimination of alcohol in women as compared to their male siblings. *Alcohol Clin Exp Res* 13:752–754, 1989.

23. Lancaster FE, Spiegel KS: Voluntary beer drinking by pregnant rats: Offspring sensitivity to ethanol and preference for beer. *Alcohol* 6:207–217, 1989.

24. Wilks J, Callan VJ, Austin DA: Parent, peer and personal determinants of adolescent drinking. *Br J Addict* 84:619–630, 1989.

25. Mankes RF, Glick SD, Van der Hoeven T, LeFevre R: Alcohol preference and hepatic alcohol dehydrogenase activity in adult Long-Evans rats is affected by intrauterine sibling contiguity. *Alcohol Clin Exp Res* 15:80–85, 1991.

26. Whichelow MJ, Erzinclioglu SW, Cox BD: A comparison of the diets of non-smokers and smokers. *Br J Addict* 86:71–81, 1991.

27. Taylor J, Harris N, Vogel WH: Voluntary alcohol and cocaine consumption in "low" and "high" stress plasma catecholamine responding rats. *Pharmacol Biochem Behav* 37:359–363, 1990.

28. Miller BA, Downs WR, Testa M: Interrelationships between victimization experiences and women's alcohol use. *J Stud Alcohol* (Suppl) 11:109–117, 1993.

29. Lancaster FE: Gender differences in the brain: Implications for the study of human alcoholism. *Alcohol Clin Exp Res* 18:740–746, 1994.

30. Jacobson M: Dependence of the developing nervous system on nutrition and hormones, in Jacobson M (ed): 1991, *Developmental Neurobiology*, 3rd ed. New York, Plenum Press, p 285.

31. Akwa Y, Sananes N, Gouezou M, *et al:* Astrocytes and neurosteroids. Metabolism of pregnenolone and dehydroepiandrosterone. Regulation by cell density. *J Cell Biol* 121:135–143, 1993.

32. Kabbadj K, El-Etr M, Baulieu E-E, Robel P: Pregnenolone metabolism in rodent embryonic neurons and astrocytes. *Glia* 7:170–175, 1993.

33. Paul SM, Purdy RH: Neuroactive steroids. *FASEB J* 6:2311–2322, 1992.

34. Majewska MD: Neurosteroids: Endogenous bimodal modulators of the $GABA_A$ receptor. Mechanism of action and physiological significance. *Prog Neurobiol* 38:379–395, 1992.

35. Prince RJ, Simmonds MA: 5B-Pregnan-3B-ol-20-one, a specific antagonist at the neurosteroid site of the GABA$_A$ receptor-complex. *Neurosci Lett* 135:273–275, 1992.
36. Demirgoren S, Majewska MD, Spivak CE, London ED: Receptor binding and electrophysiological effects of dehydroepiandrosterone sulfate, an antagonist of the GABA$_A$ receptor. *Neuroscience* 45:127–135, 1991.
37. Wu F-S, Gibbs TT, Farb DH: Pregnenolone sulfate: A positive allosteric modulator at the N-methyl-D-aspartate receptor. *Mol Pharmacol* 40:333–336, 1991.
38. Maione S, Berrino L, Vitagliano S, et al: Pregnenolone sulfate increases the convulsant potency of N-methyl-D-aspartate in mice. *Eur J Pharmacol* 219:477–479, 1992.
39. Costa E, Guidotti A: Diazepam binding inhibitor (DBI): A peptide with multiple biological actions. *Life Sci* 49:325–344, 1991.
40. Hwang BH, Lumeng L, Wu JY, Li T-K: Increased number of GABAergic terminals in the nucleus accumbens is associated with alcohol preference in rats. *Alcohol Clin Exp Res* 14:503–507, 1990.
41. Morrisett RA, Swartzwelder HS: Attenuation of hippocampal long-term potentiation by ethanol: A patch-clamp analysis of glutamatergic and GABAergic mechanisms. *J Neurosci* 13:2264–2272, 1993.
42. Bao K, Middaugh LD, Becker HC, Shepherd CL: Effects of Ro 15-4513 and ethanol on operant behavior of male and female C57BL/6 mice. *Alcohol* 9:193–198, 1992.
43. Dawson D, Archer L: Gender differences in alcohol consumption: Effects of measurement. *Br J Addict* 87:119–123, 1992.

Sex Distinctiveness in Effective Genotype

Gerald E. McClearn

Abstract. The difference between sexes in incidence and prevalence of alcohol-related problems is a central feature of alcohol research. It is inevitable that these differences will receive escalating attention as it becomes increasingly apparent that the interests of both equity and good science are served by the study of sex differences in health-related processes.

For several reasons, genetic methods promise to offer powerful tools for the elucidation of sex differences. In the first place, the determination of sex depends on a genetic mechanism. Furthermore, there is an abundant literature showing the relevance of heredity to a broad variety of alcohol-related processes. Moreover, there is evidence of major differences in genetic influences in males and females in respect to alcoholism specifically. It is important to appreciate that genetic influence on sex distinctiveness may operate through several different mechanisms, with quite different implications. The purpose of this chapter is to provide an elementary description of these different genetic routes to sex differences.

1. Introduction

In mammals, the issue of whether a given animal will be male or female is determined largely by its sex chromosome constitution. The sex chromosomes constitute one pair of the many that make up the full chromosomal complement of the individual. The other chromosomes are called *autosomes*. The full complement (autosomes plus sex chromosomes) varies from species to species. There are, for example, 23 pairs in human beings and 20 pairs in one of our favorite alcohol research surrogates, mice.

The two members of each autosomal pair are of the same size and config-

Gerald E. McClearn • Department of Biobehavioral Health and Center for Developmental and Health Genetics, Pennsylvania State University, University Park, Pennsylvania 16802.

Recent Developments in Alcoholism, Volume 12: Women and Alcoholism, edited by Marc Galanter. Plenum Press, New York, 1995

uration. Except in some anomalous circumstances, for each gene located on one chromosome of the pair, there is a counterpart gene located at the same place (or *locus*) on the partner chromosome.

In contrast to the autosomes, the sex chromosomes come in two strikingly different sizes: one large, or X, chromsome and a smaller, or Y, chromosome. Individuals with two Xs are females and individuals with one X and one Y are males. YY individuals do not occur. Only at the very tip of the X and Y chromosomes is there a small region in which comparable genes are located. Logically, it might be expected that there would be two patterns of sex differences related to sex chromosomes—one for the nonmatched genes on the X and the other for nonmatched genes on the Y. In fact, examples of the latter case are extremely rare. It appears as if there is not much genetic information, apart from male-determining factors, on the Y. However, the X chromosome seems to have the normal density of genetic information. For all of the many genes carried on the X chromosome, females have the "usual" two copies, whereas males have only one (excepting only those in the very small tip region).

2. X-Linkage

The various phenomena of X-linkage are due to this basic inequality in genetic material between males and females. For all genes in females and for autosomal genes in males, the phenomenon of dominance can reduce the prevalence of serious consequences due to possession of an "abnormal" form (or allele) of a gene. At many gene loci, it only requires one "normal" allele for adequate functioning. Thus, if an individual has both one normal and one abnormal allele at a particular locus, the manifest properties of the individual (the phenotype) will be normal. The normal allele is said to be dominant over the abnormal (recessive) one. In order for the abnormal phenotype to appear, both alleles must be abnormal. In the case of an X-borne gene, however, the male with an abnormal recessive allele does not have a normal one to compensate, and an abnormal phenotype will result. With respect to this same X-borne locus, the female will be normal unless both of her alleles are abnormal. One of the most prominent features of X-linkage, a higher prevalence in males than in females, is the consequence. In general, the likelihood of a male displaying the abnormal phenotype is simply the relative frequency of the abnormal allele in the population. For a female, the likelihood is the square of this value. Thus if the prevalence of the abnormal phenotype is 1 in 100 in males, it will be 1 in 10,000 in females.

There are also characteristic X-linked recessive transmission patterns within families. For example, there will be no father-to-son transmission because males have necessarily given their son a Y chromosome, which cannot contain the responsible allele. There can be a grandfather-to-grandson transmission, however. An affected grandfather can give his X chromosome to his daughter who will usually be normal because of a normal, dominant allele on the other X chromosome received from her mother. This daughter, however, will give her father-derived, abnormal allele-carrying X chromosome to one half of her sons. Another necessary consequence of the X-linkage system is that an affected daughter must have an affected father, but it will be rare that she has an affected mother. (All mothers of affected daughters must possess one abnormal allele, but, as noted earlier, not many will have both alleles abnormal.) Half of her maternal uncles will also be expected to be affected.

These (and other) hallmarks of X-linkage are at their most obvious when the homozygotes for the abnormal allele (those females with a "double dose") or the "hemizygous" males (with a single dose) display the affected phenotype unambiguously. This will be the case of so-called single-gene or major-gene effects, in which the genetic configuration at the locus in question has a superordinant influence, overshadowing all other possible genetic effects and environmental influences. Such circumstances typically yield categorical outcomes of "normal" and "affected." Many of the phenomena scrutinized in alcohol research are not of this nature, however, but are distributed continuously. Some of the continuity of these distributions may be due to the effects of environmental factors that can operate in a graded manner; some also may be due to the existence of a number of different relevant genetic loci, each of which has an influence on the same phenotype. (The fraction of the total phenotypic variance due to this latter class of influences is the well-recognized measure of *heritability*.)

Sex linkage might still be detectable under these circumstances. If, for example, the phenotype under study is under polygenic influence of this type, but with one of the loci on the X chromosome, then, depending on the relative influence of this locus, it might be possible to detect that the resemblance of fathers and sons may be lower than the resemblance of mothers and sons, mothers and daughters, or fathers and daughters. Obviously, however, sex-linkage identified in this way would be characteristic only of a part of that genetic determinant system, with perhaps most of the variance being generated by autosomal loci.

3. Sex Differences and Autosomal Genes

Based simply on considerations of the relative number of autosomal and X-borne loci, any observed genetically influenced sex difference is likely to be not sex-linked but sex-limited or sex-influenced. Sex-limitation is the situation in which autosomal genes are expressed only in one sex; sex-influence is the situation in which expression of the same autosomal genes is different in males than in females. The classic and oft-cited example of sex limitation is milk production in cattle. The males have all of the relevant loci but are incapable of expressing the phenotype. Pattern baldness is commonly cited as an example of sex-influenced inheritance.

Although the detailed mechanism may be poorly understood in specific cases, the general explanation of sex-limitation and sex-influence is relatively straightforward. The key notion is that genetic influences and environmental influences all feed into a common, complex causal network. Complex systems of this sort obviously present opportunities for interactions of various kinds— gene–gene, gene–environment, and environment–environment.

The primary product of any given gene thus operates in a context. If this primary gene product is an enzyme, for example, the reaction in which it participates requires a substrate, which is likely the product of some other enzyme-mediated reaction. Likewise, its product will quite probably serve as the substrate for some subsequent reaction. Furthermore, it is likely that there exist feedback controls, such as end-product inhibition, that affect the total flux in the chain. Further intricacies arise when chains of this sort converge with others to form the networks that mediate genetic influence on complex traits.[1,2]

The consequences of such a polygenic causal field will be the same in males and females, of course, if all of the participating elements in the field are the same. However, the outcome of a serial reaction or of a network process might be quite different between the sexes if some elements systematically differ between females and males. The most obvious example would be sex hormones or derived metabolites. These endocrinological differences must provide a major source of sex-limitation or sex-influence.

It is not only in the realm of biochemical processes closely coupled to primary gene products that sources of sex differences should be sought. Differential social roles and expectations can clearly have major influence. A conspicuous example relevant to the present topic is the opprobrium associated with alcohol consumption in women, particularly those born in the first half of the century. A substantial difference between men and women in the mean quantity of alcohol ingested arising from mores of this sort could well lead to different chemical contexts for the operation of autosomal genes.

Yet another possible avenue of social environmental influence, also of greater relevance to older cohorts, could be through differential occupation-related stresses. Without engaging the issue of whether worksite stresses are greater or less than homemaking stresses, it is reasonable to think that they may differ in pattern with possible differences in the prevailing endocrinological environment.

The above examples give a general basis for understanding how functioning of the same autosomal genes can give rise to different outcomes in males and females. There remains another theoretical prospect for explaining sex-limitation and sex-influence. The enormous strides taken recently in elucidating the mechanisms through which genes are turned on or off raise the possibility of differential activation of particular loci between the sexes. Thus, while the autosomal loci possessed by females and males may be equivalent, there could conceivably be considerable differences between the sexes in *effective* genotype. There is little empirical basis at present for such a conjecture, but recent developments in the identification of quantitative trait loci[3,4] make the search for differential gene activation feasible.

ACKNOWLEDGMENT. Support for ongoing research at Penn State on alcohol-related processes is provided by a gift from John Hanley and grant AA08125 from the National Institute on Alcohol Abuse and Alcoholism.

References

1. McClearn GE: Genetics, systems, and alcohol. *Behav Genet* 23(2):223–230, 1993.
2. McClearn GE, Plomin R: The search for genetic influences in alcohol-related phenotypes, in Begleiter H, Kissin B (eds): *The Genetics of Alcoholism*. New York, Oxford University Press, 1995, pp 610–659.
3. McClearn GE, Plomin R, Gora-Maslak G, Crabbe JC: The gene chase in behavioral science. *Psychol Sci* 2(4):222–229, 1991.
4. Plomin R, McClearn GE: Quantitative trait loci (QTL) analyses and alcohol-related behaviors. *Behav Genet* 23(2):197–211, 1993.

12

Sex Differences in Ethanol-Related Behaviors in Genetically Defined Murine Stocks

Byron C. Jones and Keith E. Whitfield

Abstract. Over the past 30 years, there have been a number of important developments in our understanding of the etiology and consequences of excessive drinking among humans. Probably one of the most important findings to date is that there are large individual differences among humans in appetite for alcohol and age of onset of problem drinking. We recognize this finding in at least two different alcoholic types, each with its own estimate of genetic influence. We have also come to realize that there are important differences between men and women, both in etiology of problem drinking and in the consequences of chronic alcohol use. In this chapter, the advantages and limitations of applying genetically defined animal models, primarily, selected lines and inbred strains of mice, are evaluated with examples from the literature.

1. Sex Differences in Alcohol-Related Problems in Humans

The comparison between women and men in etiology of alcohol drinking and related behavioral and pathophysiological outcomes is receiving increased attention. Some important new findings are resulting from this work; however, much remains to be clarified. For example, many researchers agree that, in the main, men consume greater amounts of alcohol and more frequently than do women.[1] This seems to be a consistent finding in North American studies including subjects from African, Hispanic, and European lineages.[2] One particularly interesting finding is that while North American women drink less than do men, those who do drink heavily are more likely to develop

Byron C. Jones and Keith E. Whitfield • Program in Biobehavioral Health, Pennsylvania State University, University Park, Pennsylvania 16802-6508.

Recent Developments in Alcoholism, Volume 12: Women and Alcoholism, edited by Marc Galanter. Plenum Press, New York, 1995

alcohol-related psychological problems.[2] More thorough cross-cultural inspection has shown that in some cultures, e.g., Sioux and Chinese, women may in actuality consume more alcohol more frequently than do isocultural men.[3,4] The contribution of genetics to drinking in women is also somewhat unclear. The work of Cloninger and colleagues[5] indicates that in humans there are at least two types of alcoholism, one that has a large genetic component and another that is more dependent on environment. The former is considered to be more prevalent in men, while the latter may be seen in both men and women. The picture is not entirely clear, however. Recent evidence suggests there may be parallel, genetic- and environment-prevalent alcoholic types for women as well as for men.[6,7]

As important as understanding the contributions of sex and genetics to the development of alcohol drinking and alcohol misuse is, recent evidence suggests that the pathophysiological consequences of chronic consumption of alcohol may be more serious in women than in men. This includes damage to liver[8,9] and brain.[10]

While there have been remarkable advances in methodology for human studies of alcoholism, the fact remains that the data are, for ethical and practical reasons, retrospective. Complementary studies in appropriate animal models may help provide a clearer picture of sex differences in alcohol consumption, problem drinking, and pathophysiology. The kinds of information gained from the animal models can indicate the biological significance of sex in alcohol-related phenotypes. Moreover, when genetically defined animals are employed in basic research, we have the powerful ability to address the importance of sex differences relative to overall genetic variability.

2. Approaches to Understanding Basic Processes Using Genetically Defined Animals

A number of behavioral and physiological criteria have been developed by researchers as partial counterparts to human-relevant outcomes. Thus, as models for alcohol ingestion, there are three widely used methods. First is the two- (or more) bottle choice test in which the animal is given a choice between water (or other solutions) and dilute ethanol solution. A second method is alcohol acceptance, which involves depriving the animal for a short period of all fluid and then presenting a dilute solution of ethanol for a finite period and measuring intake. Third, animals may be trained to press a lever that delivers an ethanol solution. Length of inability to execute the righting reflex following an anesthetic dose of ethanol is a measure of hypnotic sensitivity, and locomotion following low doses is indicative of ethanol's activating effects. A major physiological effect of ethanol on thermoregulation is easily assessed in animals, and handling-induced seizures during abstinence following a period of ethanol administration is used to study physical dependence. Studies of each of the alcohol-related phenotypes in genetically defined animals indicate most, if not all, are influenced by several genes, i.e., instead of showing pure dominance, these characteristics evince additive genetic-based variance.

Just as there are several alcohol-related phenotypes studied in animals, there are also several types of genetically defined animals. Among mammals rodents have been used more than any other order because of their abundance and short reproductive cycles. As described below, there are various types of genetically defined rats and mice. Although the laboratory mouse has been the favored species for developing genetically defined animals, there has been an increased interest recently in developing various genetically defined rats. Genetically defined animals include several types. A more complete discussion of these may be found in an overview by McClearn.[11] For this chapter, three types of genetically defined animals characterize the preponderance of the work relevant to sex differences. They are:

1. Inbred strains. Animals in this category are descended from 20 generations of brother–sister matings. This results in animals that share greater than 99% of segregating alleles—within sex.

2. Selected lines. These groups of animals result from selection in a heterogeneous stock for extreme response of animals for mating. Perhaps one of the more productive selections studies relevant to ethanol is the selection for extremes in hypnotic sensitivity in mice conducted by McClearn and Kakihana.[12] The resultant stocks, Long-Sleep and Short-Sleep mice, so named for their characteristic response to the anesthetic effects of ethanol, have been the subject for nearly 300 research reports in the literature.

3. Recombinant inbred strains. Selection for extreme response, as in the case of the Long-Sleep and Short-Sleep mice, oftentimes results in coselection for other differences. For example, Long-Sleep mice are less activated by a low dose of ethanol than are Short-Sleep mice, and the two lines show other behavioral and neurobiological differences as well.

The extent to which the differences for which selection was not performed are linked to the selected character cannot be ascertained by investigating only two lines of animals. The same is true for inbred strains that differ on a number of criteria. The way to determine the extent to which these several criteria may be associated is by developing recombinant inbred strains[13] and performing genetic correlational analysis. The development of recombinant inbred strains is actually quite simple. One makes hybrid crosses of two homogeneous strains to produce a F_1 generation. These animals are uniformly genetically heterogeneous. Members of the F_1 generation are then mated *inter se* to produce the F_2 generation, which is the first generation for which the genes segregate and reassort. Several (i.e., 25–40) families are inbred by brother–sister matings again to bring linkage groups to equilibrium and to fix the alleles as for any other inbred strain. The result is a large number of inbred strains, all of which have the same genes as the original stocks, but reassorted presumably in random fashion. Genetic correlational analysis by using strain means as the unit of analysis will now reveal which characteristics are genuinely linked and which of the apparent associations were spurious. Genetic correlational analysis is valuable not only in investigating behavior–behavior associations, but also in assessing brain–behavior associations, a particularly fruitful endeavor in pharmacogenetics.

3. Sex Differences in Alcohol-Related Behaviors in Genetically Defined Animals

In evaluating sex differences in inbred strains, selected lines, etc., it is important to address the significance of not only direction but degree of difference. For example, if in all genetically defined animal stock sex differences were in the same direction and in the same magnitude, then studies in genetically heterogeneous stocks would be just as informative. If, however, it can be shown that direction and extent of sex difference varies among genetically defined stocks, then it is likely that expression of important sex differences operate within the effective genotype as described by McClearn.[14]

3.1. Hypnotic and Hypothermic Sensitivity

In the extant literature, a consistent finding for hypnotic sensitivity is that following an anesthetic dose of ethanol, males of the Long-Sleep and Short-Sleep and derived recombinant inbreds evince longer loss of righting response than do their female counterparts.[15] When blood ethanol concentrations are measured upon regaining the righting response, however, there are no differences between the sexes.[16] This indicates that target tissue sensitivity between the sexes is equivalent, while the longer sleep times for the males probably indicate a difference from females in alcohol clearance. The sex difference in duration of loss of righting response has been replicated in the panel of recombinant inbred strains derived from the Long-Sleep and Short-Sleep selected lines.[17] Unfortunately, blood ethanol concentrations at regaining the righting response were not reported in this study. What was reported, however, but not discussed, was the variability between strains in sex differences. Among the 27 Long-Sleep × Short-Sleep recombinant inbred strains, 15 showed males with longer mean duration of loss of righting; for 8 strains, males had shorter mean duration of loss of righting; and for 4 strains, there was essentially no difference between the sexes.

Sensitivity to hypothermic effects of alcohol may be greater in females than in males in mouse lines selected for differential sensitivity to alcohol's hypothermic effects.[18] Interestingly, this sex difference was seen in the sensitive (cold), insensitive (hot), and control-unselected lines.

3.2. Effects of Ethanol on Locomotion

At low doses, ethanol tends to stimulate locomotor activity in mice while at slightly higher doses ethanol may produce locomotor inhibition.[19,20] Both effects show wide genetic-based variability. In a biometrical study of locomotor activation and inhibition, it was shown by Dudek and co-workers[19] that females were more sensitive to the locomotor activating effect of ethanol than were males. Middaugh and colleagues[22] showed that in the C57BL/6 strain males evinced greater locomotor activation at 1.5 g/kg and greater locomotor inhibition at 2.5 g/kg (both IP) than did females. Interestingly in the Dudek *et al.*[19] study, neither male nor female C57BL/6 mice evinced locomotor activation at 1.5 g/kg ethanol.

In our laboratory, we are in the final stages of analyzing locomotor activation following doses of 1.0–2.0 g/kg ethanol (IP) in the Long-Sleep by Short-Sleep recombinant inbred panel. In this study, we administered ethanol to equal numbers of male and female animals. Preliminary data analysis produce data that agree with those from Erwin *et al.*,[21] i.e., overall, females are more activated throughout the dose ranges than are males. Additionally, like the results observed in the study of hypnotic sensitivity in this recombinant inbred panel,[17] we observe wide variation in degree and direction of locomotor activation between the sexes across the recombinant inbred strains.

3.3. Ethanol Self-Administration

Consistent with most of the rodent literature, most studies of ethanol consumption in mice report higher consumption in females than in males. This is true also of inbred strains.[23] In a recent study, we investigated two-bottle choice ethanol selection in reciprocal hybrid mice derived from Long-Sleep by C57BL/10 and Short-Sleep by C57BL/10 progenitors. The purpose of the study was to investigate the cooperation between variable sensitivity to ethanol's hypnotic effects and high appetite for alcohol as shown by the C57BL/10 strain. The inbred strains differed overall in ethanol consumption, with C57 consuming more than the other two strains. Although the differences were not significant, Long-Sleep mice tended to drink more than Short-Sleep mice. As predicted, female inbred and hybrid mice consumed more ethanol (10% v/v) than did their male counterparts.

Of particular interest was our observation of sex × heterosis interaction in the Long-Sleep × C57BL/10 groups. In the females but not the males we observed significantly higher ethanol consumption in the hybrids than in either inbred strain. In the males, we observed a maternal effect in the Short-Sleep × C57 hybrids. In the hybrid males whose mothers were C57s, the animals drank quantities of ethanol comparable to C57 males. In the hybrid males whose mothers were Short-Sleep, the pattern was near total avoidance of ethanol. The observation of the sex × heterosis interaction indicated to us that the expression of probable polygenic influence on ethanol consumption is highly influenced by sex. As to whether this influence is mediated by some sort of epistatic mechanism or by the endocrine milieu, and so on, will have to be determined by further study. The maternal effect seen in the Short-Sleep × C57 hybrids is also quite intriguing, and while it is tempting to propose major influence by sex chromosomes, other factors (e.g., intrauterine environment, preweaning nest environment, etc.) may also be operative and need to be teased apart by further study.

4. Summary

For too long, examination of sex differences in preclinical psychopharmacological research has been neglected, probably because of the opinion expressed by many that the estrous/menstrual cycling of females added a "nuisance" variable. If this were true and if the timing of cycling were not controlled, then one would expect that the noise introduced would add to random error and thus decrease the power of statistical analysis. In our experience with selected lines, inbred strains, and recombinant strains, we find that error variance estimates for control and experimental treatments are comparable between males and females. Alternatively, if the stage of estrous/menstrual cycle is an important factor, then proper examination of this factor will yield important information about sex differences in alcohol-related behaviors.

There are emerging statistical techniques, called *sex limitation models,* that examine origins of sex differences in familial settings. There are three such models, one that examines total variance observed between males and females, another in which sex limitation is evidenced by different ratios for the genetic and environmental sources of variance, and a third in which different genes or different environments are operating in males compared with females.[26] These models have been explored in human twin comparisons using model-fitting techniques.[26,27] Since members of inbred strains are essentially identical twins, the application of human modeling techniques might be fruitful, especially with recombinant inbred strains.

Of the types of genetically defined mice available, recombinant inbred strains provide a unique window into the operation of different arrangements of the same genes. The immediate value of this model is that by genetic correlational analysis, the investigator is able to determine likely associations between several alcohol-related behaviors. Moreover, genetic correlational analysis is also a powerful means to investigate brain–behavior associations. For example, a recent study using the Long-Sleep × Short-Sleep recombinant inbred strains, reported significant correlations between hypnotic sensitivity and neurotensin receptors in the cortex and between locomotor activation by 1.5 g/kg ethanol and neurotensin receptors in cortex and caudate–putamen.[24] Another powerful technique for which recombinant inbred strains are well-suited is quantitative trait loci (QTL) analysis.[25] This technique correlates quantitatively evaluated phenotypes, e.g., alcohol-induced locomotor activation with polymorphic markers located on specific chromosomes, and thus indicates the general location of genes that influence the specific phenotype. Examination of sex-specific patterns of genetic correlations and QTLs will provide valuable evidence for important genetic-based sex differences in alcohol related phenotypes.

References

1. Wilsnack SC, Wilsnack RW: Epidemiology of women's drinking. *J Subst Abuse* 3:133–157, 1991.
2. Robbins C: Sex differences in psychosocial consequences of alcohol and drug abuse. *J Health Soc Behav* 30:117–130, 1989.
3. Weibel-Orlando J: Women and alcohol: Special populations and cross-cultural variations, in *Women and Alcohol: Health-Related Issues*. Rockville, MD, National Institute on Alcohol Abuse and Alcoholism, 1986, p 161.
4. Armstrong RW: Tobacco and alcohol use among urban Malaysians in 1980. *Int J Addict* 20:1803–1808, 1985.
5. Cloninger CR: Neurogenetic adaptive mechanisms in alcoholism. *Science* 236:410–416, 1987.
6. Hill SY, Smith TR: Evidence for genetic mediation of alcoholism in women. *J Subst Abuse* 3:159–174, 1991.
7. Cadoret RJ, O'Gorman TW, Troughton E, Heywood E: Alcoholism and antisocial personality: Interrelationships, genetic and environmental factors. *Arch Gen Psychiatry* 42:161–167, 1985.
8. Saunders JB, Davis M, Williams R: Do women develop alcoholic liver disease more readily than men? *Br Med J* 282:1140–1142, 1981.
9. Norton R, Batey R, Dwyer T, MacMahon S: Alcohol consumption and the risk of alcohol-related cirrhosis in women. *Br Med J* 295:80–82, 1987.
10. Mann K, Batra A, Günthner A, Schroth G: Do women develop alcoholic brain damage more readily than men? *Alcohol Clin Exp Res* 16:1052–1056, 1992.
11. McClearn GE: The tools of pharmacogenetics, in Crabbe JC Jr, Harris RA (eds): *The Genetic Basis of Alcohol and Drug Actions*. New York, Plenum Press, 1991, p 1.
12. McClearn GE, Kakihana R: Selective breeding for ethanol sensitivity: Short-Sleep and Long-Sleep mice, in McClearn GE, Deitrich RA, Erwin VG (eds): *Development of Animal Models as Pharmacogeneic Tools*. DHHS Publication No. (ADM) 81-1133. Washington, DC, US Government Printing Office, 1981, p 147.
13. Bailey DW: Strategic uses of recombinant inbred and congenic strains in behavioral genetics research, in Gershon ES, Breakfield XO, Ciaranello RD (eds): *Genetic Research Strategies for Psychobiology and Psychiatry*. New York, Boxwood Press, 1981, p 189.
14. McClearn GE: Sex distinctiveness in effective genotype, in Galanter M (ed): *Recent Developments in Alcoholism*. New York, Plenum Press, 1995, p xx.
15. Collins AC, Yeager TN, Lebsack ME, Panter SS: Variations in alcohol metabolism: Influence of sex and age. *Pharmacol Biochem Behav* 3:973–978, 1975.
16. Dudek BC, Phillips TJ: Distinctions among sedative, disinhibitory and ataxic properties of ethanol in inbred and selectively bred mice. *Psychopharmacology* 101:93–99, 1990.
17. DeFries JC, Wilson JR, Erwin VG, Petersen DR: LS × SS recombinant inbred strains of mice: Initial characterization. *Alcohol Clin Exp Res* 13:196–200, 1989.
18. Crabbe JC, Feller DJ, Dorow JS: Sensitivity and tolerance to ethanol-induced hypothermia in genetically selected mice. *J Pharmacol Exp Ther* 249:456–461, 1989.
19. Dudek BC, Phillips TJ, Hahn ME: Genetic analysis of the biphasic nature of the alcohol dose–response curve. *Alcohol Clin Exp Res* 15:262–269, 1991.
20. Erwin VG, Radcliffe RA, Jones BC: Chronic ethanol consumption produces genotype-dependent tolerance to ethanol in LS/Ibg and SS/Ibg mice. *Pharmacol Biochem Behav* 41:275–281, 1992.
21. Erwin VG, Jones BC, Radcliffe RA: Further characterization of LS × SS recombinant inbred strains of mice: Activating and hypothermic effects of ethanol. *Alcohol Clin Exp Res* 14:200–204, 1990.
22. Middaugh LD, Frackelton WF, Boggan WO, *et al*: Gender differences in the effects of ethanol on C57BL/6 mice. *Alcohol* 9:257–260, 1992.
23. Jones BC, Connell JM, Erwin VG: Appetite for and sensitivity to ethanol in C57BL by Short-Sleep and Long-Sleep mouse hybrids. *Alcohol Clin Exp Res* 14:301, 1990.
24. Erwin VG, Jones BC: Genetic correlations among ethanol-related behaviors and neurotensin

receptors in Long-Sleep (LS) × Short-Sleep (SS) recombinant inbred strains of mice. *Behav Genet* 23:191–196, 1993.

25. Plomin R, McClearn GE: Quantitative trait loci (QTL) analyses and alcohol-related behaviors. *Behav Genet* 23:197–211, 1993.

26. Neale MC, Martin NG: The effects of age, sex and genotype of self-reported drunkenness following a challenge dose of alcohol. *Behav Genet* 19:63–78, 1989.

27. Heath AC, Neale MC, Hewett JK, *et al:* Testing structural equation models for twin data using LISREL. *Behav Genet* 19:9–35, 1989.

13

Sex Differences in Mesolimbic Dopamine Responses to Ethanol and Relationship to Ethanol Intake in Rats

Betty A. Blanchard and Stanley D. Glick

Abstract. Sex differences in ethanol intake in rats suggest that there may be sex differences in brain dopamine systems believed to mediate ethanol's reinforcing properties. To test this hypothesis, we used *in vivo* microdialysis to examine changes in nucleus accumbens and striatal dopamine, DOPAC and HVA following acute administration of several doses of ethanol in male and female Long-Evans rats. Following dialysis, rats were trained to bar press for oral ethanol reinforcement. In nucleus accumbens, females showed greater increases in dopamine than males at low to intermediate doses. In striatum, both sexes showed increased dopamine at the low to intermediate doses. In addition to showing increased responsiveness to ethanol-induced mesolimbic dopamine stimulation, females consumed more ethanol than males during behavioral testing. Correlations between neurochemical measures and subsequent ethanol consumption indicated that among males, both basal and peak ethanol-induced nucleus accumbens dopamine levels were inversely related to later ethanol intake. No such relationship was observed for females. Striatal neurochemical measures were not significantly related to ethanol intake. These findings supported the hypothesis of sex differences in mesolimbic responses to ethanol and suggested that the relationship of those responses to subsequent ethanol intake may differ for males and females.

1. Introduction

Sex differences in ethanol consumption exist in several species, including humans and rodents.[1-3] In contrast to human females, who typically con-

Betty A. Blanchard • Department of Pathology and Anatomical Sciences, School of Medicine, University of Missouri, Columbia, Missouri 65212.   **Stanley D. Glick** • Department of Pharmacology and Toxicology, Albany Medical College, Albany, New York 12210.

Recent Developments in Alcoholism, Volume 12: Women and Alcoholism, edited by Marc Galanter. Plenum Press, New York, 1995

sume less alcohol than males,[1] female rodents tend to consume larger volumes of ethanol than males.[2,3] While sex differences in ethanol consumption among humans are likely to be attributable to a variety of causes, including social factors, sex differences in rodents suggest that gonadal hormones may play a modulatory role in the regulation of ethanol intake.

The mechanisms by which gonadal hormones might influence ethanol intake are unclear. One possible mechanism mediating differential ethanol intake by male and female rats may be sex differences in the reward efficacy of ethanol. The reinforcing properties of drugs of abuse, including ethanol, are believed to be closely related to the ability of those drugs to activate specific brain dopamine systems.[4-6] The mesolimbic dopamine system, which projects from the ventral tegmental area (VTA) of the midbrain to the nucleus accumbens is thought to be of particular importance in the mediation of drug reinforcement.[4-7] A number of studies have provided support for a role of dopamine in the reinforcing effects of ethanol. Low to intermediate doses of ethanol stimulate dopamine synthesis, metabolism, and turnover[8-11] and increase the firing rate of dopamine neurons in the VTA.[12] *In vivo* microdialysis studies indicate that ethanol also produces an increase in dopamine release in the nucleus accumbens.[13-17] Conversely, ethanol withdrawal decreases extracellular dopamine concentrations.[18]

Most if not all of the work examining neurochemical factors underlying ethanol reward has been done using male rats exclusively, despite the fact that females consume more ethanol than males in voluntary intake paradigms. If ethanol reward and consequently ethanol intake are related to ethanol's stimulation of mesolimbic dopamine release, then it might be predicted that females would show even greater dopaminergic responses to ethanol than males. Sex differences in ethanol intake may be related to sex differences in brain dopamine systems, just as genetic differences in dopamine systems appear to underlie some genetic differences in ethanol intake. For example, selective breeding studies have suggested that differential ethanol intake may be related to differences in basal dopaminergic activity, as well as in ethanol's effect on dopamine systems. Rats selectively bred for high alcohol preference (alcohol-preferring, or P rats) have been reported to have lower dopamine and dopamine metabolite levels than rats bred for low ethanol preference (nonpreferring, or NP rats).[19] In addition, ethanol-induced increases in dopamine metabolism were found to be greater in P than in NP rats.[10] Behavioral studies have indicated that P rats showed stimulant effects of low-dose ethanol, while NP rats did not.[20] Ethanol-induced behavioral activation is also believed to be mediated by the mesolimbic dopamine system.

We hypothesized that, similarly to genetic differences in ethanol consumption, sex differences in ethanol intake may be related to sex differences in the responsiveness of brain dopamine systems to ethanol. To begin to evaluate this hypothesis, we used *in vivo* microdialysis in combination with high-pressure liquid chromatography (HPLC) to examine mesolimbic and nigrostriatal dopamine release in response to systemic ethanol in male and female rats. Following microdialysis, some of the subjects were trained to bar press for oral ethanol reinforcement to determine the relationship between neurochemical responses to acute ethanol and subsequent ethanol intake. All animals used in the study were intact (nongonadectomized) adult Long-Evans rats.

2. Methods

2.1. In Vivo *Microdialysis*

Guide cannulae were stereotaxically placed in nucleus accumbens and in striatum, with the side for each structure balanced across animals. Several days after surgery, microdialysis probes (BAS/Carnegie Med) continuously perfused with artificial cerebrospinal fluid were lowered into the brain. Sample collection (every 20 min) began the following morning. Six baseline samples were obtained before ethanol was administered (20% v/v solution with 0.9% saline). Rats were injected intraperitoneally with 0.0, 0.25, 0.5, or 1.0 g/kg ethanol. Sample collection continued for 3 more hr, for a total of nine postinjection samples. Following microdialysis, a subgroup of rats that had received the lower doses of ethanol were allowed to recover for later ethanol self-administration testing. Those that received the higher dose of ethanol (1.0 g/kg) were sacrificed and histological analysis of the brains was performed to verify the location of the guide cannulae. Probes were tested *in vitro* prior to *in vivo* use, but because *in vitro* recovery is not quantitatively related to *in vivo* recovery,[21] all *in vivo* values are expressed as "uncorrected" dialysate concentrations. Dopamine, 3, 4-dihydroxyphenylacetic acid (DOPAC), and homovanillic acid (HVA) contents of perfusate samples were analyzed by HPLC with electrochemical detection.

2.2. *Self-Administration*

Subjects in this phase of the experiment were trained to orally self-administer ethanol in operant chambers equipped with fluid delivery systems. The procedure used to train animals to bar press for oral ethanol reinforcement was a modification of the sucrose-fading technique,[22] with saccharin substituted for sucrose. Rats were initially trained to respond for a 0.15% (w/v) saccharin solution. Once responses were established, ethanol was introduced in the saccharin solution. The concentration of ethanol was gradually increased to 10%, while the concentration of saccharin was decreased until it was eliminated. Rats were then maintained on 10% ethanol for 1 week. Following the week at 10% ethanol, a second bar was introduced into the chamber in order to assess preference for ethanol. Animals received 10% ethanol by pressing one bar and water by pressing the other. Side of presentation of ethanol was changed daily for a total of 10 days. At no time were animals food-or water-deprived. On completion of behavioral testing, rats were sacrificed and their brains examined to verify location of the guide cannulae.

3. Results

3.1. In Vivo *Microdialysis*

Baseline levels of dopamine, DOPAC, and HVA: Mean absolute levels of dopamine, DPOAC, and HVA in 15 μl of dialysate are shown in Table 1. There were no sex differences on any of these measures.

Neurochemical response to ethanol administration: For each subject, each data point was expressed as a percent of the mean baseline dialysate concentration (mean of the six preethanol injection samples; Figure 1). Rats that received 0.25 or 0.5 g/kg ethanol had significantly higher dopamine levels in nucleus accumbens than rats that received 0.0 or 1.0 g/kg ethanol. Also, females showed greater ethanol-induced dopamine release than males, regardless of dose of ethanol; these differences were seen in the first 2 hr following ethanol injection.

As in nucleus accumbens, significant increases in striatal dopamine were observed at 0.25 and 0.5 g/kg. Responses were similar for males and females. Figure 2 presents cumulative dopamine release (sum of percent of baseline levels for each postinjection sample) to facilitate the depiction of the dose–response relationship in nucleus accumbens and striatum for both males and females.

There were small increases in extracellular DOPAC and HVA in nucleus accumbens for approximately 2 hr following injection of 0.5 g/kg ethanol, but no effects on striatal DOPAC and HVA.

Table I. Mean Baseline Absolute Levels of Dopamine and Dopamine Metabolites in Dialysate Samples (pmoles/15 μl)

	Nucleus accumbens	
	Males	Females
Dopamine	0.036 ± 0.004	0.039 ± 0.001
DOPAC	16.57 ± 1.47	14.39 ± 1.62
HVA	8.49 ± 0.88	8.36 ± 1.35
	Striatum	
	Males	Females
Dopamine	0.044 ± 0.004	0.059 ± 0.008
DOPAC	25.76 ± 2.05	23.63 ± 3.03
HVA	19.98 ± 1.83	16.07 ± 2.03

Nucleus accumbens

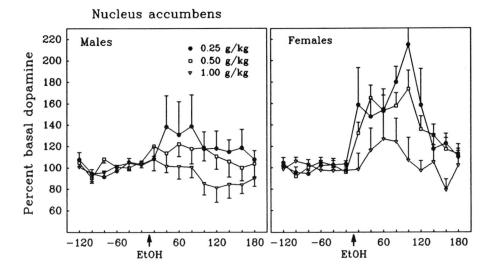

Striatum

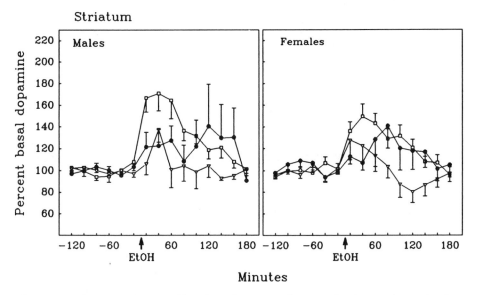

Figure 1.   Mean percentage of basal nucleus accumbens and striatum dopamine levels following 0.25, 0.5, or 1.0 g/kg ethanol for male and female rats.

3.2. Ethanol Self-Administration

Data presented in Fig. 3 represent the mean intake of ethanol (g/kg) over the last week of testing, during which time rats bar pressed to receive a 10% ethanol solution containing no saccharin. As expected, females consumed significantly greater amounts of ethanol than males. There was no sex differ-

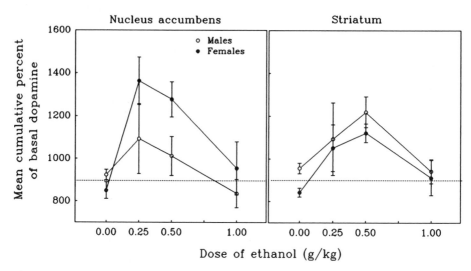

Figure 2. Mean cumulative percentage (sum of nine postethanol measures) of basal dopamine in nucleus accumbens and striatum in male and female rats following 0.0, 0.25, 0.5, or 1.0 g/kg ethanol. (A cumulative score of 900 indicates no net change from baseline over the 3-hr period, corresponding to 100% of baseline level at each of the nine postethanol measures.)

ence in ethanol preference, with both males and females showing preference ratios (volume of ethanol intake/total volume of fluid intake) of 0.70 (± 0.08). Importantly, the sex difference in intake was similar to the sex difference in neurochemical response in the nucleus accumbens, with females showing both increased extracellular dopamine in response to ethanol and higher subsequent ethanol intake relative to males.

3.3. Correlations between Baseline Neurochemical Measures and Ethanol Intake

We examined the correlations between mean intake of ethanol (10% v/v) and basal dialysate dopamine, DOPAC, and HVA in both nucleus accumbens and striatum. Among males, there was a significant inverse relationship between basal nucleus accumbens dopamine level and ethanol intake (Fig. 4). Males also showed significant correlations between DOPAC levels and subsequent ethanol intake ($r = -0.532$, $p < 0.05$) and between HVA levels and ethanol intake ($r = -0.491$, $p < 0.05$) (data not shown). There were no relationships between any of the nucleus accumbens neurochemical measures and ethanol intake among females. Neither males nor females showed significant relationships between striatal neurochemical measures and ethanol intake.

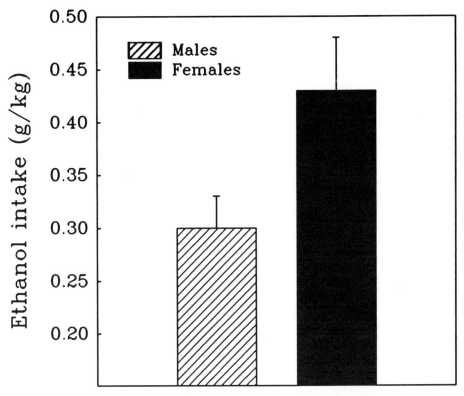

Figure 3.   Mean daily intake (g/kg) of 10% (v/v) ethanol over a 1-week period by male and female rats.

3.4. Correlations between Peak Ethanol-Stimulated Dopamine Release and Ethanol Intake

Correlations between peak dopamine response to ethanol and ethanol intake were examined only for those animals that had received 0.5 g/kg ethanol during microdialysis. (There was an insufficient number of animals that received 0.25 g/kg ethanol during microdialysis to obtain reliable correlational data.) Among males, there was a significant inverse correlation between peak absolute nucleus accumbens dopamine concentration in the dialysate and mean intake of the 10% ethanol solution (Fig. 4). There was no relationship between peak nucleus accumbens dopamine response and ethanol intake in females. As with basal levels, there were no relationships between peak striatal dopamine levels and intake in either sex. These data indicated that male rats that showed the greatest ethanol-induced dopamine release in nucleus accumbens consumed the least amount of ethanol.

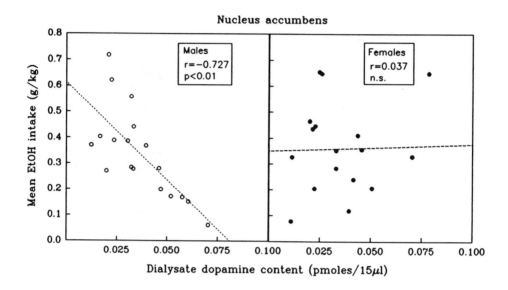

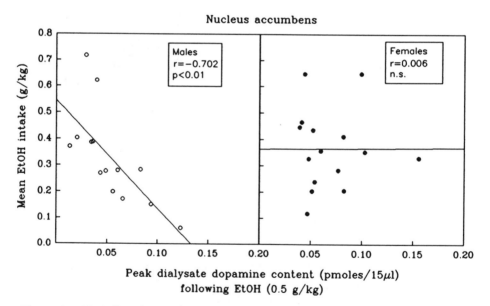

Figure 4. (Top) Correlations between basal dialysate dopamine content and subsequent ethanol intake for male and female rats. (Bottom) Correlations between peak ethanol-induced (0.5 g/kg) dopamine and subsequent ethanol intake for male and female rats.

4. Discussion

The results of the present study supported the hypothesized sex difference in ethanol-induced dopamine release. This sex difference was region specific: females showed greater extracellular dopamine levels than males in nucleus accumbens following all doses of ethanol, but there was no sex difference in striatum. Because the sex difference was region-specific, we believe that it is due at least in part to sex differences in the sensitivity of that region to ethanol. If the sex differences in ethanol-induced nucleus accumbens dopamine release were related to other factors, such as sex differences in ethanol metabolism or in brain ethanol concentrations, a similar sex difference would be predicted in the striatum as well.

These findings suggest the possibility that gonadal hormones have a modulatory influence on neurochemical response to ethanol specifically and possibly on brain reward systems in general. The nature of the putative gonadal hormone modulation of these systems has not been explored directly. Some studies have indicated that in female rats, ethanol intake varies over the estrous cycle, with intake being lowest at proestrous when estrogen levels are highest.[23,24] Such findings suggest that circulating levels of ovarian hormones in adult female rats can influence ethanol intake, possibly via cyclic variations in the responsiveness of reward systems to ethanol. The influence of androgens on ethanol-induced stimulation of dopaminergic pathways has not been examined, although effects on ethanol intake have been reported.[2] It is not known what factors underlying ethanol reward might be influenced by gonadal steroids.

It is important to note that the pattern of ethanol effects on nucleus accumbens dopamine release reflects ethanol intake patterns: females showed greater low-dose ethanol-induced enhancement of mesolimbic dopamine neurotransmission than males, as well as greater consumption of ethanol. This suggests that, in general, those animals that show greater increases in dopamine release in response to ethanol would be expected to consume greater amounts of ethanol, possibly due to greater reward efficacy of ethanol for those animals. However, the correlational data in males appears to contradict this pattern: males that showed greater ethanol-induced dopamine release consumed lesser amounts of ethanol. There is a possible reason for this apparent discrepancy between the implications of the sex difference data and those of the correlational data. Since the dose–response function for ethanol-induced dopamine release was biphasic (Fig. 2), using responses to only one dose of ethanol for the correlational study may have limited our ability to detect relationships between ethanol sensitivity of the mesolimbic dopamine system and subsequent ethanol intake. There were also relationships between basal nucleus accumbens dopamine, DOPAC, and HVA and ethanol consumption in males. Animals with lower basal dopamine and metabolite levels consumed larger quantities of ethanol than those with higher dopamine and metabolite levels. These findings are consistent with those showing that among selectively bred rats, animals bred for high ethanol intake have lower dopamine and metabolite concentrations than those bred for low intake.[19] Our data extend those findings by suggesting that not only group differences but individual differences in the mesolimbic dopamine system may be related to individual differences in ethanol intake.

In contrast to males, there appeared to be no relationship between either basal or ethanol-induced dopamine release and subsequent ethanol consumption in females. We believe that this was likely due in part to estrous variation in ethanol intake, which has been reported previously.[23,24] Hormonal variation during the estrous cycle may also influence responsiveness of the mesolimbic dopamine system to ethanol; we are currently exploring this possibility.

We have described the initial experiments performed in our attempt to understand how gonadal hormones influence the responses of the mesolimbic dopamine system to ethanol. Ongoing experiments include examining whether manipulation of gonadal hormone levels influences neurochemical responses to ethanol in both males and females. In addition, possible sex differences in changes in the mesolimbic dopamine system after chronic ethanol exposure are also being explored.

References

1. Chomak S, Collins RL: Relationship between sex-role behaviors and alcohol consumption in undergraduate men and women. *J Stud Alcohol* 48:194–201, 1987.
2. Mankes RF, Glick SD, Van der Hoeven T, Lefevre R: Alcohol preference and hepatic alcohol dehydrogenase activity in Long Evans rats is affected by intrauterine sibling contiguity. *Alcohol Clin Exp Res* 15:80–85, 1991.
3. Lancaster F, Spiegel KS: Sex differences in pattern of drinking. *Alcohol* 9:415–420, 1992.
4. Wise RA, Bozarth MA: A psychomotor stimulant theory of addition. *Psychol Rev* 94:469–492, 1987.
5. Koob GF: Drugs of abuse: Anatomy, pharmacology and function of reward pathways. *Trends Pharmacol Sci* 13:177–184, 1992.
6. Weiss F, Koob GF: The neuropharmacology of ethanol self-administration, in Meyer RE, Koob GF, Lewis MJ, Paul SM (eds): *Neuropharmacology of Ethanol: New Approaches*. Boston, Birkhauser, 1991, pp 125–162.
7. DiChiara G, Imperato A: Drugs abused by humans preferentially increase synaptic dopamine concentrations in the mesolimbic system of freely moving rats. *Proc Natl Acad Sci* 85:5274–5278, 1988.
8. Bustos G, Roth RH: Effect of acute ethanol treatment on transmitter synthesis and metabolism in central dopaminergic neurons. *J Pharm Pharmacol* 28:580–582, 1976.
9. Dar MS, Wooles WR: The effect of acute ethanol on dopamine metabolism in the striatum of mice. *J Neural Transm* 60:283–294, 1984.
10. Fadda F, Mosca E, Colombo G, Gessa GL: Effects of spontaneous ingestion of ethanol on brain dopamine metabolism. *Life Sci* 44:281–287, 1989.
11. Signs SA, Yamamoto BK, Schecter MD: *In vivo* electrochemical determination of extracellular dopamine in the caudate of freely moving rats after a low dose of ethanol. *Neuropharmacology* 26:1653–1656, 1987.

12. Brodie MS, Shefner SA, Dunwiddie TV: Ethanol increases the firing rate of dopamine neu-rons in the ventral tegmental area *in vitro. Brain Res* 508:65–69, 1990.
13. Blanchard BA, Steindorf S, Wang S, Glick SD: Sex differences in ethanol-induced dopamine release in nucleus accumbens and in ethanol consumption in rats. *Alcohol Clin Exp Res* 17:968–973, 1993.
14. DiChiara G, Imperato A: Ethanol preferentially stimulates dopamine release in the nucleus accumbens of freely moving rats. *Eur J Pharmacol* 115:131–132, 1985.
15. Imperato A, DiChiara G: Preferential stimulation of dopamine release in the nucleus accum-bens of freely moving rats by ethanol. *J Pharmacol Exp Ther* 239:219–239, 1986.
16. Wozniak KM, Pert A, Mele A, Linnoila M: Focal application of alcohol elevates extracellular dopamine in rat brain: A microdialysis study. *Brain Res* 540:31–40, 1991.
17. Yoshimoto K, McBride WJ, Lumeng L, Li TK: Alcohol stimulates the release of dopamine and serotonin in the nucleus accumbens. *Alcohol* 9:17–22, 1992.
18. Rossetti ZL, Melis F, Carboni S, Gessa GL: Marked decrease of extraneuronal dopamine after alcohol withdrawal in rats: reversal by MK-801. *Eur J Pharmacol* 200:371–372, 1991.
19. Murphy JM, McBride WJ, Lumeng L, Li TK: Contents of monoamines in forebrain regions of alcohol-preferring (P) and -nonpreferring (NP) lines of rats. *Pharmacol Biochem Behav* 26:389–392, 1987.
20. Waller MB, Murphy JM, McBride WJ, *et al:* Effect of low-dose ethanol on spontaneous motor activity in alcohol-preferring and non-preferring rats. *Pharmacol Biochem Behav* 24:617–623, 1986.
21. Glick SD, Dong N, Keller RW Jr, Carlson JN: Estimating extracellular concentrations of dopa-mine and DOPAC in nucleus accumbens and striatum using microdialysis: Relationship between *in vitro* and *in vivo* recoveries. *J Neurochem,* 62:2017–2021, 1994.
22. Samson HH: Initiation of ethanol reinforcement using a sucrose substitution procedure in food- and water-sated rats. *Alcohol Clin Exp Res* 10:436–442, 1986.
23. Forger NG, Morin LP: Reproductive state modulates ethanol intake in rats: Effects of ovariec-tomy, ethanol concentration, estrous cyclicity and pregnancy. *Pharmacol Biochem Behav* 17:323–331, 1982.
24. Morin LP, Forger NG: Endocrine control of ethanol intake by rats or hamsters: Relative contribution of the ovaries, adrenals and steroids. *Pharmacol Biochem Behav* 17:529–537, 1982.

14

Anxiolytic Effects of Steroid Hormones during the Estrous Cycle

Interactions with Ethanol

Michelle D. Brot, George F. Koob, and Karen T. Britton

Abstract. Behavioral differences in anxiety have been observed between both males and females and across the ovarian cycle in females. However, the data are not entirely consistent and the mechanisms of this potential interaction are largely unexplored. It appears that the GABA/BZ receptor complex is a site of action for steroids as well as for many anxiolytic drugs. Both natural steroids, such as progesterone and its metabolites, and synthetic steroids, such as alphaxalone, reduce anxiety-like behavior in rats. Alphaxalone also reverses the behavioral effects of potent anxiogenic agents in the conflict test of anxiety. Studies reported here found that ethanol administered to rats in different phases of the estrous cycle was more effective as an anxiolytic when hormone levels were high. The anticonflict response to chlordiazepoxide also was examined in ovariectomized and steroid-replaced female rats. Insight into the mechanisms and sites of action for these steroids can be gained from such an approach.

1. Introduction

Fluctuating levels of gonadal steroid hormones during the ovarian cycle have a variety of nonreproductive behavioral and neurobiological consequences.[1,2]

Michelle D. Brot and George F. Koob • Department of Neuropharmacology, Scripps Research Institute, La Jolla, California 92037.   **Karen T. Britton** • Department of Psychiatry, VA Medical Center and University of California, San Diego, California 92161.

Recent Developments in Alcoholism, Volume 12: Women and Alcoholism, edited by Marc Galanter. Plenum Press, New York, 1995

For example, pain sensitivity,[3,4] cognitive abilities, [5] ingestive behaviors,[6–8] and fear and anxiety[9,10] are all affected by hormonal changes. There is evidence in humans that females show a much higher incidence of depression and anxiety-related disorders,[11–13] and that female rats demonstrate anticonflict behavior during times of elevated estrogen and progesterone.[14,15] Furthermore, anxiolytic drugs have also been found to vary in effectiveness across the estrous cycle.[16] Recent research in our laboratory has focused on investigating (1) the effect on anxiety of the interaction of exogenously administered steroid hormones with the anxiolytic agent, chlordiazepoxide, and (2) whether the varying pharmacological effectiveness of anxiolytic drugs (e.g., ethanol) during the estrous cycle is mediated by an interaction with gonadal steroid hormones.

1.1. Anxiety and Alcohol Effects in Human Females

In humans, anxiety disorders occur much more frequently in females than in males,[13,17,18] and this has stimulated research on the relationship between anxiety and gonadal hormone levels across the ovarian cycle. For example, the symptoms of anxious female patients seemed to increase during the seven days prior to menstruation, according to observations made by their clinicians.[19] Premenstrual women appeared more susceptible to anxiety in an experiment in which they were exposed to electric shock that was paired with pictures of natural scenes. Their skin conductance response to stimuli was more rapid and their latency to extinction was delayed compared with women in other phases of the menstrual cycle.[9] Self-report data on anxiety collected across the menstrual cycle have indicated that more negative mood states are observed premenstrually when gonadal hormones are low.[20,21] However, better-controlled, prospective studies have been unable to document this observation.[22–24] Measurements of the blood alcohol levels (BAL) of cycling women revealed that premenstrual women consistently achieved higher peak BALs and faster absorption rates than women tested during menstruation or ovulation.[25] Another study was able to substantiate the finding that BAL was affected by gonadal hormones, although the correlations with the times during the cycle were not the same[26] and others could not demonstrate any BAL differences through the cycle.[27–29]

1.2. Gender Differences and Hormonal Effects on Anxietylike Behavior in Rats

Research using animals has also had somewhat mixed results in determining particular gender patterns of anxiety. While gender differences in tests of anxiety are frequently observed, the interpretation of these findings is not obvious. Male and female rats were found to differ in several tests of anxiety; however, these differences were not consistently in the same direction across tests[30] or across ages.[31] Therefore, it is possible that various tests of anxiety may not be measuring the same underlying phenomena. The rodent data suggested that the sex differences in fearfulness are in part dependent on estrogen levels, which diminish fearfulness.[10] However, a more recent study using the anxiety/defense test battery, which tests the rats' natural defense response to threatening stimuli, concluded that female rats are more defensive than males.[32] The effects of hormonal changes in female rats in relation to anxiety have also been examined in cycling animals. In an open field test measuring anxiety, female rats showed reduced anxietylike behavior during estrous when gonadal hormones are elevated.[33,34] Nevertheless, simply observing gender differences or attempting to correlate changes in anxiety with phases of the ovarian cycle has not provided conclusive evidence for the relationship between gonadal hormones and anxiety. Therefore, experimental approaches that manipulate levels of gonadal hormones have also been employed.

1.3. Steroid Hormone Effects on Behavior

The most common way to directly study the effects of steroid hormones on behavior involves the removal of endogenous hormones through ovariectomy, which can then be replaced with controlled administration of exogenous hormones. Using this methodology, progesterone or its active metabolites have been shown to influence motor activity,[35,36] aggression,[37] and anxiety.[14,15,38] For example, a combination of estrogen and progesterone (at concentrations that would result in estrous) causes increased anticonflict behavior that does not occur with the administration of progesterone alone.[14] Similarly, the withdrawal of progesterone increases behaviors associated with anxiety in a prod-burying paradigm.[39]

2. The γ-Aminobutyric Acid–Benzodiazepine Complex

2.1. Structure

The similarity of the purported anxiolytic effects of steroids to those caused by the traditional anxiolytic drugs such as benzodiazepines (BZ), barbiturates, and ethanol (ETOH) has led to the speculation that they may share a common mode of action within the γ-aminobutyric acid (GABA)–BZ receptor complex. This complex, pictured in Fig. 1, is a membrane protein with a chloride channel that opens and closes according to binding on its GABA receptor site. The complex is also composed of sites to which BZs, barbiturates, and picrotoxinlike convulsant drugs bind. These then interact allosterically within this receptor complex to regulate $GABA_A$ receptor chloride ion conductance (reviewed in Olsen et al.[40]).

2.2. Neurosteroid Binding

There is also evidence that there are specific receptor sites on the GABA complex for neuroactive steroids, which supports the concept that steroid

GABA Receptor Complex

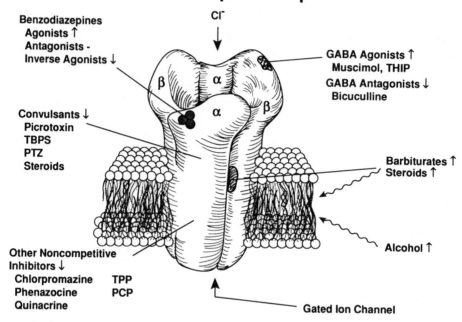

Benzodiazepines
Agonists ↑
Antagonists -
Inverse Agonists ↓

Cl⁻

GABA Agonists ↑
Muscimol, THIP

GABA Antagonists ↓
Bicuculline

Convulsants ↓
Picrotoxin
TBPS
PTZ
Steroids

β   α
    α   β

Barbiturates ↑
Steroids ↑

Alcohol ↑

Other Noncompetitive
Inhibitors ↓
Chlorpromazine   TPP
Phenazocine   PCP
Quinacrine

Gated Ion Channel

Figure 1. Schematic model of the GABA$_A$ receptor complex. This model does not intend to show the precise subunit assembly or location of the various recognition sites associated with the subunits. The arrows indicate the enhancement (↑) or reduction (↓) of GABAergic function by a variety of agents. Abbreviations: GABA, γ-aminobutyric acid; THIP, 4,5,6,7-tetrahydroisoxazolo [5,4-c]pyridin-3-ol; TBPS, t-butylbicyclophos-phorothionate; PTZ, pentylene tetrazole; TPP, tetraphenylphosphonium; and PCP, phencyclidine. (Redrawn with permission from Schwartz.[81])

hormones and their metabolites may directly modulate GABA activity through a nongenomic action at the membrane.[41-42] Studies in cell culture that examine the structural importance of the different receptor subunits for various ligands to activate the GABA-gated Cl⁻ current revealed that GABA modulation by diazepam was dependent on the GABA$_A$ receptor structure, whereas binding by neurosteroids such as allopregnanolone appeared independent of the type of subunit present in the receptor.[44] The neurosteroid binding probably occurred at a site in the transmembrane domain of the receptor, a highly conserved region in all six possible subunits of the GABA$_A$ receptor.

2.3. Interaction with Steroids

Studies that have examined the interaction between steroid hormones and the GABA–BZ receptor *in vivo* indicate that ovarian hormones appear to modulate the GABA–BZ receptor complex by binding at the steroid site. In the majority of studies of ovariectomized rats, estradiol administration leads to an increase of BZ binding sites in various brain areas,[45–47] while progesterone also leads to an increase in BZ sites with the distribution more limited to the amygdala and hippocampus.[45,48] An upregulation of GABA receptors has also been demonstrated in response to progesterone exposure in ovariectomized rats. Surprisingly, perhaps, both GABA receptors and BZ sites appear not to be influenced by the hormonal changes through the rat estrous cycle.[49,50] The BZ receptor number and affinity were also similar among male, female, and ovariectomized female groups,[50] although sex differences in BZ binding have been reported in one strain of rats.[51]

3. The Effects of Synthetic Steroids on Anxiety Mechanisms

3.1. The Conflict Test

The Geller-Seifter conflict test is a well-known paradigm for assessing the anxiolytic actions of drugs and has been used effectively in our lab for years to demonstrate the behavioral antianxiety properties of BZs and alcohol.[52–54] The conflict procedure involves an operant multiple schedule, consisting of three components: a pure reward component (unpunished component), time-out component, and a conflict component (punished component). During the unpunished component, rats are rewarded with a 45-mg Noyes food pellet on a random interval 30-sec reinforcement schedule. The time-out component has no shock or food reinforcement associated with lever pressing. In the punished component, rats simultaneously receive both food reward and foot shock punishment on a continuous reinforcement schedule. The shocks are delivered through stainless steel bars on the floor and they increase in intensity in increments of 0.15 mA to a maximum of 3.3 mA. Each phase of the test has light cues uniquely associated with that component so the animal can determine the consequences of lever pressing. A testing session consists of two cycles of a 5-min reward period, a 2-min time-out, and a 2-min conflict period presented in succession, giving a total daily session duration of 18 min in the conflict boxes (see Table I). Using these procedures, ETOH in the intoxicating dose range reliably produces a dose-dependent release of punished responding as reflected in an increase in lever pressing during the conflict component. These same doses produce dose-dependent decreases in responding during the unpunished component which presumably reflects the acute motor-debilitating effects of ETOH.

3.2. Alphaxalone

Synthetic steroids as well as naturally occurring hormones can be administered exogenously to intact animals to study their effects on anxiety-related

Table I. Outline of the Modified Geller-Seifter Multiple Schedule Conflict Test for Anxiety[a]

Component	Length	Discriminitive stimulus	Contingency
Random interval	5 min	Chamber dark	RI 30 sec. for food alone
Time-out	2 min	Houselight on	None operative
Conflict	2 min	Houselight and lever lights flashing	Continuous reinforcement for food and incremental shock

[a]The multiple schedule of the Geller-Seifter modified conflict test consists of three components. A testing session is composed of two 9-min cycles, giving a total daily session duration of 18 min. Rats are tested in soundproof operant chambers equipped with stainless steel bars on the floor through which electric shock is delivered on the conflict component of the test. The shock consists of a scrambled constant current, biphasic square wave and is incremental to a maximum of 3.3 mA.

behaviors. In a recent study, the effects of the synthetic steroid anesthetic alphaxalone were tested in intact male rats in the Geller-Seifter conflict test and the elevated plus maze.[55] Alphaxalone resembles a progestogenic steroid and is particularly interesting because it has been demonstrated to have differential analgesic effects on male and female rats.[56] When alphaxalone was injected intraperitoneally (IP) to produce analgesia, it was observed that the male rat required approximately four times more alphaxalone than the female rat. Further testing revealed that this sex difference is age-dependent, cannot be accounted for by different metabolic clearance rates, and appears to be estrogen-dependent. When male rats were castrated and replaced with chronic estrogen, the dose of alphaxalone required was similar to that of female rats.

3.3. Anxiolytic Activity of Alphaxalone

Both the naturally occurring progesterone metabolite allopregnanolone and the synthetic steroid anesthetic alphaxalone have been demonstrated to increase the binding of flunitrazepam to BZ binding sites, to enhance muscimol binding to GABA receptor sites, and to potentiate GABA-mediated chloride ion uptake.[42,57,58] However, their mechanisms of action are as yet unknown. To characterize the behavioral properties of alphaxalone and its sites of action, alphaxalone and several ligands of the GABA receptor complex were examined in two behavioral tests of anxiety. In the conflict test, alphaxalone produced an increase in punished responding similar to that observed with the BZ agonist chlordiazepoxide (CDP) at doses of 2–8 mg/kg (Fig. 2). In the plus maze, alphaxalone dose-dependently increased open arm time, although it only became significant at the highest dose tested (8 mg/kg).[55] A lack of interaction of an 8 mg/kg dose of alphaxalone with various BZ and GABA receptor ligands on the conflict test indicated that alphaxalone was probably producing its anxiolytic effects at a binding site other than the BZ or picrotoxin sites on the GABA–BZ complex. For example, doses of 3–12 mg/kg

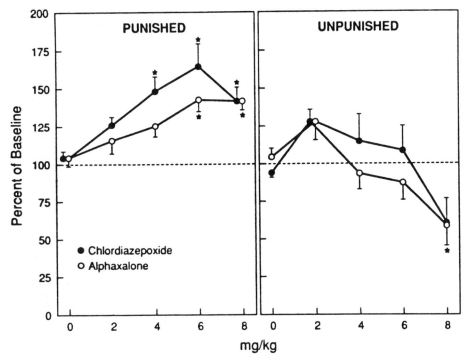

Figure 2. The effect of alphaxalone and chlordiazepoxide on punished (conflict) and unpunished (random interval) responding in an operant conflict test. Results are expressed as percentage of baseline responding from previous 2 days (mean ± SEM). For alphaxalone, $n = 6$ except for 2 mg/kg ($n = 5$) and 8 mg/kg ($n = 7$). For chlordiazepoxide, $n = 6$ except for 0 and 6 mg/kg ($n = 5$) and 8 mg/kg ($n = 7$). *Significantly different from vehicle, ANOVA followed by Dunnett's test, $p<0.05$. (Taken with permission from Britton et al.[55])

of Ro 15-1788, a BZ antagonist, and doses of 5–15 μg/kg of IPPO, a picrotoxin ligand, were ineffective in reversing the anticonflict effects of alphaxalone. Likewise, as shown in Fig. 3, bicuculline and picrotoxin did not significantly antagonize the increase in punished responding displayed in the alphaxalone alone group, nor did either drug have an effect on its own.

This finding is consistent with the results of Rodriguez-Sierra et al.,[14,15] who showed that progesterone acts as an anxiolytic agent in the lick suppression and conflict tests; however, its mechanism of action appears to be independent of the BZ receptor since CDP did not enhance progesterone's effects.

3.4. Alphaxalone Reverses Stress Response

In response to stressful stimuli, the levels of naturally occurring steroids such as progesterone, deoxycorticosterone, and their metabolites have been

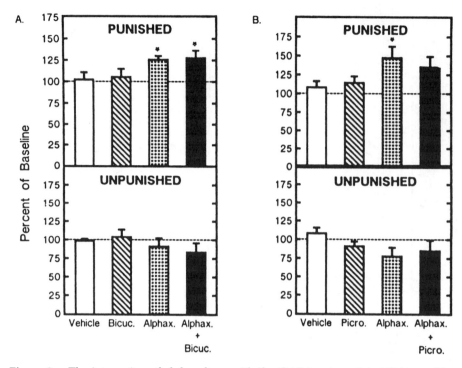

Figure 3. The interaction of alphaxalone with the GABA antagonists (A) bicuculline and (B) picrotoxin on rates of responding in an operant conflict test. Values expressed as percentage of baseline responding from previous 3 days (mean ± SEM). For A, vehicle ($n = 6$), Bicuc. and Alphax alone ($n = 7$), interaction ($n = 9$); for B ($n = 7$) all groups. *Significantly different from vehicle controls, Dunnett's, $p < 0.05$. The interaction of alphaxalone vs. bicuculline or picrotoxin was not significant. (Taken with permission from Britton et al.[55])

shown to increase.[59–61] Since these steroids also bind with a high affinity to $GABA_A$ receptors, it is possible that they may be endogenous modulators of central $GABA_A$ receptors. Although the physiological significance of these steroids in modulating the stress response is unknown, more of a role could be indicated if they were shown to reverse the effects of induced and natural stressors. In fact, alphaxalone was able to reverse the stress response induced by corticotropin-releasing factor (CRF) administration in the conflict test and induced by a forced swim in the plus maze test.[62] The CRF was infused intraventricularly at 0.5-μg dose, which is known to produce anxiogeniclike or "proconflict" effects in the conflict test. In the conflict test, alphaxalone significantly reversed the anxiogenic effect of CRF at the 3- and 6-mg/kg doses (Fig. 4). Likewise, a swim stress typically decreases the open arm time of rats on the plus maze; however, this reduction was abolished when the stress was followed by an injection of 3 or 6 mg/kg of alphaxalone. The effects of alphaxalone are typical of classical anxiolytic drugs such as CDP and ETOH, which

PUNISHED RESPONDING

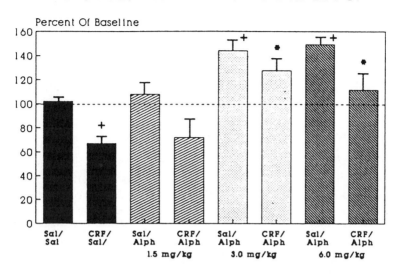

Percent Of Baseline

UNPUNISHED RESPONDING

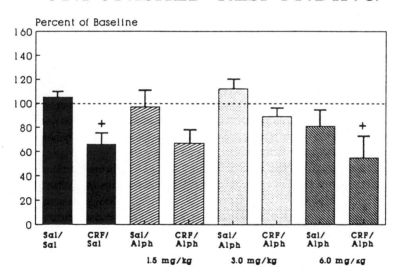

Percent of Baseline

Figure 4. Effect of alphaxalone (1,3, or 6 mg/kg, IP) on CRF-induced (0.5 μg, ICV) suppression of punished and nonpunished responding in the conflict test. Hatched bars, 1.5 mg/kg alphaxalone; stippled bars, 3.0 mg/kg alphaxalone; dark hatched bars, 6.0 mg/kg alphaxalone. Values are expressed as a percent of baseline responding from previous 3 days (mean ± SEM). Sal/Sal ($n = 21$), CRF/Sal ($n = 16$), Sal/Alph 1.5 mg/kg, CRF/Alph 3.0 mg/kg ($n = 6$), Sal/Alph 3.0 and 6.0, CRF/Alph 1.5 and 6.0 ($n = 7$). *Significantly different from CRF/Sal groups; †significantly different from vehicle control. ANOVA, Newman-Keuls, $p < 0.05$. (Taken with permission from Britton *et al.*[62])

also reverse CRF's response-suppressing effects in the conflict test.[63,65] The results of this study raise the possibility that there is an interaction between the GABA–BZ and CRF binding sites.

4. The Role of Gonadal Steroids in the Effects of Ethanol and Anxiolytic Drugs during the Estrous Cycle

4.1. Sex Differences in the Anxiolytic Effects of Ethanol

4.1.1. Humans. The mechanisms through which ovarian hormones may be having anxiolytic effects and whether a synergistic action with ETOH or other anxiolytic agents would produce a heightened relaxation are of some interest. Ethanol's stress-reducing properties have been consistently demonstrated in human,[65–67] as well as animal research.[53,68] In studies of college students, several reports have determined that there are differences between women and men on various measures related to anxiety and alcohol intake, although the results are often contradictory. These include self-reported reduced anxiety in women who believed they drank alcohol but not in men,[69] in contrast to less self-disclosure in women who expected alcohol but increased self-disclosure in men.[70] Among alcoholic women, more reported drinking to alleviate anxiety and more were binge drinkers than their male counterparts.[71] Another report studying depressed and nondepressed students found that although depressed men drank the most alcohol, both nondepressed women and depressed men had substantially reduced depression scores after drinking.[72] However, a study that examined the drinking patterns of high-anxiety and low-anxiety college students found significant differences in alcohol consumption between the two groups, no differences in frequency, and no differences between male and female subgroups.[73]

4.1.2. Rats. While changes in self-reported anxiety have been used to explore this effect in humans, animal research has needed to rely on behavioral and physiological indices of anxiety reduction. In a more naturalistic anxiety test using a brief exposure to a cat as an unconditioned stimulus, rats respond with defensive behavior that can last 24 hr or more. When administered in this test, ETOH appeared to inhibit the fear on certain activities; however, the effects of the ETOH were relatively minimal. Instead, large sex differences in defensive behavior were discovered, with male rats showing reduced reactivity to the fear-inducing stimulus in comparison with female rats.[74] In another study, male rats trained to voluntarily consume a 5% ETOH solution showed an approximately 50% decrease in ETOH intake following the administration of estrogen while female rats showed a 73% decrease with virtually no effect on food intake.[75]

4.1.3. Other Anxiolytics. In addition, the effectiveness of diazepam and serotonergic anxiolytics vary as a function of both gender and the phase of the estrous cycle. Proestrous females demonstrate a high sensitivity to the anxiolytic effects of diazepam in the defensive burying test compared with metestrous females, which have low hormone levels, or males.[16] The administration of diazepam to mice at estrous or diestrous was more anxiolytic at these times than during the rest of the cycle.[76]

4.2. Effects of Ethanol Vary during the Rat Estrous Cycle

In a preliminary study, the anxiolyticlike effects of ETOH were tested through the rats' estrous cycle to determine whether there was a differential sensitivity to ETOH at the different phases of the cycle. Female Wistar rats were trained on the modified Geller-Seifter conflict test until they achieved a stable baseline. Vaginal smears, in which cell samples are taken from the inner surface of the vagina with a cotton swab, were performed daily and the stage of each rat's estrous cycle was noted. The study proceeded with rats that demonstrated at least one complete ovarian cycle, consisting of 3 days—proestrous, estrous, and metestrous or diestrous, which were collapsed into one unit since there are low levels of ovarian hormones at these stages. Each morning for the 4 days of one cycle, between 8 and 9 AM, rats were vaginally smeared, injected with 1 ml/kg saline, and tested in the conflict paradigm. During the subsequent cycle, the rats were randomly injected at different stages of their cycle with 10% ETOH (0.75 g/kg) and then tested in the conflict test. The data were analyzed by examining the ETOH conflict scores of the same animals in relation to the saline injection conflict scores from the previous estrous cycle. A two-factor repeated-measures ANOVA showed a significant main effect of cycle ($F = 3.9$) and of drug ($F = 20.2$), but no interaction ($F = 2.0$). Subsequent simple comparisons in the saline and ETOH groups revealed that the saline groups were the same across the estrous cycle, while a significant difference in responding to ETOH existed between the estrous and combined met- and diestrous conditions (Fig. 5). The estrous females were more sensitive to the effects of ETOH, and thus showed an enhanced anticonflict response.

These results are consistent with data by Fernández-Guasti and Picazo[16] that demonstrated a greater sensitivity to diazepam's anxiolytic effects in proestrous females with higher hormone levels than in metestrous females. In addition, behavioral data have indicated that during proestrous or after the administration of progesterone and estrogen to ovariectomized rats there is a reduction in anxiety levels,[77] and the exogenous administration of these hormones also results in increased GABAergic transmission.[78–80] Together, these data suggest that during a period of high hormonal levels there is an increase in GABAergic activity, and this may account for the higher sensitivity to the anxiolytic drugs.

4.3. The Interaction of Steroid Hormones and Chlordiazepoxide in Anticonflict Behavior

To further investigate this phenomenon and to explore whether estrogen and progesterone replacement in ovariectomized rats would enhance the anx-

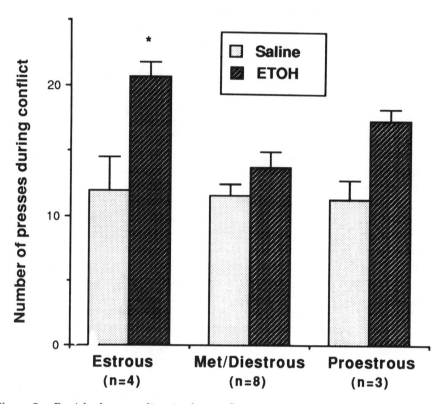

Figure 5. Punished responding in the conflict test across the estrous cycle in rats injected with saline and compared with the same rats' responding after a 0.75 g/kg ETOH injection the following cycle. *Estrous group significantly different from met/diestrous, ANOVA followed by Scheffe test, $p < 0.05$.

iolytic effects of CDP, ovariectomized rats were injected with estrogen subcutaneously (SC) (2 μg/day) each morning for 5 days, and on the fifth day the rats received 500 μg progesterone SC 4 hr prior to conflict testing. The other half of the rats were injected with saline in place of each hormone injection. On the day of the conflict test, half of the hormone-treated rats were injected with 5 mg/kg CDP and the other half with saline IP 30 min prior to testing. Likewise, half of the ovariectomized females were administered CDP and half were given saline. A two-factor ANOVA indicated an overall effect of drug treatment ($F = 14.4$) but no effect of hormone administration ($F = 0.6$) and no interaction ($F = 1.3$). Although not significant, it appeared that there was an mild interaction between CDP and the ovarian hormones since the differences between the hormone-treated saline group and the hormone-treated CDP group were greater than in the ovariectomized groups (Fig. 6).

These results are also consistent with the results of Rodriguez-Sierra *et*

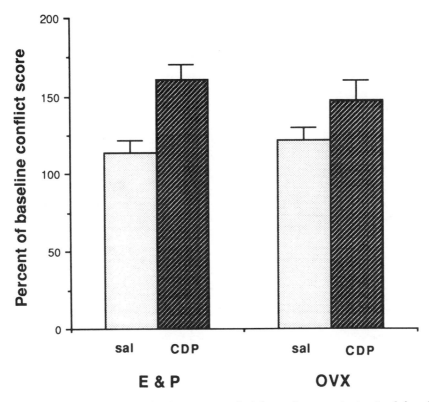

Figure 6. The effect of gonadal hormones administered to ovariectomized female rats on punished responding following saline or 5 mg/kg chlordiazepoxide (CDP). For estrogen and progesterone and ovariectomized (ovx) rats given saline, $n = 9$. For E and P rats given CDP, $n = 7$, and for ovx rats given CDP, $n = 8$.

al.,[14,15] who showed that while progesterone alone had anxiolytic effects, it was unlikely to be acting via the BZ receptor since CDP did not enhance progesterone's effects. However, the lack of anxiolytic effect in the hormone-treated saline group differs from the findings of Fernández-Guasti and Picazo,[77] who reported that the administration of these two ovarian hormones together resulted in anxiolyticlike behavior.

5. Conclusions

These preliminary findings lend support to the hypothesis that steroid hormone levels can differentially modify anxiety mechanisms and the actions of anxiolytic agents. The mechanisms for these interactions and precisely where they are having their effects remain to be determined. A likely site for their modulatory action would be at the steroid site on the GABA–BZ receptor complex. Future studies with specific agonists and antagonists for the receptors at this site will yield substantial new information and help to tease apart the interactions occurring at this complex that influence anxiety.

References

1. Van Haaren F, Van Hest A, Heinsbroek RPW: Behavioral differences between male and female rats: Effects of gonadal hormones on learning and memory. *Neurosci Biobehav Rev* 14:23–33, 1990.
2. Beatty WW: Gonadal hormones and sex differences in nonreproductive behaviors in rodents: Organizational and activational influences. *Behav Neural Biol* 12:112–163, 1979.
3. Ratka A, Simpkins JW: Effects of estradiol and progesterone on the sensitivity to pain and on morphine-induced antinociception in female rats. *Horm Behav* 25:217–228, 1991.
4. Bodnar RJ, Romero MT, Kramer E: Organismic variables and pain inhibition: Roles of gender and aging. *Brain Res Bull* 21:947–953, 1988.
5. Williams CL, Meck WH: The organizational effects of gonadal steroids on sexually dimorphic spatial ability. *Psychoneuroendocrinology* 16:155–176, 1991.
6. Cohen IT, Sherwin BB, Fleming AS: Food cravings, mood, and the menstrual cycle. *Horm Behav* 21:457–470, 1987.
7. Bowen DJ, Grunberg NE: Variations in food preference and consumption across the menstrual cycle. *Physiol Behav* 47:287–291, 1990.
8. Weizenbaum F, Benson B, Solomon L, Brehony K: Relationship among reproductive variables, sucrose taste reactivity and feeding behavior in humans. *Physiol Behav* 24:1053–1056, 1980.
9. Van Der Molen GM, Merckelbach H, Van Den Hout MA: The possible relation of the menstrual cycle to susceptibility to fear acquisition. *J Behav Ther Exp Psychiatry* 19:127–133, 1988.
10. Gray JA: Sex differences in emotional behaviour in mammals including man: Endocrine basis. *Acta Psychologica* 35:29–49, 1971.
11. Robins LN, Helzer JE, Weissman MM, *et al*: Lifetime prevalence of specific psychiatric disorders in three sites. *Arch Gen Psychiatry* 41:949–958, 1984.
12. Amenson CS, Lewinsohn PM: An investigation into the observed sex difference in prevalence of unipolar depression. *J Abnorm Psych* 90:1–13, 1981.
13. Emmelkamp PMG: *Phobic and Obsessive Compulsive Disorders: Theory Research and Practice.* New York, Plenum Press, 1982.
14. Rodriguez-Sierra JF, Hagley MT, Hendricks SE: Anxiolytic effects of progesterone are sexually dimorphic. *Life Sci* 38:1841–1845, 1986.
15. Rodriguez-Sierra JF, Howard J, Pollard GT, Hendricks SE: Effect of ovarian hormones on conflict behavior. *Psychoneuropharmacology* 9:293–300, 1984.
16. Fernández-Guasti A, Picazo O: The actions of diazepam and serotonergic anxiolytics vary according to the gender and the estrous cycle phase. *Pharmacol Biochem Behav* 37:77–81, 1990.
17. Vázquez-Barquero JL, Diez Manrique JF, Muñoz J, *et al*: Sex differences in mental illness: A community study of the influence of physical health and socio demographic factors. *Soc Psychiatry Psychiatr Epidemiol* 27:62–68, 1992.
18. Barlow DH: *Anxiety and Its Disorders: The Nature and Treatment of Anxiety and Panic.* New York, Guilford Press, 1988.
19. Breier A, Charney DS, Heninger GR: Agoraphobia with panic attacks. *Arch Gen Psychiatry* 43:1029–1036, 1986.
20. May R: Mood shifts and the menstrual cycle. *J Psychosom Res* 20:125–130, 1975.
21. Wilcoxon LA, Schrader SL, Sherif CW: Daily self-reports on activities, life events, moods and somatic changes during the menstrual cycle. *Psychosom Med* 38:399–417, 1976.

22. Slade P: Premenstrual emotional changes in normal women: Fact or fiction? *J Psychosom Res* 28:1–7, 1984.

23. Rubinov DR, Roy-Byrne P: Premenstrual syndromes: Overview from a methodological perspective. *Am J Psychiatry* 141:163–172, 1984.

24. Halbreich U, Endicott J: Methodological issues in studies of premenstrual changes. *Psychoneuroendocrinology* 10:15–32, 1985.

25. Jones B, Jones M: Alcohol effects in women during the menstrual cycle. *Ann NY Acad Sci* 273:567–587, 1976.

26. Zeiner A, Kegg P: Menstrual cycle and oral contraceptive effects on alcohol pharmacokinetics in Caucasian females. *Alcohol Clin Exp Res* 4:233–237, 1980.

27. Hay W, Nathan P, Heermans H, Frankenstein W: Menstrual cycle, tolerance, and blood alcohol level discrimination ability. *Addict Behav* 9:67–77, 1984.

28. Brick J, Nathan P, Westrick E, *et al:* The effects of menstrual cycle on blood alcohol levels and behavior. *J Stud Alcohol* 47:472–477, 1986.

29. Freitag WJ, Adesso VJ: Mood effects of alcohol and expectancies across the menstrual cycle. *Alcohol* 10:291–298, 1993.

30. Johnson AL, File SE: Sex differences in animal tests of anxiety. *Physiol Behav* 49:245–250, 1991.

31. Imhof JT, Coelho ZMI, Schmitt ML, *et al:* Influence of gender and age on performance of rats in the elevated plus maze apparatus. *Behav Brain Res* 56:177–180, 1993.

32. Blanchard RJ, Blanchard DC, Weiss SM: Ethanol effects in an anxiety/defense test battery. *Alcohol* 7:375–381, 1990.

33. Anderson EE: The sex hormones and emotional behavior: I. The effect of sexual receptivity upon timidity in the female rat. *J Genet Psychol* 56:149–158, 1940.

34. Burke AW, Broadhurst PL: Behavioral correlates of the oestrous cycle in the rat. *Nature* 209:223–224, 1966.

35. Dhar V, Stark R, Kraulis I, Murphy BEP: Contrasting effects of 5α- and 5 β-pregnane-3,20-dione on the motor activity of ovariectomized rats. *J Steroid Biochem* 26:577–580, 1987.

36. Heinsbroek RPW, VanHaaren F, VandePoll NE: Effects of progesterone on open field behavior of food deprived ovariectomized female rats. *Physiol Behav* 43:779–782, 1988.

37. Fraile IG, McEwen BS, Pfaff DW: Comparative effects of progesterone and alphaxalone on aggressive, reproductive and locomotor behaviors. *Pharmacol Biochem Behav* 30:729–735, 1988.

38. Bitran D, Hilvers RJ, Kellogg CK: Anxiolytic effects of 3α-hydroxy-5α(B)-pregnane-20-one: Endogenous metabolites of progesterone that are active at the GABA$_A$ receptor. *Brain Res* 561:157–161, 1991.

39. Gallo MA, Smith SS: Progesterone withdrawal decreases latency to and increases duration of electrified prod burial: A possible rat model of PMS anxiety. *Pharmacol Biochem Behav* 46:897–904, 1993.

40. Olsen RW, Sapp DM, Bureau MH, *et al:* Allosteric actions of CNS depressants including anesthetics on subtypes of the inhibitory GABA$_A$ receptor-chloride channel complex. *Ann NY Acad Sci* 625:145–154, 1991.

41. Gee KW: Steroid modulation of the GABA/benzodiazeprine receptor-linked chloride ionophore. *Mol Neurobiol* 2:291–317, 1988.

42. Majewski MD, Harrison NL, Schwartz RD, *et al:* Steroid hormones metabolites are barbiturate-like modulators of the GABA receptor. *Science* 232:1004–1007, 1986.

43. Smith SS, Waterhouse BD, Chapin JK, Woodward DJ: Progesterone alters GABA and glutamate responsiveness: A possible mechanism for its anxiolytic action. *Brain Res* 400:353–359, 1987.

44. Puia G, Vicini S, Seeburg PH, Costa E: Different sites of action of neurosteroids and benzodiazepines on natural and recombinant GABA$_A$ receptors, in Biggio G, Concas A, Costa E (eds): *GABAergic Synaptic Transmission.* New York, Raven Press, 1992, pp 103–110.

45. Canonaco M, Valenti A, Tavolaro R, *et al:* Differential modulation of [3H]flunitrazepam binding in female rat brain by sex steroid hormones. *Eur J Pharmacol* 160:95–99, 1989.

46. Pérez J, Zucchi I, Maggi A: Estrogen modulation of the GABA receptor complex in the central nervous system of the rat. *J Pharmacol Exp Ther* 244:1005–1010, 1988.

47. Wilkinson M, Bhanot R, Wilkinson DA, Brawer JR: Prolonged estrogen treatment induces changes in opiate, benzodiazepine, and β-adrenergic binding sites in female rat hypothalamus. *Brain Res Bull* 11:279–281, 1983.

48. Schumacher M, Coirini H, McEwen BS: Regulation of high-affinity GABA$_A$ receptors in the dorsal hippocampus by estradiol and progesterone. *Brain Res* 487:178–183, 1989.

49. Harmon M, Goetz C, Euvrard C, *et al:* Biochemical and functional alterations of GABA receptors during chronic estradiol treatment. *Brain Res* 279:141–152, 1983.

50. Wilson MA: Influences of gender, gonadectomy, and estrous cycle on GABA/BZ receptors and benzodiazepine responses in rats. *Brain Res Bull* 29:165–172, 1992.

51. Shephard RA, Nielson EB, Broadhurst PL: Sex and strain differences in benzodiazepine receptor binding in Roman rat strains. *Eur J Pharmacol* 77:327–330, 1982.

52. Koob GF, Strecker RE, Bloom FE: Effects of naloxone on the anticonflict properties of alcohol and chlordiazepoxide substance. *Subst Alcohol Actions Misuse* 1:447–457, 1980.

53. Britton KT, Ehlers CL, Koob GF: Ethanol antagonist, Ro-4513, is not selective for ethanol. *Science* 239:648–649, 1987.

54. Koob GF, Britton KT, Britton D, *et al:* Destruction of the locus coeruleus or dorsal noradrenergic bundle does not alter release of punished responding by ethanol and chlordiazepoxide. *Physiol Behav* 33:479–485, 1984.

55. Britton KT, Page M, Baldwin H, Koob GF: Anxiolytic activity of steroid anesthetic alphaxolone. *J Pharmacol Exp Ther* 258:124–129, 1991.

56. Fink G, Sarkar DK, Dow RC, *et al:* Sex difference in response to alphaxalone anaesthesia may be oestrogen dependent. *Nature* 298:270–272, 1982.

57. Gee KW, Change W, Brinton RE, McEwen BS: GABA-dependent modulation of Cl-ionophore by steroids in the rat brain. *Eur J Pharmacol* 136:419–423, 1987.

58. Morrow AL, Suzdak PD, Paul SM: Steroid hormone metabolites potentiate GABA receptor-mediated chloride ion flux with nanomolar potency. *Eur J Pharmacol* 142:483–485, 1987.

59. Ladisch W: Influence of stress on regional brain serotonin metabolism after progesterone treatment and upon plasma progesterone in the rat. *J Neural Transm* 36:33–42, 1975.

60. Schamblen M, Biglieri E: Deoxycorticosterone production and regulation in man. *J Clin Endocrinol Metab* 34:695–703, 1972.

61. Purdy RH, Morrow AL, Moore PH, Paul SM: Stress-induced elevations of γ-aminobutyric acid type A receptor-active steroids in the rat brain. *Proc Natl Acad Sci* 88:4553–4557, 1991.

62. Britton KT, McLeod S, Koob GF, Hauger R: Pregnane steroid alphaxalone attenuates anxiogenic behavioral effects of corticotropin releasing factor and stress. *Pharmacol Biochem Behav* 41:399–403, 1992.

63. Britton KT, Koob GF: Ethanol reverses the proconflict effect of corticotropin releasing factor. *Regul Pept* 16:315–320, 1986.

64. Britton KT, Morgan J, Rivier J, Koob GF: Chlordiazepoxide attenuates CRF-induced response suppression in the conflict test. *Psychopharmacology* 86:170–174, 1985.

65. Capell H, Herman CP: Alcohol and tension reduction. *Q J Stud Alcohol* 33:33–64, 1972.

66. Pohorecky LA: The interaction of alcohol and stress. A review. *Neurosci Biobehav Rev* 5:209–229, 1981.

67. Polivy J, Schuenemen AC, Carlson K: Alcohol and tension reduction. *J Abnorm Psychol* 85:595–600, 1976.

68. Koob GF, Braestrup C, Britton KT: The effects of FG7142 and Ro15-1788 on the release of punished responding produced by chlordiazepoxide and ethanol in the rat. *Psychopharmacology* 90:173–178, 1986.

69. De Boer MC, Schippers GM, Van Der Staak CPF: Alcohol and social anxiety in women and men: Pharmacological and expectancy effects. *Addict Behav* 18:117–126, 1993.

70. Abrams DB, Wilson GT: Effects of alcohol on social anxiety in women: Cognitive versus physiological processes. *J Abnorm Psychol* 88:161–173, 1979.

71. Dunne FJ, Galatopoulos C, Schipperheijn JM: Gender differences in psychiatric morbidity among alcohol misusers. *Compr Psychiatry* 34:95–101, 1993.

72. Berger BD, Adesso VJ: Gender differences in using alcohol to cope with depression. *Addict Behav* 16:315–327, 1991.
73. Kalodner CR, Delucia JL, Ursprung AW: An examination of the tension reduction hypothesis: The relationship between anxiety and alcohol in college students. *Addict Behav* 14:649–654, 1989.
74. Blanchard RJ, Blanchard DC, Weiss SM: Ethanol effects in an anxiety/defense test battery. *Alcohol* 7:375–381, 1990.
75. Messiha FS: Steroidal actions and voluntary drinking of ethanol by male and female rats. *Prog Biochem Pharmacol* 18:205–215, 1981.
76. Carey MP, Billing AE, Fry JP: Fluctuations in responses to diazepam during the oestrous cycle in the mouse. *Pharmacol Biochem Behav* 41:719–725, 1992.
77. Fernández-Guasti A, Picazo O: Changes in anxiety levels along the various phases of the estrous cycle. Submitted.
78. O'Connor LH, Nock B, McEwen BS: Regional specificity of gamma-aminobutyric acid receptor regulation of estradiol. *Neuroendocrinology* 47:473–481, 1988.
79. Peréz J, Zucchi I, Maggi A: Sexual dimorphism in the response of the GABAergic system to estrogen administration. *J Neurochem* 47:1798–1803, 1986.
80. Turner JP: Potentiation of the GABA analogue muscimol by physiologically occurring steroids. *Br J Pharmacol* 87:148P, 1986.
81. Schwartz RD: The GABA$_A$ receptor-gated ion channel: Biochemical and pharmacological studies of structure and function. *Biochem Pharmacol* 37:3369–3375, 1988.

III

Behavior and Treatment Issues

Alfonso Paredes, Section Editor

Overview

Alfonso Paredes

The lifetime prevalence of alcohol dependence among persons aged 15 to 54 years is 8.2% for women and 20.1% for men.[1] Although females seem to be less at risk than males, this does not justify the lack of information about alcohol problems in women which until recently was characteristic in the scientific literature. Nixon[2] notes that until slightly more than 10 years ago, the issue of female alcoholism was seldom mentioned in the research literature. Women, sex, or gender was not even indexed in Jellineck's classic book *The Disease Model of Alcoholism*.[3] To a great extent, the literature on alcoholism was written from a male perspective, leading to extrapolations and unverified assumptions. The complex relationships between alcohol and gender were often explained with simple theories, when multivariate analyses could have been applied to elucidate how clusters of variables operate to increase or reduce the risks of problem drinking.[4] Much new information is becoming available. This is exemplified by the review chapters of this book, including the contributions to this section.

The mechanisms responsible for gender differences in alcoholism risk are poorly understood. This understanding will be necessary to address more effectively the problem as it affects women. Adequate explanations require data gleaned from different vantage points. This section presents information from three different perspectives by researchers with considerable experience in the area. The interrelationships between women, alcohol, and sexuality are examined first, followed by a chapter on cognitive performance and recovery in women alcoholics, and then by a chapter discussing the development of alcohol treatment services for women. In the following paragraphs, I will

Alfonso Paredes • Residential Treatment Center, West Los Angeles Veterans Administration Medial Center, University of California School of Medicine, Los Angeles, California 90024.

Recent Developments in Alcoholism, Volume 12: Women and Alcoholism, edited by Marc Galanter. Plenum Press, New York, 1995

outline some of the highlights in these chapters. This may encourage the reader to attend closely to the important material in this section.

The chapter entitled "Women, Alcohol, and Sexuality" by Linda J. Beckman and Kimberly T. Ackerman indicates that, from the perspective of sexual behavior, studies on its relationships with alcohol use have been stimulated by the emergence of AIDS as a major health problem and by the increasing public response to violence against women. The high frequency of alcohol use by perpetrators and victims during sexual assaults is a well-known fact. This has increased the concern for new information that may explain such behavior.

The interactions between sexual behavior and alcohol in women are complex. In this area many assumptions are made without adequate validation. It is noted that there are significant discrepancies between the assumed effects of alcohol on sexual responsiveness in females and the physiological effects. These effects are actually suppressed or decreased rather than stimulated. Women appear to have internalized commonly held views such as the assumed sexually arousing effects of alcohol. The expectancies may have an influence on how alcohol effects are interpreted.

Sexual dysfunction seems to play a role in alcohol dependence since this problem is more prevalent among alcoholic women than in nonalcoholics. It is suggested that some women alcoholics may use alcohol to relieve symptoms of sexual dysfunction. Sexual trauma appears to play a role as a risk factor in alcoholism. There is a strong association between incest during childhood, sexual abuse, and alcohol dependence. In regard to alcohol and violence, women who experience sexual assault or rape are often the victims of intoxicated offenders. Women with histories of sexual assault report drinking more than those without such history. Sexual assaults may be related to male expectations regarding the effects of alcohol in women. Males may feel that drinking makes women more receptive, interpreting drinking in dating situations as indicative of a woman's willingness to have sex.

Sara Jo Nixon and Susan Wagner Glenn, in their chapter entitled "Cognitive Psychosocial Performance and Recovery in Female Alcoholics," have provided a review of the literature and shared their considerable research experience on this topic. The attempt to contrast the findings in male populations with those in women is a particularly challenging task given that women have been understudied and undertreated. Despite this limitation, several interesting trends emerge. The characteristics of alcohol-related problems in males and females show significant differences. Males are more likely to experience difficulties in psychosocial adjustment variables regarding, for example, work or school performance. They are more likely to face vehicular charges and legal problems and experience medical difficulties. Females, on the other hand, are more likely to report psychological problems, such as depression, in association with the use of alcohol. Particularly striking is the preexistence of depression as a prominent symptom before drinking becomes a problem. Women are more vulnerable to physical and verbal conflicts and more likely to be diagnosed as having an affective disorder.

There is considerable similarity in the nature and degree of cognitive impairment in males and female alcoholics despite the fact that women report shorter length and lesser amounts of alcohol use. Like males, they exhibit a range of cognitive deficits well described by the researchers team. These deficits seem to recover slowly and incompletely following a predictable sequence. For example, verbal deficits recover first, followed by complex abstract function and problem solving, and lastly perceptual motor skills. Interestingly, cognitive physiological correlates such as visual evoked potentials do not seem to parallel the improvements assessed through neuropsychological testing.

Anatomical and functional changes related to heavy alcohol use have been well documented with new imaging techniques. So far these deficits have not been found to differ in male and female alcoholics. Data on women are relatively scarce, however.

The clinical course of alcohol dependence does not seem to differ between the sexes, but the protective factors are different. Marital status is associated with a low risk of relapse in men but not in women. Strikingly, the proportion of women who seem to be able to resume some drinking without severe consequences is much larger than among their male counterparts.

Laura Schmidt and Constance Weisner, in the chapter entitled "The Emergence of Problem-Drinking Women as a Special Population in Need of Treatment," have reviewed the emergence of treatment programs to address problem drinking in women. The demand for gender-sensitive treatment has increased. This is reflected by the substantial number of specialized treatment units for women that have been created within the last few years. From the philosophy of programs some critical postures have emerged vis-à-vis concepts such as "codependency" and "enabling." These terms have been criticized because they reflect traditional stereotypes such as the "housewife who drinks to relieve boredom" or the woman who "drinks to relieve work stress." Much more work is still ahead to address the stereotypes that exist regarding alcohol and women. There is, for example, a need to better study occupations that may create social conflicts or resources that weaken or strengthen the adverse consequences of women's drinking behavior.

It is noted that, as is the case with other alcohol issues, many of the arguments about alcohol-related problems in women and their appropriate treatment have been influenced by sociopolitical considerations rather than empirical data.

The authors point out interesting challenges facing researchers. For instance, the following question is raised: Are the conventional indicators of alcohol problems in women valid? Perhaps new indicators more appropriate to women's experience need to be devised. It is also noted that the effectiveness of special treatment approaches for women awaits validation. Studies on therapies especially designed for women are almost nonexistent. In spite of these limitations, there has been a governmental trend to increase the support of treatment for women in specialized gender-oriented programs. The access of women to treatment has improved. This development provides deserved political recognition to the problems affecting women, but it may have led to a fragmentation of health care systems.

Last, we must heed an important challenge: diseases that affect women disproportionally are less likely to be studied, women are less likely to be included in clinical trials, and they are less likely to be senior investigators conducting the trials.[5] This is a situation that obviously requires addressing.

References

1. Kessler R, McGonagle K, Zhao Z, *et al:* Psychiatric disorders in the United States. *Arch Gen Psychiatry* 51:8–19, 1994.
2. Nixon SJ: Typologies in women, in Galanter M (ed): *Recent Developments in Alcoholism*. New York, Plenum Press, 1993, vol 11, pp 305–323.
3. Jellineck EM: *The Disease Model of Alcoholism*. New Brunswick, Hillhouse Press, 1960.
4. Wilsnack RW, Wilsnack SC: Women, work, and alcohol: Failures of simple theories. *Alcohol Clin Exp Res* 16:172–179, 1992.
5. Angell M: Caring for women's health—What is the Problem. *N Engl J Med* 329:271–272, 1993.

Women, Alcohol, and Sexuality

Linda J. Beckman and Kimberly T. Ackerman

Abstract. Alcohol consumption increases subjective sexual desire, arousal, and pleasure for many women, although it lowers physiological arousal. Despite the general belief that alcohol disinhibits female sexual behaviors, alcohol leads to changes in sexual behavior only for a minority of women. Expectancies about the effects of alcohol on sexual behavior may be important mediators of the alcohol–sexual behavior linkage. There also is a relationship between overall alcohol consumption and risky sexual behavior for women, but when alcohol use at or preceding individual instances of sexual activity is examined, there is no association in the majority of studies. Alcohol use by both perpetrators and victims has been implicated in instances of sexual victimization. Heavy alcohol consumption and alcohol problems in women are associated with heightened risk of childhood incest, sexual assault, and sexual dysfunction.

The last ten years have witnessed a dramatic increase in some areas of research involving alcohol and sexual behavior in women, while other areas have remained dormant. Most notably, the devastating scourge of AIDS since the early 1980s and the recent rise in the United States in the percentage of AIDS cases involving heterosexual transmission have led to a focus on the role of alcohol in promoting risky sexual behavior. Second, an increasing awareness of the high incidence of violence against women and the frequent presence of alcohol consumption among both perpetrators and victims of sexual assault have resulted in a burgeoning series of studies that attempt to better understand the role of alcohol in incidents of rape and incest. Finally, research on alcohol-related expectancies, beliefs, and attributions that grew rapidly in the early to middle 1980s has continued to grow, albeit at a reduced rate. In contrast, the study of alcohol and female sexual arousal, responsiveness, and dysfunction and of sexual behavior in specific subgroups

Linda J. Beckman and Kimberly T. Ackerman • California School of Professional Psychology, Los Angeles Campus, Alhambra, California 91803-1360.

Recent Developments in Alcoholism, Volume 12: Women and Alcoholism, edited by Marc Galanter. Plenum Press, New York, 1995

of women, with the exception of those at high risk for HIV, has remained sparse.

The purpose of this chapter is to review and critique recent research on women, sexuality, and alcohol from all of the above areas. In this review we emphasize research that has been published since Wilsnack's excellent 1984 review.[1] Sexuality is one area in which women are not expected to be like men. Although to some extent women have been ignored in research in this area, it is widely accepted that gender differences in sexuality and sexual behavior exist. For instance, a recent meta-analysis of gender differences in sexuality[2] reported that men and women show differences in both the incidence of specific types of sexual behavior (e.g., masturbation), with men reporting higher levels, and sexual attitudes, with men having more permissive attitudes toward casual sex. Similarly, with regard to sexual violence, it is widely recognized that women are more often the victims of abuse rather than the perpetrators. While at times differences between women and men will be discussed, it is not our purpose to examine gender differences in alcohol consumption and sexual behavior. Rather, this chapter reviews the empirical literature and clinical research on alcohol consumption and sexuality for women, a group whose alcohol consumption and sexuality have (separately and jointly) too frequently been ignored in the research literature.

The research on women, alcohol, and sexuality presents a series of conflicting views, unanswered questions, and methodological problems. Definitions of alcohol abuse and alcohol consumption vary in different studies and almost all studies of alcoholism in women are studies of women in treatment and/or recovery. Few studies of nonalcoholic and nonproblem drinking in women have examined dose–response relationships in a systematic way. Definitions that attempted to discern problem drinking and alcoholism for men sometimes have been poorly adapted to measure the patterns of drinking exhibited by women. Definitions of sexual dysfunction, sexual assault, rape, and incest have fluctuated across studies, making cross-study comparisons problematic. In many earlier studies only these terms (e.g., have you even been *raped?*) were presented to participants. Only in more recent studies have definitions been more precise, focusing on specific situations and behaviors.

Sexuality is a multidimensional concept. When examining alcohol use and female sexuality, we find the following dimensions most appropriate: (1) physiological sexual responsiveness; (2) subjective feelings of sexuality, that is, subjective arousal, desire, and enjoyment; (3) expectancies about alcohol and sexuality; sexual behaviors, that is, types and frequency of sexual acts including coerced sex and sexual behaviors that heighten risks of AIDS and other sexually transmitted diseases (STDs); and (4) sexual partners, including the number and type of partners. Each dimension interacts with other dimensions and more than one dimension may have a specific effect; for instance, number of sexual partners is itself a risk factor for STDs and AIDS.

1. Alcohol Use, Physiological Sexual Arousal, and Sexual Feelings

For women a discrepancy exists between the reported effects of alcohol use on sexual responsiveness and physiological indices of these effects. Generally women report that alcohol at least in moderate amounts has positive effects on sexual feelings, yet laboratory studies suggest that alcohol suppresses physiological sexual responsiveness in women. Level of alcohol consumption has been found to be negatively associated with vaginal blood flow[3] and positively associated with the time to achieve orgasm during masturbation.[4] As consumption increased, women in the Malatesta *et al.*[4] study also reported increased difficulty in having an orgasm and decreased organismic intensity. What is surprising is that in all of these studies, women's *self-reports* reveal greater sexual arousal and sexual pleasure with increasing blood alcohol levels.

The reputed aphrodisiac effects of alcohol for women have been widely accepted for thousands of years in Western society. The results of many survey studies, as well as the laboratory studies discussed above, suggest that women have internalized such views. Many contemporary women without alcohol problems report in surveys and other nonlaboratory studies that they experience increased sexual desire, feelings, and arousal and decreased sexual inhibitions when drinking.[1,5,6] For instance, Beckman[5] found that for women without a history of alcoholism or other psychiatric disorder, 29% reported they desired intercourse more after alcohol consumption and 32% reported they enjoyed intercourse more after drinking. In a recent national survey of women's drinking in the United States, Wilsnack *et al.*[7] found that 59% of light- and moderate-drinking women and 68% of heavy-drinking women stated that alcohol sometimes or usually resulted in less sexual inhibition.

Method of data collection may have an effect on results. In a study of 69 female volunteers aged 18 to 34, the retrospective questionnaire data indicated that alcohol enhanced female sexuality, while results from daily diaries kept over two to three menstrual cycles suggested that drinking had little effect on sexuality.[8] Apparently, women expect alcohol to affect sexuality. Therefore, they report these effects when retrospectively reporting on frequency or presence of behavior over a considerable time period, whereas daily reports, which are less subject to distortion due to beliefs about alcohol and sexuality, show no association.

And what of the effects of alcohol on sexuality among women who are alcohol abusers? Do the expected effects of alcohol serve as a reason for drinking for these women? Beckman[5] found that alcoholic women were more likely to report increased sexual desire, enjoyment, and activity after drinking compared with both women without drinking problems and women with other psychiatric problems. Other studies of alcoholic women suggest that responses to alcohol may be bimodal, with approximately equal proportions indicating that drinking has positive and negative effects on sexual arousal and performance.[9] Interestingly, Jenson[10] found that 50% of alcoholic women believed that alcohol relieved their sexual problems, usually problems of lack of sexual desire, even though 25% of these women identified as having sexual dysfunctions. Klassen and Wilsnack[6] report that heavier-drinking women in their national survey were more likely to indicate that alcohol consumption sometimes or usually made them feel less inhibited sexually. They interpret these findings as suggesting that expectations of disinhibition of sexuality might serve as a motive for drinking for some women.

Several explanations have been put forth to explain the discrepancy between reported and actual effects of alcohol on female sexual responsiveness and desire including: (1) both pharmacological (through effects on cognitive functioning) and psychological disinhibition[11]; (2) the presence of a generalized state of physiological arousal that women interpret as sexual arousal[1]; (3) social learning theory[12]; and (4) expectations about how alcohol will affect sexual feelings and behavior that lead to psychological disinhibition.[1,11]

2. Alcohol Use and Sexual Behavior

Generally, when "disinhibition" as a consequence of alcohol use is discussed major interest is in the disinhibition of behavior rather than feelings. Alcohol could directly disinhibit behavior through its physiological and expectancy effects or alcohol could heighten sexual feelings which in turn could lead to changes in sexual behavior.

A global relationship between overall frequency or quantity of alcohol use and overall frequency of sexual behavior in women does exist. Women who drink more heavily may evidence more "nontraditional" sexual behaviors, including premarital intercourse, masturbation to orgasm, and admitted homosexual feelings.[6]

It is commonly believed that young women, particularly those in new or casual relationships, are more likely to engage in sexual behavior after they consume alcohol. However, whereas the literature clearly suggests that alcohol use, at least in moderate amount, increases feelings of sexual arousal and desire and decreases feelings of inhibition for some groups of women, much less evidence supports its disinhibition of women's sexual behavior. Feelings about sex—sexual desires and urges—that may be enhanced through alcohol use are not necessarily reflected in behavior. In fact, in a daily diary study, alcohol consumption by women was inversely related to female-initiated sexual activity.[8] Only 22% of respondents in the national sample of women's drinking reported ever becoming more "sexually forward" when drinking and only 8% stated they became "less particular in choice of sexual partners."[6] Other studies indicate that relative equal percentages of women think alcohol consumption has positive and negative effects on sexual performance,[9] and still others find no differences in sexual activity between alcoholic and nonalcoholic women.[13]

2.1. Alcohol Use and Risky Sexual Behavior

Women now constitute the fastest growing group likely to contract AIDS and the proportion of adolescent girls who have become infected is "worryingly high."[14] Moreover, minority women have been disproportionally affected by the AIDS epidemic; the number of reported AIDS cases associated with heterosexual transmission has been steadily increasing, and these cases occur more frequently in women than men.[14] Two major risky sexual behaviors are nonuse of condoms and vaginal or anal intercourse with multiple partners. Although use of condoms has increased among US women since 1985, most investigators concur that the majority of adolescents and young adults at risk do not use condoms regularly during intercourse.[15]

The literature supports a relationship between overall alcohol use and engaging in risky sexual behaviors. Persons who drink more heavily have more sexual partners and less frequently use condoms.[16] While few studies focus specifically on women, a recent investigation[17] provides indirect evidence that alcohol use is associated with risky sexual behavior in women. This representative survey of 968 households in the San Francisco Bay area in 1988–89 strongly supports problem drinking as a risk factor for STDs. Female problem drinkers were approximately 4.5 times more likely to have had an STD even when all other potential risk factors (e.g., age, drug use) were controlled. Problem drinking heightened risk of STDs more than did a history of multiple sexual partners. It is noteworthy that among women, two drinking variables—frequent bar going and high-volume drinking—were important contributors to a history of a high number of sexual partners when other factors were controlled. Thus, these two variables indirectly contribute to risk of HIV and other STDs.

When the relationship between risky sexual behaviors and the use of alcohol immediately preceding or at the time of sexual contract is retrospectively reported for a specific time period, the trend is for alcohol consumption and risky sex to be associated. In many cases, this association may be attributable to uncontrolled third variables. For instance, in a survey of the San Francisco Bay area, a strong relationship was found for women, and men as well, between frequency of alcohol consumption in conjunction with sexual activity and the frequency of sexual risk-taking, but the relationship disappeared when total amount of sexual activity was taken into account.[18]

When women are asked about alcohol use associated with discrete sexual events, results are mixed, with most studies showing no differences in unprotected sex between drinking and nondrinking sexual encounters.[16] In one study[19] of adolescents, however, drinking prior to specific instances of intercourse (first intercourse with most recent partner and first instance of intercourse) increased the likelihood of risky sex. These effects remained significant after controlling for age, race, and pattern of alcohol use and were similar for girls and boys. In contrast, the only two studies that have used a daily diary method to examine the relationship between alcohol use and sexual behavior on the individual incident level[8,20] did not support a positive association between alcohol use and risky sexual practices. Harvey and Beckman[8] reported no relationship between coitus-dependent contraceptive use and alcohol consumption, whereas Leigh[20] found that for sex with new partners there was a trend toward more safe sex when drinking occurred.

3. Expectancies about Alcohol Consumption and Sexual Behavior in Women

The psychological disinhibitory effects of alcohol on sexual functioning at least for a subgroup of women may be due to socially learned expectations. Crowne and George[11] define alcohol expectancies as beliefs regarding alcohol's influence on behavior as well as beliefs regarding its effect as a mediating variable on social judgments. As Cooper *et al.*[21] have pointed out, if alcohol provides an "anticipatory excuse" for engaging in risky sexual behaviors, individuals who engage in such behaviors should show a combination of specific beliefs about its excuse-giving properties. The *belief* that alcohol has been consumed appears to have had no effect on sexual arousal for women.[22] However, more specific social expectancies about the effects of alcohol on sexuality, sexual desire, and sexual behavior may play a significant causal role in the association between alcohol consumption and risky sex.[18]

A key question is does the expectancy that drinking leads to less inhibition influence women's drinking in a sexual or potentially sexual situation. The literature suggests that expectancies about the effects of alcohol on sexual feelings and behavior motivate drinking for some women. Klassen and Wilsnack[6] interpret their findings as suggesting that this expectation may serve as a motive for drinking, and women in our sexually repressed society may use alcohol to counteract the sexual suppression that they experience. Kline[23] found no evidence of gender differences in expectancies for sexual enhancement; but for women the belief that alcohol enhances sexuality was associated with social rather than solitary drinking, which is to be expected if drinking disinhibits sexual behavior since sex is a social act.

Leigh[24] recently studied sexual-related alcohol expectancies in a community sample of adults aged 18 to 50 in San Francisco. Heavier drinkers more strongly endorsed positive beliefs about the effects of alcohol on sexual responsiveness (e.g., enhances sexual experience, decreases nervousness). She found an interaction between negative sexual attitudes (i.e., more guilt about sex, nervousness, etc.) and alcohol expectancies among heterosexual women. Women with negative sexual attitudes and strong expectancies drank the most during their last sexual encounter. Also, women with stronger alcohol expectancies were twice as likely to initiate sexual activity as women with weaker expectancies. Her results suggest that expectancies are most likely to motivate drinking in women in need of an excuse for sexual disinhibition.

More research is needed on identification of individual differences that moderate the association between expectancies and sexual feelings and behaviors for women. It is possible that negative sexual attitudes, nervousness about sexual encounters, poor interpersonal communication skills, certain types of sexual dysfunction, past sexual experiences, and heavy alcohol consumption may help explain the association or lack of association between alcohol expectancies and the "disinhibition" of sexual behavior.

4. Alcohol Use and Sexual Dysfunction

Despite some alcoholic women's beliefs about the positive effects of alcohol consumption on female sexual functioning, there is a "dark side" of the effects of alcohol on women's sexual and reproductive functioning. Alcoholic women are often characterized as having sexual problems including "frigidity," anorgasmia, dyspareunia, and vaginismus.[25] Most of the evidence supporting this view has been gleaned from clinical studies that lack adequate controls. There are, however, a number of studies involving nonalcoholic or other psychiatric control groups.[7,13,26,27] For the most part, the present analysis only touches on the earlier clinical studies that lack control groups, focusing instead on the control group and recent national survey results.

Types of female sexual dysfunction include low sexual desire, difficulties in sexual arousal, primary organismic disorder, secondary organismic disorder, vaginismus (contractions of the vagina that interfere with intercourse and can make it impossible to achieve intercourse), and dyspareunia (painful intercourse). Clinical studies suggest that lack of sexual interest and sexual inhibition in alcoholic women ranges between 23 and 100%.[1] Rates of primary and secondary organismic dysfunction combined range from about 15 to 64%.[1] Most studies do not report rates of vaginismus or dyspareunia separately nor do they report on difficulties in sexual arousal distinct from organismic dysfunction. Two exceptions are Hammond et al.[28] and Murphy et al.[9] Hammond et al.[28] reported that 12% of their sample of 44 alcoholic outpatients reported vaginismus on 50% or more of sexual encounters and 7% reported dyspareunia 95% or more of the time. Murphy et al.[9] found that only 2% of their sample reported vaginismus on 50% or more of sexual occasions and 6% reported dyspareunia on 50% or more of occasions. These rates are considerably below rates of problems of sexual desire (23% and 30%, respectively) and primary or secondary organismic dysfunction (54% and 28%, respectively).

Although rates of sexual problems and sexual dysfunction of alcoholics in treatment appear to be higher than for the general population, the sociodemographic characteristics of alcoholic women in treatment do not mirror those of the general population. Therefore, studies that have included control groups of demographically similar nonalcoholic women are particularly important when trying to establish an association between alcohol use and sexual dysfunction. Pinhas[26] compared 34 alcohol and 34 nonalcoholic women matched on age, ethnicity, education, socioeconomic status, marital status, and religious preference. Using a standardized questionnaire she found that alcoholic women reported more guilt surrounding sexual behaviors and sexuality than did the nonalcoholic women. In a second study,[27] 35 middle-class white alcoholic women were compared with 35 white nonalcoholic women matched on age, education, marital status, and religious preference. Over 85% of the alcoholic women reported that they had experienced at least one type of sexual dysfunction while they were drinking, while 59% of the control group women reported any sexual dysfunction. As in other studies the most common sexual problems were lack of sexual interest, lack of sexual arousal or pleasure, and difficulty in reaching an orgasm.

A final control group study[13] compared 55 women alcoholics and a control group of 54 nonalcoholics that were selected using a snowball technique and matched on age, marital status, number of children, social class, and education. Their standardized questionnaire was based on Helen Singer Kaplan's[29] theory of disorders of sexual desire. They found that alcoholic women were more likely to have negative attitudes toward sexuality (one of their indices of a sexual desire disorder) including severe feelings of depression linked to sexuality and a decrease in sexual desire over time. Alcoholic women also were more likely to evidence antecedents of sexual desire disorders, hypothesized by Kaplan: prematurely turning off sexual feelings with inhibiting thoughts and avoiding intimate situations that may involve sex; greater difficulty in communication with one's partner about sexuality; greater hostility toward and from partner; and more fear of physical contact and sexual anxiety. Differences between the two groups in the expected effects of alcohol on sexual enhancement, sexual relaxation, and alcohol as a substitute for sexual satisfaction support the conclusion that alcoholic women appear more likely to self-medicate by using alcohol in the face of sexual problems.

One major issue not answered by these studies is the causal relationship between alcohol consumption and sexual dysfunction. It frequently is assumed that excessive alcohol use precedes development of female sexual dysfunction; but, as suggested above, sexual difficulties may also precede and cause alcohol abuse. Two small clinical studies[27,30] have provided information on the retrospectively reported temporal relationship between alcohol use and sexual dysfunction. Both report that a large percentage of women experienced sexual dysfunction preceding their problem drinking and reported sexual dysfunction increases after problem drinking begins.

The Wilsnack et al.[31] 5-year follow-up of the 1981 national survey of women's drinking provides important data on the temporal interrelationship between drinking practices and sexual dysfunction. Interviews were conducted with two groups of women who had participated in the 1981 survey: 143 identified as problem drinkers and 157 nonproblem drinkers. Among women who were problem drinkers in 1981 the best predictor of chronic problem drinking in 1986 was level of sexual dysfunction (defined as lack of sexual interest, vaginismus, primary or secondary organismic disorder) reported in 1981. This effect was upheld when age was controlled and other demographic, personality, social–environmental, and life history event were entered into the multiple regression equation. In contrast, sexual dysfunction in 1981 did not predict the onset of alcohol problems among women in the nonproblem drinker group by 1986. These findings suggest that women problem drinkers use alcohol to cope with sexual dysfunction, but retrospective reports that sexual dysfunction precedes problem drinking are not supported. Of course, 5 years is a relatively short time period for problem drinking to develop and may not be sufficient to evaluate this relationship. It is noteworthy, however, that in the 1981 survey[6] there was little relationship between level of alcohol consumption and sexual dysfunction; a curvilinear relationship suggested that moderate drinking may have a facilitating effect on sexual functioning. There remains a need for prospective, longitudinal research that examines the relationships between women's heavy and problem drinking and types of sexual dysfunction.

5. Sexual Orientation

Among variation in sexuality involves sex of partner. The percentage of women alcoholics who report having had one or more homosexual experience varies widely, ranging from 4 to 45%.[1] The figures vary by sample characteristics and year of data collection, with more recent studies generally reporting higher levels of homosexual experience. This reported change may be due to changing attitudes about the provision of sensitive information involving sexual behavior rather than to an actual increase in homosexual experience. The above figures include women who describe themselves as bisexual or as having had one or more same-sex experience as well as those who self-define as lesbian. For instance, although 20% of the women alcoholics in Beckman's[5] study reported at least one same-sex sexual experience, only 6% considered themselves homosexual and 3% identified as bisexual. Beckman's[5] study was one of the few with multiple control groups of women. In this study the alcoholic women were more likely to have had a homosexual experience than the "normal" nontreatment controls, but they did not differ significantly from the psychiatric treatment control group.

In the few studies of women alcoholics[5,27,32] in which the percentage of women who self-identify as lesbians as differentiated from bisexual is calculated, the range is from 2 to 29%, a figure higher than the 2–3% of women estimated to be lesbian in the general population.[33]

When a complementary approach is adopted and the rate of alcohol abuse among homosexuals is examined, clinical studies and community surveys both suggest high rates of alcohol problems in female and male homosexuals.[1] In community surveys the rates of alcohol problems among lesbians and gay men have been estimated at as much as 30%, a rate much higher than that of the general population.[34–36] Additionally, the percentage of abstainers in the homosexual community is half that found in the general population, 14% versus 29%, respectively.[37]

A criticism of research looking at homosexual populations and alcohol use is that samples are selected mainly from bars and drinking establishments. Thus the rates of reported alcohol use and abuse may be overestimated. In a large study ($N = 3400$) in an urban setting, McKirnan and Peterson[37] distributed surveys through a large homosexual-oriented newspaper, advertisements in mainstream publications, groups serving the homosexual community, and large events within the homosexual community. Only 5% of their respondents learned about the survey in a bar setting. Responses from this homosexual sample were compared with results from a 1979 national general population survey, but apparently comparisons were not adjusted for demographic and other differences between the two samples. Usage of alcohol by the homosexual sample was higher than in the general population and homosexual women and men were much more similar in drinking patterns and rates of alcohol problems than were women and men in the general population sample. Heavy drinking, defined as over 60 drinks a month, was not found to be higher in homosexuals, but they reported a higher rate of alcohol-related problems. What is most interesting is that lesbians had identical rates of alcohol problems as men homosexuals and there was a large difference in problem prevalence between lesbians and general population women (23% vs. 8%). At every age group, lesbians reported alcohol-related problems that exceeded those of heterosexual women, although differences were greatest at ages 26 to 40. The authors concluded that these differences in alcohol-problem prevalence may be due to psychosocial and cultural factors related to lower role responsibilities of lesbian women compared with their heterosexual counterparts in more traditional social environments. The levels of reported alcohol problems remain relatively stable with age for lesbian women but decrease dramatically for heterosexual women. It is assumed that as they get older many heterosexual women have increased role responsibilities associated with marriage and children which leads to a decrease in their alcohol consumption and as a consequence a lower rate of alcohol-related problems.

Lesbians may drink for different reasons and develop alcohol problems through different pathways than heterosexual women. They may drink as a way of coping with the stigma and discrimination that they experience as lesbians or, for some, the stress of attempting to appear straight to family or co-workers. There is evidence suggesting that lesbians receive less support from families than do heterosexual women. Mays et al.[32] found that African-American alcoholic women who are lesbian or bisexual received less social support for treatment entry from family and from male sources than did heterosexual black women alcoholics. Lesbians also may drink for social and cultural reasons that reflect the lifestyle of certain groups of lesbians.[37] Heavy-drinking norms exist in many lesbian communities and lesbians may congregate in occupations in which drinking is part of the lifestyle, expected of those who wish to attain success. Important issues for future research include the effects, if any, of the recent national emphasis on health and curtailment of consumption in some environments (e.g., if you intend to drive) on the lesbian community; drinking patterns of subgroups of lesbians who maintain different lifestyles; and the interactions of environmental stress (including stigma and discrimination), quality of social support, and coping strategies on the consumption and alcohol problems of lesbian women.

6. Sexual Violence against Women

Before 1980, there were few published data on alcohol use and abuse as a precursor, concomitant, or consequence of sexual violence toward women. In the last 10–15 years the extent to which many women suffer sexual abuse and violence at the hands of a drinking perpetrator has been recognized, and researchers have attempted to understand the complex relationships between alcohol use and violence against women. Most theories consider alcohol consumption or alcohol abuse in victim or perpetrator as an antecedent or contributor to sexual abuse.

6.1. Incest and Childhood Sexual Abuse

The first national study of childhood sexual victimization reported a rate of 27% for women.[38] Moreover, these estimates are probably low due to underreporting. There are only occasional references in the literature on childhood incest (or other childhood sexual abuse) to its role in the development of alcohol abuse in women,[39] and studies of women alcohol abusers that examine history of childhood incest or other sexual abuse are still rare. The literature in this area suggests a strong association between childhood incest and sexual abuse and the development of alcohol abuse. The prevalence rates for a history of incest among alcoholic women range from 12% to 85%[27,39] and vary according to the population being studied (i.e., AA meetings, treatment facility women). Most authors note that the rates of incest reported by alcoholic women are significantly higher than rates reported in the general population. The few studies[27,40–43] that compare the prevalence of childhood incest in alcoholic and nonalcoholic women controls support this finding. In a recent study, Miller et al.[41] determined that not only did alcoholic women in treatment have higher rates of childhood sexual and physical abuse than women in a general population, they also had more childhood sexual and physical abuse than women receiving mental health services who had no alcohol problems. The findings persisted even after demographic characteristics and parents' drinking practices were controlled. The Wilsnack and Klassen[44] national survey also suggested a strong association between childhood sexual abuse and problem drinking.

The personality profile of the women incest survivor bears a striking resemblance to that of the alcoholic woman. Hurley,[39] in a review of the literature on women and incest and women and alcohol, illustrates the commonalities when these two areas of research are juxtaposed. For example, the alcoholic woman tries to conceal her drinking problem while the incest survivor frequently tries to conceal her incest experience. Both have a chaotic disruptive childhood and both groups frequently exhibit acting-out behavior during adolescence that results in school difficulties, drinking behavior, and "promiscuity." Finally, the alcoholic woman as well as the incest survivor experiences difficulties related to sexual functioning and development of intimacy. These common characteristics frequently are hypothesized as significant for the development of alcoholism in women.

The increased rate of childhood sexual victimization reported among women alcoholics may be a consequence of the instability—often associated with parental alcoholism—frequently reported in their family of origin. Incest that occurs within the context of the alcoholic family is usually a result of the alcoholic father's behavior. Additionally, incest has also been shown to occur when an alcoholic mother is unavailable to her husband. As a result, her husband may turn to the daughter for the support and love he once received from his wife. A recent dissertation[45] on adult adjustment of daughters of alcoholics found that incest was more likely to have occurred when the mother was the alcoholic parent.

As Hurley[39] has noted, an important question is why some female incest survivors become alcoholic and others do not. In a small qualitative study using a semistructured interview with ten alcoholic and nine nonalcoholic incest survivors, both groups reported difficulties with sex and intimacy.[46] The alcoholic incest survivors more often complained of sexual inhibition, lack of orgasm, and low sexual arousal and used alcohol to medicate these feelings and to lower sexual inhibition. In contrast, nonalcoholic incest survivors identified their major sexual problem as a lack of interest in sex and as a result tended to avoid sex.

A complementary approach has been to compare alcoholic women who do or do not have histories of childhood incest. Retrospective clinical studies report that alcoholic incest survivors experienced sexual dysfunction more frequently.[39] Although limited by their retrospective methodology, these studies suggest that for this subgroup of women sexual dysfunction and alcohol problems may develop in tandem. For incest survivors, as for other women with sexual dysfunction, alcohol may be used to self-medicate sexual difficulties *or* other modes of functional or dysfunctional coping may be invoked. The development of alcoholism or alcohol abuse is most likely for those women who self-medicate with alcohol. The high rates of sexual dysfunction found in incest survivors may be an intervening variable that explains their high rates of alcohol abuse (and alcoholic women's high rates of childhood incest).

Finally incest experiences of alcoholic women and nonalcoholic women have been compared. Findings suggest that chemically dependent women report a younger age at first sexual incident[42]; longer duration of abuse[27,42]; and more violent abuse.[27]

Studies of childhood incest and alcohol abuse have been limited by varying definitions of incest, lack of appropriate theoretical models, and failure to examine variations in incest experience that may be linked to level of adult adjustment and type of substance abuse or other psychiatric problems in adulthood. Important variables may include the age at which incest first occurred, type and severity of abuse, relationship of the perpetrator, the length of time that the abuse occurred, whether the woman disclosed the experience, and the reaction when she disclosed (i.e., was she believed). More studies are needed that link variation in childhood incest experiences to drinking patterns and problems and examine personal characteristics and social environments that protect childhood incest survivors from development of drinking problems and promote their healthy adult adjustment.

6.2. Sexual Assault and Alcohol Consumption

Researchers who focus on sexual assault have a difficult time with definitions. As reported by Abbey et al.[47] legal definitions of rape and sexual assault can vary by state or by the particular legal enforcement organization. As a result of the variation in definitions of sexual assault and rape, prevalence rates must be interpreted with caution. In most cases an underestimation of the behavior in question is likely. Abbey et al.[47] utilized the term sexual assault to describe any nonconsensual sexual contact, including penetration, whereas the term rape is reserved for sexual behaviors that involve penetration.

It is estimated that 50% of rapes are associated with alcohol use by perpetrator, victim, or both.[47–49] The direction of the relationship between alcohol and sexual assault cannot be clearly delineated. What can be stated is that women who experience sexual assault or rape are often the victims of intoxicated offenders.[49] In a national study 60% of women respondents reported that someone who was drinking had become "sexually aggressive" toward them.[6] Additionally, research suggests many women who have a history of alcohol abuse or who drink heavily concomitantly have a history of sexual assault. Wilsnack[1] reported that 30 to 75% of women alcoholics have experienced incest or adult sexual assault. Kilpatrick[50] reported that sexual assault victims were more likely than nonsexual assault victims to have a substance abuse disorder, and in a paper presented by Abbey,[48] women who had histories of sexual assault drank more than women who had never been sexually assaulted. It is possible that women who abuse alcohol or other drugs or who simply are heavier drinkers are at a higher risk for sexual assault or rape because of their lifestyles. Further research is needed to determine the temporal ordering between sexual assault and heavy or problem drinking in adult women and to examine if such temporal relationships are causal ones.

Sexual assault is most common in younger women[51] (late adolescence to early adulthood). Many women that fall into this age group are students on college campuses. Alcohol consumption is a major part of college life. Reported rates of alcohol consumption on college campuses is higher than in the general population and college women have been shown to be at increased risk for acquaintance rape.[47]

6.2.1. Acquaintance Rape. Acquaintance rape is very common on American college campuses. From 15 to 30% of college women report they have experienced acquaintance rape, usually at the hands of a fellow student.[47] Frequently, alcohol use is associated with acquaintance rape either by the assailant, the victim, or both. Kanin[52] found that the second strongest factor of acquaintance rape was excessive alcohol use by college men. Koss and Dinero[53] concurred that alcohol use was one of the strongest predictors of assault on college women victims. College women who have been sexually assaulted had more frequent alcohol consumption and drank more frequently during consensual sex than college women who had not experienced assault.[47]

Abbey[54] proposed seven explanations for the relationship between alcohol consumption and date rape on college campuses, three related to the male perpetrator and four related to the female victim. Many of these explanations are also applicable for the relationship between alcohol use and other kinds of sexual assault and to other victim populations.[47] Explanations for the relationship between acquaintance rape and alcohol consumption for men include: (1) expectancies about the effects of alcohol; (2) misperception of women's intentions; and (3) the use of alcohol as a valid excuse for forced sexual interactions. Men's beliefs about the effects of alcohol can result in a self-fulfilling prophecy that concludes in what they believe to be consensual sex but legally is defined as acquaintance rape. Males expect alcohol to disinhibit behavior, especially sexual behavior, and these expectancies shape postdrinking behavior. The effects of alcohol on the cognitive system also can decrease a man's ability to accurately interpret a woman's intentions in a drinking environment.

Studies suggest that men interpret a variety of female behaviors including use of alcohol in dating situations as more indicative of a woman's willingness to have sex than do women.[47] Men's beliefs about the types of women that consume alcohol can increase the risk of date rape in women. Garcia and Kushnier[55] asked college students to rate a female student's sexuality based on three factors: academic performance, attractiveness, and drinking behavior. The female students who were attractive, drank, and had a low academic record were rated as more sexual than any of the other combination of the three variables of characteristics of females students. In another study, George et al.[56] used a vignette depicting a woman on a date consuming alcoholic or nonalcoholic drinks to examine perceived sexual availability. They found that a woman who drank on a date was rated as more sexually predisposed, more sexually available, and more like to engage in foreplay and intercourse than a nondrinking female date. This study varied only women's drinking behavior, not that of their male partners, and did not include sexual aggression as a part of the vignette. Thus it appears that in college situations just the fact that a female student drinks can put her at risk.

Men are socialized to believe that if they wait long enough and persist hard enough, the woman's resistance to their sexual advances will eventually break down. The use of force in a sexual encounter often is consistent with male socialization practices in the United States, and men may use alcohol as a justification for their use of force. Koss *et al.*[57] surveyed thousands of undergraduates and found that 25% of college men surveyed admitted to sexually aggressive behavior, with 75% of them using alcohol or drugs prior to the incident.

Abbey[54] proposed four explanations regarding women that affect the relationship between alcohol use and date rape: (1) poor sending and receiving of sexual cues; (2) a diminished coping response due to the effects of the alcohol on the cognitive system; (3) existing stereotypes about women and drinking; and (4) an enhanced sense of responsibility. Much research on women's feelings, cognitions, and behaviors that may influence the relationship between alcohol and acquaintance rape focuses on the perception of enhanced responsibility. In a study in which college students given vignettes about a college woman who had been raped after a party, the woman was perceived as more responsible for the rape if she had been drinking but the male attacker was held less responsible if he had consumed alcohol.[58] A more recent study[59] that focused on judgments about an acquaintance rape scenario is one of the few that sampled young adults over 21 rather than only college students. The findings did not support the above contention that the woman is held more responsible if she had been drinking at the time of the rape. Their results show that acquaintance rape is not judged as negatively when both parties have been drinking and is judged more severely when only the victim was drinking. The beliefs held regarding the role that alcohol consumption, both by the assailant and victim, has on judgment, responsibility, and behavior may encourage harsh or lenient prosecution of offenders. In addition, the counseling and support offered victims may be influenced by such beliefs about the responsibility of the victim who consumes alcohol, and the involvement of alcohol in the assault may result in blaming the victim who is in need of help.

The social context in which drinking occurs can have differential effects on expectations and drinking patterns.[60] College women and men have been shown to use and abuse alcohol for different reasons. It has been suggested that women may use alcohol to increase feelings of worth, reduce feelings of anxiety in social situations, and help them feel better about themselves. If these are some of the underlying factors involved in college women's drinking behavior, Abbey's[54] proposed explanations for the relationship between alcohol and date rape can be further understood. The drinking woman in a more relaxed state sends sexual cues that confound with a man's expectations of a woman who drinks and can increase the risk of rape against a women who needed the drink to better enable herself to function socially. While the woman may view alcohol as helping her in social situations, in contrast it may be doing just the opposite. This is consistent with Brown *et al.*[61] who, in studying self-report expectancies, found that women expected more global positive changes from drinking, while men expected more arousal and aggression.

Although most research on acquaintance rape involves college populations, more broadly defined populations occasionally have been studied. It is unfortunate that more attention has not been given to other groups of women, particularly poverty-level women in urban settings who are believed to be at greatest risk for sexual assault. Distinctions have been made in the literature regarding the degree of relationship between perpetrator and victim and how these affect sexual assault patterns. Marital status has been found to be a mediating variable between alcohol consumption and violence against women.[62] For married women, a violent assault is usually preceded only by her spouse's drinking behavior, while for an unmarried women her own participation in drinking is more likely to be found when there was an assault. This implies that a married women may be viewed by her husband as property. She does not require any "loosening up" through alcohol consumption on her part in order for him to have sex with her. A man may feel more entitled to sexual behavior from an intimate partner than from a partner with whom he is less intimate. On the other hand, the unmarried woman requires more effort. If the perpetrator can get her drunk, he then may have his way. The consumption of alcohol by the man, in many cases, contributes to an excuse for his behavior. Morgan[63] argues that the connection between disinhibition as a prerogative of power and drinking behavior can be used to uphold male domination over women; that is, the man is believed to have the right to his drinking (and sexually violent) behavior. Morgan's thesis is supported by several studies showing that men with stronger beliefs in traditional gender roles are more likely to commit sexual assault.[47] Beliefs about the negative effects of alcohol on disinhibition allows men to invoke alcohol consumption as an excuse for sexual violence against their partners.

7. Conclusions

The 1980s and 1990s have produced new information about women, alcohol, and sexuality, partially answering some questions and raising others. We know that alcohol use and abuse by women and their partners are associated with heightened risk of sexual dysfunction, childhood incest, and sexual assault. At the same time alcohol use may increase subjective sexual desire, arousal, and pleasure and in certain cases may "disinhibit" female sexual behavior. The research literature would benefit from: (1) studies that disentangle the causal pathways involved in the association of alcohol and sexuality and examine varying causal explanations for the relationships that exist; (2) studies based on theory, including theories of adolescent and adult development; (3) a focus on subgroups of women diverse in cultural values, racial/ethnic group, social class and socioeconomic status, age, and sexual orientation; (4) behaviorally based definitions of sexual behavior and instruments that use these definitions[64] which are employed in multiple studies and with different populations so that findings are comparable across studies; and (5) new modes of data collection such as daily diaries that may be provide more reliable and valid measures of sexual feelings and behaviors. Only through continued, careful investigation that is both rigorous and creative will we further develop a knowledge base, valuable for enhancing the sexual functioning of women and their partners, preventing sexual abuse and assault, and perhaps limiting drinking problems in women.

ACKNOWLEDGMENT. The authors would like to thank S. Marie Harvey and Lana Simon for their comments and assistance in preparation of earlier versions of sections of this chapter.

References

1. Wilsnack SC: Drinking, sexuality, and sexual dysfunction in women, in Wilsnack SC, Beckman LJ (eds): *Alcohol Problems in Women: Antecedents, Consequences, and Intervention.* New York, Guilford Press, 1984, pp 189–227.
2. Oliver MB, Hyde JS: Gender differences in sexuality: A meta-analysis. *Psychol Bull* 114:29–51, 1993.
3. Wilson GT, Lawson DM: Effects of alcohol on sexual arousal in women. *J Abnorm Psychol* 85:587–594, 1976.
4. Malatesta VJ, Pollack RH, Crotty TD, *et al:* Acute alcohol intoxication and female orgasmic response. *J Sex Res* 15:101–107, 1982.
5. Beckman LJ: The reported effects of alcohol on the sexual feelings and behavior of women alcoholics and nonalcoholics. *J Stud Alcohol* 40:491–498, 1979.
6. Klassen AD, Wilsnack SC: Sexual experience and drinking among women in a US national survey. *Arch Sex Behav* 15:363–392, 1986.
7. Wilsnack SC, Klassen AD, Wilsnack RW: Drinking, sexual experience, and reproductive dysfunction among women in a 1981 national survey. Paper presented at the 14th Annual Medical-Scientific conference of the National Alcoholism Forum, Houston, Texas, April 1983.
8. Harvey SM, Beckman LJ: Alcohol consumption, female sexual behavior and contraceptive use. *J Stud Alcohol* 47:327–332, 1986.
9. Murphy WD, Coleman E, Hoon E, *et al:* Sexual dysfunction and treatment in alcoholic women. *Sex Disabil* 3:240–255, 1980.
10. Jensen SB: Sexual function and dysfunction in younger married alcoholics: A comparative study. *Acta Psychiatr Scand* 69:543–549, 1984.
11. Crowne LC, George WH: Alcohol and human sexuality: Review and integration. *Psychol Bull* 105:374–386, 1989.
12. Wilson GT: Alcohol and human sexual behavior. *Behav Res Ther* 15:239–252, 1977.
13. Heiser K, Harmann U: Disorders of sexual desire in a sample of women alcoholics. *Drug Alcohol Depend* 19:145–157, 1987.
14. Erhardt EA: Trends in sexual behavior and the HIV pandemic. *Am J Public Health* 82:1459–1461, 1992.
15. De Buono BA, Ziner SH, Daamen M, *et al:* Sexual behavior of college women in 1975, 1986 and 1989. *N Engl J Med* 322:821–825, 1990.

16. Leigh BC, Stall R: Substance use and risky sexual behavior for exposure to HIV: Issues in methodology, interpretation, and prevention. *Am Psychol* 48:11023–1034, 1993.
17. Ericksen KP, Trocki KF: Behavioral risk factors for sexually transmitted diseases in American households. *Soc Sci Med* 34:843–853, 1992.
18. Leigh BC: The relationship of substance use during sex to high risk sexual behavior. *J Sex Res* 27:199–213, 1990.
19. Cooper ML, Pierce RS: Sex differences in alcohol use and sexual risk-taking. Paper presented at annual meeting of the American Psychological Association, San Francisco, August 1991.
20. Leigh BC: Alcohol consumption and sexual activity as reported with a diary technique. *J Aborm Psychol* 103:491–493, 1993.
21. Cooper ML, Skinner JB, George WH: Alcohol use and sexual risk-taking among adolescents: Methodological approaches for addressing causal issues. In Seminara D, Pawlowski A, Watson R (eds): *Alcohol, Immunomodulation, and AIDS*. New York, Alan R. Liss, 1990.
22. Wilson GT, Lawson DM: Expectancies, alcohol and sexual arousal in women. *J Abnorm Psychol* 87:358–367, 1978.
23. Kline RB: The relation of alcohol expectancies to drinking patterns among alcoholics: Generalization across gender and race. *J Stud Alcohol* 51:175–182, 1990.
24. Leigh BC: The relationship of sex-related alcohol expectancies to alcohol consumption and sexual behavior. *Br J Addict* 85:919–928, 1990.
25. Pinhas V: Sexual dysfunction in women alcoholics. *Med Aspects Hum Sex* 21:97–101, 1987.
26. Pinhas V: Sex guilt and sexual control in women alcoholics in early sobriety. *Sex Disabil* 3:256, 1980.
27. Covington SS: Sexual experience, dysfunction, and abuse: A descriptive study of alcoholic and nonalcoholic women. PhD dissertation, Union Graduate School, Cincinnati, Ohio, 1982.
28. Hammond DC, Jorgensen GQ, Ridgeway DM: Sexual adjustment of the female alcoholic. Salt Lake City Alcohol and Drug Abuse Clinic, University of Utah, unpublished manuscript, 1979.
29. Kaplan HS: *Disorders of Sexual Desire*. New York, Simon & Schuster, 1979.
30. Sholty MJ: *Female Sexual Experience and Satisfaction as Related to Alcohol Consumption*. Baltimore, Alcohol and Drug Abuse Program, 1979.
31. Wilsnack SC, Klassen AD, Schur BE, *et al:* Predicting onset and chronicity of women's problem drinking: A five-year longitudinal analysis. *Am J Public Health* 81:305–318, 1991.
32. Mays VM, Beckman LJ, Oranchak E, *et al:* Perceived social support for help-seeking behaviors of black heterosexual and homosexual women alcoholics. *Psychol Addict Behav*, 1994.
33. Janus SS, Janus CL: *The Janus Report on Sexual Behavior*. New York, Wiley, 1993.
34. Fifield I: On my way to nowhere: Alienated, isolated, drunk. Los Angeles Gay Community Services Center, 1975.
35. Lohrenz LJ, Connelly JC, Coyne L: Alcohol problems in several Midwestern homosexual communities. *J Stud Alcohol* 39:1959–1963, 1978.
36. Lewis CE, Shagir MT, Robins E: Drinking patterns in homosexual and heterosexual women. *J Clin Psychiatry* 43:277–278, 1982.
37. McKirnan DJ, Peterson PL: Alcohol and drug use among homosexual men and women: An epidemiology and population characteristics. *Addict Behav* 14:545–553, 1989.
38. Finkelhor D, Hotaling G, Lewis IA, *et al:* Sexual abuse in the national survey of adult men and women: Prevalence, characteristics, and risk factors., *Child Abuse Negl* 14:19–28, 1990.
39. Hurley DL: Women, alcohol, and incest: An analytical review. *J Stud Alcohol* 52:253–268, 1991.
40. Rohsenow DJ, Corbett R, Devine D: Molested as children: A hidden contribution to substance abuse? *J Subst Abuse Treat* 5:13–18, 1988.
41. Miller BA, Downs WR, Testa M: Interrelationships between victimization experiences and women's alcohol use. *J Stud Alcohol Suppl* 11:109–117, 1993.
42. Schaefer S, Evans S, Sterne M: Incest among women in recovery from drug dependency: Correlation and implication for treatment. Proceedings of the Thirty-fourth International

Congress on Alcoholism and Drug Dependence, Calgary, Alberta, Canada, August 1985, pp 268–269.

43. Swett C, Cohen C, Surrey J, *et al:* High rates of alcohol use and history of physical and sexual abuse among women outpatients. *Am J Drug Alcohol Abuse* 17:49–60, 1991.

44. Wilsnack SC, Klassen AD: Childhood sexual abuse and problem drinking in a US national sample of women. Paper presented at Women's Issues related to Alcohol Abuse and Violence Conference, University of Illinois at Chicago, College of Nursing, September 1992.

45. Erhard AV: Effects of sex of alcoholic parent, family functioning and compensatory support on adult adjustment of daughters of alcoholics. Unpublished PhD dissertation, California School of Professional Psychology, Los Angeles, 1993.

46. Hurley DL: Incest and the development of alcoholism in adult female survivors. *Alcohol Treat Q* 7:41–56, 1990.

47. Abbey A, Thomson L, McDuffie D: Alcohol's role in sexual assault, in Watson RR (ed): *Drug and Alcohol Abuse Reviews.* Clifton NJ, Humana Press, 1992, vol 4.

48. Abbey A, Ross LT, McDuffie D: Alcohol and sexual assault. Paper presented at the 121st annual meeting of the American Public Health Association, San Francisco, October 1993.

49. Koss MP: Hidden rape: Sexual aggression and victimization in a national sample of students in higher education, in Burgess AW (ed): *Rape and Sexual Assault.* New York, Garland, 1988, pp 3–25.

50. Kilpatrick DG: Violence as a precursor of women's substance abuse: The test of the drugs-violence story. Paper presented at the annual meeting of the American Psychological Association, Boston, August 1990.

51. Koss MP: The underdetection of rape: Methodological choices influence incidence estimates. *J Soc Issues* 48:61–76, 1992.

52. Kanin EJ: Date rapists. *Arch Sex Behav* 14:219–231, 1985.

53. Koss MP, Dinero TE: Discriminant analysis of risk factors for sexual victimization among a national sample of college women. *J Consult Clin Psychol* 57:242–250, 1989.

54. Abbey A: Acquaintance rape and alcohol consumption on college campuses: How are they linked? *J Am Coll Health* 39:165–169, 1991.

55. Garcia LT, Kushnier K: Sexual inferences about female targets: The use of sexual experience correlates. *J Sex Res* 23:252–272, 1987.

56. George WH, Gournic SJ, McAfee MP: Perceptions of postdrinking female sexuality: Effects of gender, beverage choice, and drink payment. *J Appl Soc Psychol* 18:1295–1317, 1988.

57. Koss MP, Gidycz CA, Wisniewski N: The scope of rape: Incidence and prevalence of sexual aggression and victimization in a national sample of higher education students. *J Consult Clin Psychol* 55:162–170, 1987.

58. Richardson D, Campbell JL: Alcohol and rape: The effect of alcohol on attributions of blame for rape. *Pers Soc Psychol Bull* 8:468–476, 1982.

59. Norris J, Cubbins LA: Dating, drinking, and rape: Effects of victim's and assailant's alcohol consumptions on judgments of their behavior and traits. *Psychol Women Q* 16:179–191, 1992.

60. Thombs DL, Beck KH, Mahoney CA: Effects on social context and gender on drinking patterns of young adults. *J Counsel Psychol* 1:115–119, 1993.

61. Brown SA, Goldman MS, Inn A, *et al:* Expectations of reinforcement from alcohol: Their domain and relation to drinking patterns. *J Am Coll Health* 36:123–129, 1980.

62. Permanen K: *Alcohol and Human Violence.* New York, Guilford Press, 1991.

63. Morgan P: Women and alcohol: The disinhibition rhetoric in an analysis of domination. *J Psychoactive Drugs* 19:129–133, 1987.

64. Koss MP, Oros CJ: Sexual experiences survey: A research instrument in investigating sexual aggression and victimization. *J Consult Clin Psychol* 50:455–457, 1982.

16

Cognitive Psychosocial Performance and Recovery in Female Alcoholics

Sara Jo Nixon and Susan Wagner Glenn

Abstract. Female alcoholics experience greater affective symptomatology and are more frequently labeled with comorbid psychiatric diagnoses than male alcoholics. Subgroups of male and female alcoholics with antisocial symptomatology are strikingly similar across behavioral, psychosocial, and alcohol and drug use variables. Relative to controls, female alcoholics manifest deficits in standard neuropsychological testing as well as efficiency of information processing, interpersonal problem solving, neurophysiological measures, and neurophysiological assessment. The deficits are quite similar to those of male alcoholics. However, females may manifest a differential susceptibility to alcohol given the females' comparatively shorter drinking careers. There are no overall sex differences in relapse rates following treatment, although various personal and environmental factors play gender-specific roles in outcome. Patterns of recovery function with abstinence are similar for male and female alcoholics.

1. Introduction

Alcohol abuse has long been known to have detrimental cognitive, psychological, and social consequences.[1,2] Until the late 1970s, most of these conclusions were drawn from studies using male alcoholics and/or a clinical literature based largely on case studies. Empirical studies were limited to male subjects for a variety of reasons including the fact that there were limited treatment facilities for women and that relatively few women sought treatment for alcohol abuse/dependence.

The picture has changed dramatically over the past 15 years. Recognizing that the effects of alcohol abuse on women constitute a major threat to the

Sara Jo Nixon and Susan Wagner Glenn • Department of Psychiatry and Behavioral Sciences, University of Oklahoma Health Sciences Center, Oklahoma City, Oklahoma 73104.

Recent Developments in Alcoholism, Volume 12: Women and Alcoholism, edited by Marc Galanter. Plenum Press, New York, 1995

well-being of individual women as well as a significant public health issue, a number of groups have initiated studies that include and/or focus on female alcoholics. Women now constitute approximately one fourth or more of the clients seeking inpatient treatment.[3,4] The willingness of these women to participate in alcohol studies has enabled clinicians and researchers to significantly improve their understanding of the etiology and consequences of alcohol abuse and dependence.

Alcohol abuse and dependence is a multifaceted problem, regardless of sex. Other chapters in this volume address a host of issues including epidemiology, health, drinking patterns, and metabolism as they apply to women. This chapter focuses on cognitive performance, psychological and social functioning, relapse, and recovery. However, it is important to recognize that these processes are not truly independent. For example, a woman's cognitive functioning will be affected not only by her alcoholic status, but also by factors such as general health. Given this interaction, it is to be expected that some degree of redundancy will exist between this and other chapters.

The remainder of the chapter is divided into five sections. The next section (Section 2) addresses psychosocial functioning in female alcoholics. Section 3 discusses the cognitive processes compromised with chronic alcohol abuse. Because of the role of cognitive and psychosocial functioning on relapse, Section 4 considers the literature on prediction of relapse. Section 5 reviews findings relevant to the process of cognitive recovery. Finally, Section 6 provides a brief summary.

2. Psychosocial Functioning

2.1. Psychological/Psychiatric and Social Problems

Gender differences in the negative consequences associated with substance use have been noted in both general population and alcoholic samples. For instance, Robbins[5] examined data from the National Household Survey on Drug Abuse (NHSDA) sponsored by the National Institute on Drug Abuse (NIDA) and the National Institute on Alcohol Abuse and Alcoholism (NIAAA). This survey involved interviewing over 8000 individuals over the age of 12 in households across the contiguous United States. These analyses revealed that males were more likely than females to have experienced each of the 17 psychosocial problems related to alcohol and other substance abuse over the past year. Additional analyses using both factor and item analyses indicated that the patterns of problems were different for the sexes. Males experienced more social/behavioral problems associated with substance use. These problems included more trouble at school or on the job, impaired driving, financial difficulties, trouble with the law, and requiring emergency medical help.

Females, on the other hand, reported more intrapsychic problems. Of particular significance was the increased incidence of depression associated with substance use. It is interesting that women also reported greater vulnerability than men to arguments and fights as a result of substance use.

Studies with alcoholic samples have produced similar results with males generally reporting more alcohol-related problems overall, although women report more negative psychological or intrapsychic problems.[3,6-8] A recent study by Ross,[9] however, failed to replicate these findings. Consistent with previous work she found that males reported more alcohol-related problems, but only if issues of chronicity, antisocial personality, and employment were not controlled. If these factors were controlled, there were no sex differences in the reported alcohol-related problems. After controlling for these factors, females exhibited *more* symptoms of alcohol dependence.

There has been a long-standing interest in the comorbidity of alcohol and other psychiatric disorders.[10-15] Current estimates suggest that as many as 37% of the individuals who meet criteria for a lifetime diagnosis of alcohol abuse also meet criteria for another psychiatric disorder.[16]

Of particular interest to clinicians and researchers has been the role that affective state, in particular depression, may play in the etiology, course, and outcome of alcoholism.[12-13,17-19] Petty[12] in a review of the literature, found that between 10 and 30% of the alcoholics in any one study also suffer from depression. This review also indicated that not only were female alcoholics more likely to have a preexisting depression, they were also more likely to develop depression following heavy drinking.

The importance of the depressive disorders in female alcoholism has been reinforced in a number of studies.[20-23] For instance, in an early study, Schuckit and colleagues[24] found that they could successfully subtype female alcoholics on the basis of whether the alcoholism was primary or secondary in regard to the presence of an affective disorder. This work suggested significant differences between those alcoholics who had developed alcoholism in conjunction with a preexisting affective disorder (secondary alcoholics) versus those whose alcoholism was not preceded by such diagnoses. In a follow-up study using this classification scheme, female alcoholics with an affective disorder experienced better outcomes than did those with primary alcoholism.[25] This finding of improved outcome in depressed versus nondepressed female alcoholics has been supported in later work conducted by Rounsaville and colleagues.[26]

It has been suggested that not only does the prevalence of depression in female alcoholics differ from that with males, but also that the pattern of development and role of causal factors in the comorbidity differs.[22,27-30] Specifically, as noted previously, it has been observed that depression is more likely to precede the development of alcoholism in women than in men.[22] Furthermore, it has been suggested that familial/genetic factors may play a more significant role in the comorbidity of the two disorders for women than for men.[29]

To clarify this latter issue, Kendler *et al.*[31] conducted a twin study of the comorbidity of alcoholism and major depression in women. Their findings, based only on a female sample, were quite interesting. First, consistent with some studies[19] but not others,[32] these authors found that familial factors contributed significantly to the comorbidity of major depression and alcoholism.

Second, the degree to which genetic factors accounted for the comorbidity was dependent on the narrowness of definitions. That is, as alcoholism was more narrowly defined, the role of genes in accounting for the comorbidity increased (range 57 to 100%). To the contrary, as major depression was more narrowly defined, the comorbidity was increased, but not due to genetic factors. Rather, in this case, the increase was due to higher environmental correlations (range 0 to 43%).

Third, the environmental factors that contributed were not shared familial environmental factors. These common environmental factors did not contribute to the development of alcoholism or depression. On the other hand, individual-specific environmental factors did substantially increase comorbidity.

In summary, there is a wealth of literature that suggests that female alcoholics are more likely to receive a secondary psychiatric diagnosis, that this diagnosis will be one of affective disorder, and that the familial/genetic component for this comorbidity is substantial.[21-23] However, other work suggests there are no gender differences in the prevalence of either affective or other psychiatric disorders in alcoholic samples.[8] Furthermore, it has been suggested that the increased rates of psychiatric diagnoses in female alcoholics may, in fact, reflect a sociocultural bias. Helzer and Pryzbeck[22] propose that the increased rate of dual diagnosis in these samples occurs because of the perceived deviance of being both female and alcoholic. That is, because it is considered more deviant for a female as opposed to a male to be alcoholic, it may be expected that there would be a stronger association between alcoholism and other psychiatric diagnoses (i.e., other deviance) in women.

2.2. Behavioral Disorders

Antisocial personality disorder (ASP) has most generally been associated with male as opposed to female alcoholism.[21,23,33] Characteristics associated with ASP such as impulsivity, risk-taking, and criminal activity have been used in conjunction with certain drinking variables such as age of symptom onset to categorize alcoholic subtypes under several classification schemes.[33-36] Recent work indicates that at least some of these characteristics also exist in female alcoholics and may provide a useful means of subtyping female as well as male alcoholics.[36-38]

Lex and colleagues'[37] pilot work with female driving under the influence (DUI) offenders offers an interesting starting point. Using a system similar to Cloninger's type I/II typology,[33] she found that this group could be subtyped on the basis of age of onset of alcohol-related legal problems (before or after

25). Once separated, these groups differed in age, age of first drink, and age for regular drinking, with the younger-onset group reporting significantly younger ages. Although the groups did not differ in their overall Michigan Alcohol Screening Test (MAST) scores,[39] preliminary item analyses suggest the younger-symptom group does experience greater inability to abstain (a characteristic generally assigned to type II or male-limited alcoholism). It is important to note that the sample size in this study was extremely small ($n = 12$). Finally, 75% of the sample was family history positive (FH+) for alcoholism. Thus, it is impossible to separate this potential confound.

Glenn and Nixon[38] also investigated the incidence of type I/II symptoms and age of alcoholism onset in a sample of alcoholic women. In the course of the study, they applied three different classification schemes to a sample of 51 alcoholic women. Their data indicated that the most effective means of categorizing women was on the basis of age of symptom onset (before or after the age of 25) regardless of type[33] of symptom. They found that early symptom onset (ESOs) subjects were significantly more anxious and reported more antisocial symptomatology and lower socialization scores than did late symptom onset (LSO) subjects. They also reported greater use of cocaine but less use of benzodiazepines. ESOs were also less well educated and had greater job instability. These data and others suggest that assuming that ASP symptomatology does not apply to a substantial number of female alcoholics is inaccurate. Attempts to develop appropriate treatment and intervention must consider this reality.

A history of childhood behavioral disorders (CBDs) has also been associated with adult male alcoholism.[40-42] A rather extensive literature indicates that a significant number of male alcoholics report increased symptoms of attention deficit disorder (ADD) and conduct disorder (CD).[34,41,43] Work in our laboratory has generally confirmed this finding.[44] Two recent studies conducted in our laboratory examined sex differences in CBDs in alcoholics and community controls.

The first study examined ASP symptomatology, CBDs, affective state, and cognitive performance.[45] Consistent with previous work, alcoholics reported more antisocial behaviors, more CBDs, greater affective symptomatology, and poorer cognitive performance. Perhaps surprisingly, there were no sex main effects or group × sex interactions on the behavioral or affective factors. The interaction of ASP, CBDs, and cognitive performance is discussed in the next section.

In the second study currently in preparation, alcoholics and community controls were asked to complete not only the childhood symptom checklist used in the study above,[46] but also the Utah questionnaire for both childhood (ADD) and residual attentional deficit disorder (ADDRT).[47] These data are preliminary but provide groundwork for further development.

As expected, alcoholics reported significantly more CBDs than controls. Surprisingly, but consistent with the previous study, there were no sex differences. This pattern was consistent whether one considered endorsement of items on the Utah childhood symptom checklist or Tarter and co-workers' childhood symptom checklist.[46]

However, the pattern was different when ADDRT was considered. On this measure, not only was there was a significant group effect ($p = 0.0001$), but there was also a significant sex effect ($p = 0.002$) and a sex × group interaction that approached significance ($p = 0.07$). A review of the main effect means showed that females reported more ADDRT symptoms than did males. The cell means for the interactions revealed that the ordering of symptoms reported from highest to lowest was female alcoholics, male alcoholics, female controls, and male controls.

Given this pattern, a follow-up preliminary analysis of the specific items was conducted. This analysis proved useful in clarifying potential reasons for this interaction. Specifically, it revealed that females (collapsed across group) were more likely to endorse those items related to distractibility, mood changes, and depressive symptomatology.

By group, however, the pattern differed considerably. Control women endorsed more items than men only when those items related to mood changes and depressive symptomatology. Compared with alcoholic men, alcoholic women endorsed significantly more items related to mood changes, depressive symptomatology, distractibility, disorganization or being sloppy, and being anxious and/or easily flustered. Notice that neither group of women endorsed more items related to verbal or behavioral impulsivity, temper, or destructive behavior. This picture of increased affective symptomatology in female alcoholics is consistent with the majority of work with alcoholic samples. These data raise the important point that symptom checklists and similar materials must be carefully analyzed by item or factor, if accurate interpretations are to be made. Specifically, if item analyses had not been conducted on these data, the conclusion could have been drawn that women and in particular alcoholic women experienced more ADDRT than do men. The follow-up analyses clarified the results and produced a more consistent interpretation.

3. Cognitive Performance

3.1. Neuropsychological and Cognitive Tasks

The cognitive impairment associated with long-term, chronic alcohol abuse is well documented.[1,2] These deficits include problems in visual–spatial processing, perceptual–motor skills, learning–memory, and abstraction and problem solving. Many of the earlier studies employed standard neuropsychological assessments with the goal being to localize the neurotoxic effects of alcohol.[48] Overall, this literature has revealed considerable similarity in the nature and degree of cognitive impairment in male and female alcoholics, even though female alcoholics typically report shorter and/or less severe drinking histories.[49]

The broad spectrum of functions that may be impaired has led some researchers to approach cognitive studies from a slightly different perspective. Specifically, recent studies have incorporated a variety of tasks and dependent variables to ascertain the nature of the underlying cognitive *processes* impaired in both male and female alcoholics.[50–55]

Glenn and Parsons[51] examined speed–accuracy trade-offs in samples of male and female alcoholic and control subjects. They used a battery of tests which included assessments of visual–spatial processing, perceptual–motor skills, learning and memory, and abstraction–problem solving. Their data indicate male and female alcoholics are equally impaired relative to controls on an efficiency ratio (accuracy–time). In a later investigation,[52] they found that alcoholics were inferior to controls in time, accuracy, and efficiency in four areas of cognitive functioning: verbal skills, problem solving, learning and memory, and perceptual–motor skills. Consistent with previous work, the alcoholic group did not show sex differences despite the shorter drinking histories of the female sample (10 years vs. 13 years for male alcoholics). However, it might be noted that male and female alcoholics did not differ on drinking measures that incorporate both quantity and frequency indices.

Nixon and Parsons[54] applied the concept of cognitive efficiency in a different way. Extrapolating from others,[56,57] they defined efficiency as the ability to ignore irrelevant information while attending to relevant, accurate information. Within this definition, speed–accuracy trade-offs are only one of a variety of dependent variables. Using the plant task,[58,59] they tested the hypothesis that alcoholics were less efficient problem solvers. This task is an ecologically valid task patterned after Piagetian tasks for abstract thought. It requires that subjects isolate the variable from among three which might be responsible for the health of a group of plants. The data revealed that alcoholics were inferior to controls in being able to *isolate* but not *identify* the relevant variable. That is, alcoholics knew that the relevant variable was relevant, but they could not separate its effect from the potential effect of the other variables. Consistent with more traditional assessments, there was no group × sex interaction.

In a second study using an ecologically valid task, male and female alcoholics and controls were compared on their ability to address interpersonal problem situations.[60,61] Consistent with previous work with male alcoholics,[62] this study indicated that alcoholics, regardless of sex, were significantly inferior in their usual or "typical" responses to such situations. They were not inferior, however, in their ability to generate the "best" responses to these situations. Consistent with work on sex differences in interpersonal relations, females were superior to males in the "best" response condition. There was no group × sex interaction. Interestingly, a measure of self-efficacy was also obtained during the task. There were no group, sex, or group × sex differences on this measure. Thus, poor self-efficacy in such situations cannot account for the group differences. This study suggests a type of behavioral inefficiency in both male and female alcoholics; they were able to generate the better response to a difficult situation, but apparently unable to enact that response.

3.2. Neurophysiological Assessments

There is now a rather large literature describing anatomical and functional brain changes associated with alcoholism.[63–65] These data suggest significant changes across a wide array of measures including decreased white matter, increased ventricular size, abnormal EEG, and reduced amplitude and/or increased latencies in components of the event related potentials (ERPs). A complete review is beyond the scope of this chapter.[1,66] Despite the importance of these data, it should be noted that few of these types of studies have included women, or at least sufficient numbers, for statistical analysis. The data that are available are somewhat inconsistent.

For example, Parsons et al.[67] found significant neuropsychological impairment for both male and female alcoholics relative to community controls. However, deficits in neurophysiologic performance (ERPs) were observed only for the male alcoholics. Although the females reported shorter drinking histories, this difference could not account for the absence of effects.

In contrast, Jacobson's[68] earlier work on anatomical changes in females had revealed ventricular enlargement and sulcal widening in female alcoholics. In a separate study, he observed similar brain shrinkage in female and male alcoholics compared with controls, even though females reported lower peak alcohol consumption.[69]

Mann et al.[70] also investigated brain shrinkage in male and female alcoholics using computerized tomography (CT). Consistent with Jacobson's studies, male and female alcoholics showed equivalent degrees of brain shrinkage despite fewer years of alcoholic drinking in the female sample (m = 3.8 years, SD = 2.7 vs. m = 9.2, SD = 7.0).

Thus, the data regarding neurophysiological measures in female alcoholics are sparse. In general, however, the available data suggest that females are differentially susceptible to the negative effects of alcohol on such variables.[49]

3.3. Contributing Factors

Obviously, factors in addition to sex and alcoholic status may also affect cognitive and psychosocial skills. Of particular interest in alcohol research has been the putative role of a family history of alcoholism (FH+). Studies often, but not always,[71] find significant differences on cognitive and psychosocial measures between FH+ and FH— nonalcoholic subjects.[72]

However, this pattern is not consistently observed in alcoholic subjects.[43,73,74] It appears that FH and alcoholic status have additive rather than interactive effects; that is, alcoholics typically perform more poorly than controls and FH+ subjects often but not always perform more poorly than FH-subjects.

The overall consensus regarding health and psychosocial variables as well as neurocognitive measures is that FH and sex are not interactive. That is, the effect of a positive FH is similar for males and females.[74–76] It should be noted that because of the higher proportion of female alcoholics reporting positive family histories,[21,77,78] studies separating female alcoholics into FH+ and FH- have been difficult to conduct. In our own work, recruiting largely from inpatient facilities across the state, we have observed fewer than perhaps ten FH- alcoholic women over the past 3 years.

There is continued interest in the role that CBDs and/or ASP may play in influencing neurocognitive skills in alcoholics.[45,79–82] Despite the intuitive appeal of this line of research, the results have been mixed. Some studies have suggested increased cognitive deficits in individuals with these behavioral traits.[79,81,82] Others, however, have failed to obtain similar results.[80]

As we have seen previously, generalization of these data is restricted due to paucity of female subjects. One study that did include both male and female subjects obtained an interesting pattern. Hesselbrock and colleagues[80] found that male alcoholics with ASP performed *better* than their non-ASP alcoholic counterparts. Female alcoholics with ASP, however, performed *more poorly* than non-ASP females.

Recent work in our laboratories suggests that the relation between CBDs, ASP symptomatology, and psychosocial and cognitive performance will be difficult to clearly define.[45,61,83] For example, consistent with most literature, earlier symptom onset is associated with less socialization and more antisocial tendencies in female alcoholics (see Section 2.2). This finding has now been replicated in a sample of male alcoholics.[83] However, when the relation between age of symptom onset and cognitive performance was examined, no significant effects were observed.[83]

On the other hand, data from the Glenn et al.[45] study previously discussed in Section 2.2 suggest that CBDs are directly related to adult cognitive performance.[45] Specifically, this study found that the best predictor of cognitive performance, regardless of sex or group assignment, was CBD.

As described in Section 2.2, a later study (in preparation) used the same questionnaire as Glenn et al. and added the Utah questionnaires for ADD and ADDRT. This study produced a different pattern of results. In particular, neither CBDs nor ADD significantly predicted overall cognitive efficiency. In fact, the only significant predictor of cognitive efficiency was group assignment ($p = 0.002$; alcoholic vs. control); although ADDRT approached significance ($p = 0.06$). Sex was also not a significant variable.

In summary, there remains a significant need to examine factors that may affect cognitive and psychosocial performance in alcoholics. However, work to date, using both male and female alcoholics, suggests that the effects (if present) of at least some of these variables are similar in the two sexes. Furthermore, these data indicate that factors such as FH, childhood behavioral disorders, and/or residual attention deficits cannot account for differences between alcoholics and controls, regardless of sex.

4. Prediction of Relapse

Gender differences regarding recidivism rates following alcoholism treatment are somewhat controversial and easily misinterpreted. As pointed out by Nathan and Skinstad[84] and Schuckit and Winokur,[25] alcoholic women appear to be both undertreated and understudied. Sokolow et al.[85] reported that female alcoholics were easier to track during the follow-up period, but there were no sex differences in treatment outcome. Similarly, reviews by Annis[86] and Vannicelli[87] suggest no sex-related differences in outcome. However, other studies suggest that females have either a better outcome[88] or a poorer one compared with males.[89,90]

In general, recent reports indicate that men and women benefit from treatment at comparable rates. In a short-term follow-up study comparing males and females completing alcoholism treatment, O'Connor et al.[92] report that women experienced a shorter period of alcoholism prior to entering treatment (16 years vs. 19 years), but had similar rates of treatment failure relative to men (53% vs. 43%). Further, although women were more likely to be poor and reported similar drinking patterns and quantities as men, they were less likely to be homeless, uninsured, or have legal problems as a result of their alcohol abuse.

In a long-term follow-up study, DeSoto et al.[93] tracked alcoholics post-treatment for a varying number of years for a 4-year period and assessed drinking patterns, symptom severity, and occupational and psychosocial functioning. They found that in the first year following treatment, relapse rates for both men and women were fairly high (45–55%), but that this dropped drastically in subsequent years and remained similar for both sexes (see Fig. 1). For subjects who had been abstinent for more than 5 years at the time of the initial study, the relapse rates reached 0% (no relapses in 108 subjects).

General severity of physical symptoms also followed a decreasing curvilinear pattern. They, too, were strikingly similar for men and women. Correlations between relapse and symptom severity were near significant ($p = 0.07$). The best predictor of relapse, however, proved to be the duration of abstinence ($p < 0.0001$), with the probability of relapse decreasing as the amount of time since treatment increased.

Continued abstinence was associated with employment status for both men and women. From 18 to 22% showed an increase in employment status, 70–78% remained in the same general employment category, and 4–8% reported a decrease in job status or unemployment during the 4-year follow-up period. The authors conclude that the course of recovery in abstinent alcoholics—as measured by severity of symptoms, probability of relapse, and work history—was essentially the same for men and women. Furthermore, although recovery is most remarkable in the first years after treatment, it is an ongoing process in which measurable progress continues for at least 10 years.

Although the basic rate of relapse appears to be similar between male and female alcoholics, several gender-related factors have been identified that

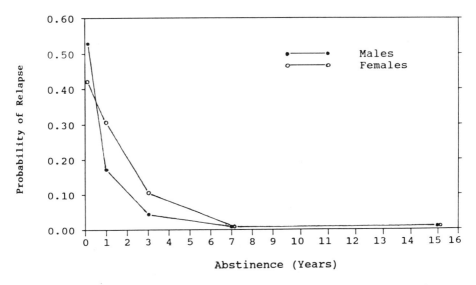

Figure 1. Long-term relapse rates in male and female alcoholics. Reprinted by permission from C. B. DeSoto, W. E. O'Donnell, and J. L. DeSoto, "Long-Term Recovery in Alcoholics," *Alcoholism: Clinical and Experimental Research*, Vol. 3, No. 5, pg. 695. Copyright 1989 Williams and Wilkins.

may be influential in outcome. Weisner and Schmidt[94] report that female alcohol abusers were more likely than men to experience greater symptom severity and to seek treatment from nonalcohol specific health care settings, particularly mental health settings. This differential use of treatment resources may influence both the type of treatment received as well as the benefit derived from treatment in terms of relapse prevention.

In a review of outcome studies utilizing controlled drinking and abstinence as separate possible outcomes following treatment, Rosenberg[95] suggested that female alcoholics who do not remain completely abstinent may be more able to achieve controlled drinking without progression to uncontrolled drinking than male alcoholics. Consistent with this conclusion, Schuckit and Winokur[25] found that nearly 50% of "good outcome" female alcoholics were able to successfully resume uncomplicated social drinking patterns. This figure is substantially higher than the 8–10% of male alcoholics reportedly able to maintain controlled social drinking in other studies.[96,97]

Moos *et al.*,[98] in an extensive study of male and female alcoholics in treatment and in the 6 months following, found that marital status played an interesting role in treatment process and outcome. At both intake and follow-up interviews, married patients (male and female) were less impaired on all criteria except social functioning compared with unmarried patients. In terms of outcome, however, being married was associated with better outcome for men but poorer outcome for women. Abstinence rates were 45% for married men, 42% for unmarried women, 18% for unmarried men, and 28% for married women. The authors postulate that this interaction between marital status, gender, and outcome may be due to the large percentage of married female alcoholics who reported living with a heavy drinker (spouse) during the follow-up period.

The researchers also found that women showed better treatment outcome when the treatment programs were structured, based on a medical model, and consisted of more lectures and films than group therapy sessions. Men, on the other hand, had better outcomes when treatment was less structured and focused on personal problem orientation in a group discussion setting. Attendance at outpatient aftercare was associated with general improvement in all areas of functioning for men. However, it was associated with a lower likelihood of abstaining, higher depression, and fewer social activities for women. Moos et al.[98] concluded that both treatment and posttreatment environmental factors had a greater influence on relapse for women than men. They suggest that treatment and life context factors may be especially important for understanding the process of relapse and remissions among women.

The relation between affective disturbances, alcoholism, and outcome is not well defined, but may have differential sex effects as well. Rounsaville et al.[26] completed extensive psychiatric evaluations on alcoholics during treatment and after 1 year. They found that for men, poor outcome was associated with additional diagnoses of major depression, ASP, or drug abuse. For women, having major depression was associated with better outcome in terms of drinking-related measures, while ASP and drug abuse were associated with poorer outcome. The authors hypothesize that females with primary alcoholism and no affective disorder may represent a form of alcoholism which has heavier genetic and environmental influences.

Babor et al.[99] further characterize potential differences in outcome between female alcoholics with and without psychiatric symptoms in their description of type A and type B alcoholics. In 12- and 36-month follow-up sessions, type A female alcoholics were found to demonstrate later onset, less severe dependence, less previous treatment for alcohol problems, fewer alcohol-related physical and social consequences, less psychopathological dysfunction, and better outcome than type B alcoholics. The same typological distinctions were identified for both male and female alcoholics. These data highlight the need for continued investigation and delineation of the role of psychiatric symptoms in relapse.

In an effort to identify specific prognostic factors in treatment outcome, we interviewed male and female alcoholics immediately following the completion of inpatient alcoholism treatment and again 14 months later.[100] At the follow-up session, subjects were identified as resumers ($n = 41$; 28 males and 13 females) or abstainers ($n = 62$; 30 males and 32 females) on the basis of drinking histories obtained in the interview and reports from subjects an collaterals contacted during the interval period. Five factors identified from the initial interview period were investigated for their ability to predict subsequent resumer or abstainer status: depressive symptomatology, psychosocial maladjustment, previous treatment history, neuropsychological performance, and ADD symptoms. Significant sex differences were found for psychosocial maladjustment, previous treatment history, and depressive symptomatology, with females receiving higher scores on each of the three variables. There were, however, no sex × drinking status interactions. Therefore, males and females were combined for further analyses.

Those subjects who became resumers over the study performed significantly more poorly than abstainers on the neuropsychological performance index and scored significantly higher than abstainers on depressive symptomatology, pretreatment psychosocial maladjustment, and ADD at the first interview. In addition, resumers manifested a trend toward higher previous treatment scores.

In multiple regression equations, depressive symptomatology proved to be the best predictor of resumer–abstainer status, followed by psychosocial maladjustment, previous treatment, neuropsychological performance, and ADD (the only factor not statistically significant in the equation). Discriminant function analyses using the five variables resulted in 75% correct classification of resumers and abstainers. Importantly, the statistical model correctly classified 76% of males and 82% of females, demonstrating the similarity of predictive variables across gender.

In conclusion, relapse rates overall appear to be similar for male and female alcoholics. There are certain factors, however, such as marital status, treatment style, symptom severity, and depressive symptomatology, which may contribute to sex-related differences in the process of relapse and remission. Prognostic factors have delineated the predictive power of depression, psychosocial functioning, cognitive performance, and ADD in identifying those patients (both male and female) who may be most likely to relapse.

5. Recovery

The prospect of reversibility of alcohol-related deficits in neuropsychological and psychosocial functioning is an exciting one that has implications for both the scientific community and for providing alcoholics with realistic expectations for future goals. This section will discuss current evidence for recovery of neuropsychological and psychosocial functioning as well as structural changes with abstinence.

Fabian and Parsons[101] examined recovery of cognitive functioning in abstinent female alcoholics using both an independent groups design of long-term and short-term sober alcoholics and controls and a longitudinal design in which the short-term alcoholics were followed from detoxification for 21 months. Neuropsychological factors of (1) problem-solving, abstracting, and perceptual motor and perceptual spatial skills, (2) verbal skills, (3) memory for spatial relations, and (4) set-shifting flexibility were assessed. Comparison of long-term (mean, 48 months sober), short-term (mean, 30 days sober), and

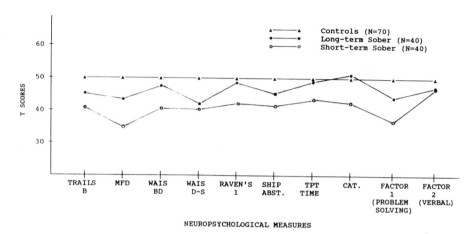

Figure 2. Comparison of nonalcoholic female controls, short-term sober alcoholic females, and long-term sober alcoholic females on neuropsychological tests (Trails B, Trail-Making Test, Part B; MFD, Memory for Designs; WAIS-BD, WAIS Block Design; WAIS D-S, WAIS Digit Symbol; Raven's 1, Raven's Progressive Matices, Set 1; Ship. Abst., Shipley Abstracting Age; TPT Time, Tactual Performance Test Time; Cat., Halstead Category Test) and overall measures of impairment (Factor 1 and Factor 2).

controls revealed significant differences on only the problem-solving factor (factor 1). Individual comparisons revealed that the long-term sober alcoholics performed intermediate to the other two groups, performing better than the short-term sober alcoholics, but not as well as the controls. Differential impairment and recovery of specific cognitive functions were assessed by examining the individual tests within the factor 1 (Fig. 2).

In the longitudinal design, two factors were used to examine recovery over 21 months: factor 1 was the same as the factor 1 in the first study; factor 2 was composed of strictly verbal measures. No differences between alcoholics and controls were found for factor 2. On factor 1, the alcoholics significantly improved from test to retest, but remained inferior to controls. Division of alcoholics into resumers and abstainers indicated that resumers performed more poorly than abstainers at both test and retest and accounted for much of the overall group differences found relative to controls. In analyzing the individual tests composing each factor, the authors again point out the possibility of differential recovery rates of various cognitive abilities. They suggest that verbal abilities, if impaired at all, recover most rapidly, followed by complex abstracting and problem-solving skills, and lastly by perceptual motor skills, which remain impaired for many months following treatment.

In a direct comparison of recovery of function in male and female alcoholics, Parsons et al.[102] compared neuropsychological performance in alcoholics and controls over a 14-month period. Alcoholics who remained abstinent during the follow-up period performed better than resumers at both test and retest. However, abstainers failed to perform as well as controls. Both abstainers and controls improved significantly over time. This pattern demonstrates that the primary cause of improvement was due to practice effects rather than reversibility of alcohol-related deficits. In this study there was no differential recovery of specific neuropsychological functions; alcoholics were impaired relative to controls on all four of the cognitive performance factors. Also, there were no significant sex differences; males and females followed similar courses of neuropsychological performance over time.

In the same subjects, Glenn et al.[103] found no improvement in alcoholics' cognitive functions as measured by electrophysiological measures of visual evoked potentials. Alcoholics who remained abstinent demonstrated amplitudes and latencies that were intermediate to relapsed alcoholics and controls, particularly N200 and P300. There was no significant improvement in abstainers over time, nor were there any significant sex differences in the lack of demonstrable recovery.

Recovery of psychosocial function was alluded to in the discussion of the DeSoto et al.[93] study in the previous section. In that study, males and females who remained abstinent showed significant, similar increases in employment status over a 10-year period. Parsons et al.[102] reported that alcoholics who relapsed in a 14-month period showed an increase in already moderately elevated depression scores at follow-up. Alcoholics who remained abstinent, however, showed significantly lower depression scores at test and at retest than resumers.

Moos et al.[98] examined stably remitted alcoholics (abstinent or drinking at a much reduced rate), relapsed alcoholics (resumed heavy drinking), and community controls at 2- and 10-year follow-up. At 2 years, stably remitted alcoholics demonstrated modest improvement over time. Specifically, they showed greater self-confidence, less depression and anxiety (equal to that of controls), increased family cohesion and family activities, and increased coping responses compared with relapsed alcoholics. At 10 years, stably remitted alcoholics reported less anxiety and depression, fewer days of hospitalization, greater family income, greater family cohesion and family organization, and fewer negative life events than the relapsed alcoholics. There were no significant differences between the three groups on other occupational, social, family functioning, work environment, or coping variables. The authors concluded that the average 10-year course of treated alcoholics is one of "modest improvement" in psychosocial functioning. With the exception of the sex differences in outcome related to marital status (married men and unmarried women have greater rates of abstinence at 6 months), there were relatively few sex-specific differences in the course of psychosocial recovery with abstinence.

Data providing support for potential reversibility of alcohol-induced structural brain changes have begun to accumulate with the advent of CT and MRI scans. Trends toward reversal in cerebral atrophy seen by CT have been reported for alcoholics abstinent for 30 to 152 weeks.[104–106] Jacobson[68] compared recently detoxified alcoholics, Alcoholics Anonymous (AA) members sober an average of 5 years, and controls to assess changes in CT scans with abstinence. Male AA members' CT scans were intermediate between alcoholics and controls, but only the cortical sulci widening was significantly less than that of current alcoholics. Female AA members also showed intermediate CT indices relative to female comparison groups, with no CT differences between AA members and controls and significant differences between current alcoholics and AA members on ventricle–brain ratio (VBR) and Sylvian fissure widening. Reduction of VBR (a measure of decreasing ventricular size) between alcoholics and AA members was 33.1% for females and 15% for males, with the reported duration of abstinence for female AA members half that of their male counterparts. Jacobson concluded that female alcoholics were more vulnerable to both structural changes and cognitive deficits with a shorter duration of alcohol abuse. However, females also showed the greater amount and rate of recovery with abstinence.

In summary, although evidence exists for recovery of alcohol-induced deficits, it does not appear to be complete compared with nonalcoholic controls. Residual deficits in abstinent alcoholics in neuropsychological function, electrophysiological measures, psychological and social/occupational function, and anatomic markers demonstrate the pervasive nature of alcoholic deficits as well as the protracted course of recovery.

No definitive sex differences in recovery have been consistently reported, reflective of both the general similarities between recovering male and female alcoholics and the need for further study of greater numbers of females in alcoholic research. Clearly evident in the recovery literature, however, is the primary importance of abstinence. In each of the studies discussed, recovery was markedly greater for alcoholics who remained abstinent or who greatly reduced consumption compared with alcoholics who resumed drinking even if at lower than pretreatment levels. Further studies investigating the potential role of factors such as premorbid variables, family history, and psychopathology may provide additional information on the process of relapse and recovery in both male and female alcoholics.

6. Summary and Conclusion

In summary, female alcoholics experience more significant affective symptomatology and shorter drinking histories. Excluding these important differences, male and female alcoholics are remarkably similar. The degree and pattern of cognitive impairment is very similar as is the apparent influence of factors such as FH and CBDs. Predictors of relapse and patterns of recovery are also similar for the sexes. These summary statements should not be interpreted as saying that differences do not exist. Obviously they do. One of the more critical differences is the differential susceptibility to alcohol's negative psychosocial and cognitive effects experienced by females. It is possible that some of the increased risk, particularly for psychosocial problems, occurs not because of inherent differences in the sexes, but rather because of society's differential response to female alcoholism.

Future research must support the strides made over the last 10 to 15 years; our commitment to the study of gender issues must continue. This focus is critical not solely because it directly impacts our understanding of female alcoholics, but also because it enhances our understanding of alcoholism, regardless of sex.

References

1. Hunt WA, nixon SJ (eds): *Alcohol-Induced Brain Damage* (Research Monograph 22). Rockville, MD, National Institutes on Alcohol Abuse and Alcoholism, 1993.
2. Parsons OA, Butters N, Nathan PE (eds): *Neuropsychology of Alcoholism: Implications for Diagnosis and Treatment*. New York, Guilford, 1987.
3. US Department of Health and Human Services: Seventh Special Report to the US Congress on Alcohol and Health. Rockville, MD, National Institute on Alcohol Abuse and Alcoholism, 1990.
4. National Council on Alcoholism and Drug Dependence: Treatment for alcoholism and other drug addictions. *NCADD Amethyst* 1:3, 1993.
5. Robbins C: Sex differences in psychosocial consequences of alcohol and drug abuse. *J Health Soc Behav* 30:117–130, 1989.
6. Hasin DS, Grant BF, Weinflash J: Male/female differences in alcohol-related problems: Alcohol rehabilitation patients. *Int J Additct* 23:437–448, 1988.
7. Morrissey ER, Schuckit MA: Drinking patterns and alcohol-related problems in a population of alcohol detoxification patients: Comparison of males and females, in Galanter M (ed): *Current Alcohol*. New York, Gruen, Stratton, 1980, vol 7, p 465.
8. Ross HE, Glaser FB, Stiasny S: Sex differences in the prevalence of psychiatric disorders in patients with alcohol and drug problems. *Br J Addict* 83:1179–1192, 1988.
9. Ross HE: Alcohol and drug abuse in treated alcoholics: A comparison of men and women. *Alcohol Clin Exp Res* 13:810–816, 1989.
10. Cowley DS: Alcohol abuse, substance abuse, and panic disorder. *Am J Med* 92(1A):41–48, 1992.
11. Kushner MG, Sher KJ, Beitman BD: The relation between alcohol problems and the anxiety disorders. *Am J Psychiatry* 147:685–695, 1990.
12. Petty F: The depressed alcoholic: Clinical features and medical management. *Gen Hosp Psychiatry* 14:258–264, 1992.
13. Ries R: Clinical treatment matching models for dually diagnosed patients. *Rec Adv Addict Disord* 16:167–175, 1993.
14. Roy A, DeJong J, Lamparski D, et al: Mental disorders among alcoholics: Relationship to age of onset and cerebrospinal fluid neuropeptides. *Arch Gen Psychiatry* 48:423–427, 1991.
15. Booth BM, Yates WR, Petty F, Brown K: Patient factors predicting early alcohol-related readmissions for alcoholics: Role of alcoholism severity and psychiatric co-morbidity. *J Stud Alcohol* 52:37–43, 1991.
16. Regier DA, Farmer ME, Rae DS, et al: Comorbidity of mental disorders with alcohol and other drug abuse: Results from the Epidemiologic Catchment Area (ECA) study. *J Am Med Assoc* 264:2511–2518, 1990.
17. McMahon RC, Davidson RS: An examination of depressed vs. nondepressed alcoholics in inpatient treatment. *J Clin Psychol* 42:177–184, 1986.
18. Murphy GE: *Suicide in Alcoholism*. New York, Oxford University Press, 1992.
19. Roy A, DeJong J, Lamparski D, et al: Depression among alcoholics: Relationship to clinical and cerebrospinal fluid variables. *Arch Gen Psychiatry* 48:428–432, 1991.

20. Bedi AR, Halikas JA: Alcoholism and affective disorder. *Alcohol Clin Exp Res* 9:133–134, 1985.
21. Gomberg ESL: Women and alcohol: Use and abuse. *J Nerv Ment Dis* 181:211–219, 1993.
22. Helzer JE, Pryzbeck TR: The co-occurrence of alcoholism with other psychiatric disorders in the general population and its impact on treatment. *J Stud Alcohol* 49:219–224, 1988.
23. Hesselbrock MN, Meyer RE, Keener JK: Psychopathology in hospitalized alcoholics. *Arch Gen Psychiatry* 42:1050–1055, 1985.
24. Schuckit M, Pitts FN Jr, Reich T, *et al:* Alcoholism. I. Two types of alcoholism in women. *Arch Gen Psychiatry* 20:301–306, 1969.
25. Schuckit MA, Winokur G: A short term follow up of women alcoholics. *Dis Nerv Sys* 33:672–678, 1972.
26. Rounsaville BJ, Dolinsky ZS, Babor TF, *et al:* Psychopathology as a predictor of treatment outcome in alcoholics. *Arch Gen Psychiatry* 44:505–513, 1987.
27. Von Knorring AL, Cloninger CR, Bohman M, Sigvardsson S: An adoption study of depressive disorders and substance abuse. *Arch Gen Psychiatry* 40:943–950, 1983.
28. Wender PH, Kety SS, Rosenthal D, *et al:* Psychiatric disorders in the biological and adoptive families of adopted individuals with affective disorders. *Arch Gen Psychiatry* 43:932–929, 1986.
29. Winokur G, Coryell W: Familial alcoholism in primary unipolar major depressive disorder. *Am J Psychiatry* 148:184–188, 1991.
30. Coryell W, Winokur G, Keller M, *et al:* Alcoholism and major depression: A family study approach to co-existing disorders. *J Affect Disord* 24:93–99, 1992.
31. Kendler KS, Heath AC, Neale MC, *et al:* Alcoholism and major depression in women: A twin study of the causes of cormorbidity. *Arch Gen Psychiatry* 50:690–698, 1993.
32. Cloninger CR, Reich T, Wetzel R: Alcoholism and affective disorders: Familial associations and genetic models, in Goodwin DW, Erickson CK (eds): *Alcoholism and Affective Disorders: Clinical, Genetic and Biochemical Studies.* New York, Spectrum, 1979, pp 57–86.
33. Cloninger CR: Neurogenetic adaptive mechanisms in alcoholism. *Science* 236:410–416, 1987.
34. Alterman A, Tarter R: An examination of selected typologies: Hyperactivity, familial, and antisocial alcoholism, in Galanter M (ed): *Recent Developments in Alcoholism.* New York, Plenum Press, 1986, vol 4, pp 169–189.
35. Irwin M, Schuckit M, Smith TL: Clinical importance of age at onset in Type 1 and Type 2 primary alcoholics. *Arch Gen Psychiatry* 47:320–324, 1990.
36. Nixon SJ: Typologies in women, in Galanter M (ed): *Recent Developments in Alcoholism.* New York, Plenum Press, 1993, vol 11, pp 305–323.
37. Lex BW, Sholar JW, Bower T, Mendelson JH: Putative Type II alcoholism characteristics in female third DUI offenders in Massachusetts: A pilot study. *Alcohol* 8:283–287, 1991.
38. Glenn SW, Nixon SJ: Applications of Cloninger's subtypes in a female alcoholic sample. *Alcohol Clin Exp Res* 15:851–857, 1991.
39. Selzer ML: The Michigan Alcohol Screening Test: The quest for a new diagnostic instrument. *Am J Psychiatry* 127:1653–1658, 1971.
40. Pihl RO, Peterson JB: Attention-deficit hyperactivity disorder, childhood conduct disorder, and alcoholism: Is there an association? *Alcohol Health Res World* 15:25–31, 1991.
41. Tarter RE: Developmental behavior—genetic perspective of alcoholism etiology, in Galanter M (ed): *Recent Developments in Alcoholism.* New York, Plenum Press, 1991, vol 9, pp 71–85.
42. Wood D, Wender PH, Reimherr FW: The prevalence of attention deficit disorder, residual type, or minimal brain dysfunction in a population of male alcoholic patients. *Am J Psychiatry* 140:95–98, 1983.
43. Hesselbrock V, Bauer LO, Hesselbrock MN, Gillen R: Neuropsychological factors in individuals at high risk for alcoholism, in Galanter M (ed): *Recent Developments in Alcoholism.* New York, Plenum Press, 1991, vol 9, pp 21–40.
44. DeObaldia R, Parsons OA, Yohman R: Minimal brain dysfunction symptoms claimed by primary and secondary alcoholics: Relation to cognitive functioning. *Intern J Neurosci* 20:173–182, 1983.
45. Glenn SW, Errico AL, Parsons OA, *et al:* The role of antisocial, affective, and childhood behavioral characteristics in alcoholics' neuropsychological performance. *Alcohol Clin Exp Res* 17:162–169, 1993.

46. Tarter RE, McBride H, Buonpane N, Schneider DU: Differentiation of alcoholics. *Arch Gen Psychiatry* 34:761–768, 1977.
47. Wood D, Reimherr F, Wender P, Johnson G: Diagnosis and treatment of minimal brain dysfunction in adults. *Arch Gen Psychiatry* 33:1453–1460, 1976.
48. Parsons OA: Neuropsychological consequences of alcohol abuse: Many questions—some answers, in Parsons OA, Butters N, Nathan PE (eds): *Neuropsychology of Alcoholism: Implications for Diagnosis and Treatment.* New York, Guilford, 1987, pp 153–175.
49. Glenn SW: Sex differences in alcohol-induced brain damage, in Hunt WA, Nixon SJ (eds): *Alcohol-Induced Brain Damage* (Research Monograph No. 22). Rockville, MD, National Institute on Alcohol Abuse and Alcoholism, 1993, pp 195–212.
50. Beatty WW, Katzung VM, Nixon SJ, Moreland VJ: Problem-solvinging deficits in alcoholics: Evidence from the California Card Sorting Test. *J Stud Alcohol* 54:687–692, 1993.
51. Glenn SW, Parsons OA: The role of time in neuropsychological performance: Investigation and application in an alcoholic population. *Clin Neuropsychol* 4:344–354, 1990.
52. Glenn SW, Parsons OA: Neuropsychological efficiency measures in male and female alcoholics. *J Stud Alcohol* 53:546–552, 1992.
53. Nixon SJ: Application of theoretical models to the study of alcohol-induced brain damage, in Hunt WA, Nixon SJ (eds): *Alcohol-Induced dBrain Damage* (Research Monograph 22). Rockville, MD, National Institute on Alcohol Abuse and Alcoholism, 1993, pp 213–228.
54. Nixon SJ, Parsons OA: Alcohol-related efficiency deficits using an ecologically valid test. *Alcohol Clin Exp Res* 15:601–606, 1991.
55. Smith ME, Oscar-Berman M: Resource-limited information processing in alcoholism. *J Stud Alcohol* 53:514–518, 1992.
56. Simon HA, Kaplan CA: Foundations of cognitive science, in Posner MI (ed): *Foundations of Cognitive Science.* Cambridge, MA, MIT, 1989, pp 1–48.
57. Sternberg RJ: Toward a triarchic theory of human intelligence. *Behav Brain Sci* 7:269–315, 1984.
58. Erwin JE, Hunter JJ: Prediction of attrition in alcoholic aftercare by scores on the embedded figures test and two Piagetian tasks. *J Consult Clin Psychol* 52:354–358, 1984.
59. Kuhn D, Brannock J: Development of the isolation of variables scheme in experimental and "natural experiment" contexts. *Dev Psychol* 13:9–14, 1977.
60. Jones SL, Lanyon RI: Relationship between adaptive skills and outcome of alcoholism treatment. *J Stud Alcohol* 42:521–525, 1981.
61. Nixon SJ, Tivis R, Parsons OA: Interpersonal problem-solvingin in male and female alcoholics. *Alcohol Clin Exp Res* 16:684–687, 1992.
62. Patterson BW, Parsons OA, Schaeffer KW, Errico AL: Interpersonal problem solving in alcoholics. *J Nerv Ment Dis* 176:707–713, 1988.
63. Harper CG, Kril JJ: Neuropathological changes in alcoholics, in Hunt WA, Nixon SJ (eds): *Alcohol-Induced Brain Damage* (Research Monograph 22). Rockville, MD, National Institute on Alcohol Abuse and Alcoholism, 1993, pp 39–69.
64. Pfefferbaum A, Rosenbloom M: In vivo imaging of morphological brain alterations associated with alcoholism, in Hunt WA, Nixon SJ (eds): *Alcohol-Induced Brain Damage* (Research Monograph 22). Rockville, MD, National Institute on Alcohol Abuse and Alcoholism, 1993, pp 71–87.
65. Porjesz B, Begleiter H: Neurophysiological factors associated with alcoholism, in Hunt WA, Nixon SJ (eds): *Alcohol-Induced Brain Damage* (Research Monograph 22). Rockville, MD, National Institute on Alcohol Abuse and Alcoholism, 1993, pp 89–120.
66. Charness ME: Brain lesions in alcoholics. *Alcohol Clin Exp Res* 17:2–11, 1993.
67. Parsons OA, Sinha R, Williams HL: Relationships between neuropsychological test performance and event-related potentials in alcoholic and nonalcoholic samples. *Alcohol Clin Exp Res* 14:746–755, 1990.
68. Jacobson R: Female alcoholics: A controlled CT brain scan and clinical study. *Br J Addict* 81:661–669, 1986.
69. Jacobson R: The contributions of sex and drinking history of the CT brain scan changes in alcoholics. *Psychol Med* 16:547–559, 1986.

70. Mann K, Batra A, Gunthner A, Schroth G: Do women develop alcoholic brain damage more readily than men? *Alcohol Clin Exp Res* 16:1052–1056, 1992.

71. Bates ME, Pandina RJ: Familial alcoholism and premorbid cognitive deficit: A failure to replicate subtype differences. *J Stud Alcohol* 53:320–327, 1992.

72. Galanter M (ed): *Recent Developments in Alcoholism: Children of Alcoholics,* vol 9. New York, Plenum Press, 1991.

73. Parsons OA: Impaired neuropsychological cognitive functioning in sober alcoholics, in Hunt WA, Nixon SJ (eds): *Alcohol-Induced Brain Damage* (Research Monograph No. 22). Rockville, MD, National Institute on Alcohol Abuse and Alcoholism, 1993, pp 173–194.

74. Sinha R, Parsons OA, Glenn SW: Drinking variables, affective measures and neuropsychological performance: Familial alcoholism and gender correlates. *Alcoholism* 6:77–85, 1989.

75. Glenn SW, Parsons OA: Alcohol abuse and familial alcoholism: Psychological correlates in men and women. *J Stud Alcohol* 50:116–127, 1989.

76. Glenn SW, Parsons OA, Stevens L: Effects of alcohol abuse and familial alcoholism on physical health in men and women. *Health Psychol* 8:325–341, 1989.

77. Kosten TR, Rounsaville BJ, Kosten TA, Merikangas K: Gender differences in the specificity of alcoholism transmission among the relatives of opioid addicts. *J Ment Nerv Dis* 179:392–400, 1991.

78. Lisansky ES: Alcoholism in women: Social and psychological concomitants. I. Social history data. *Q J Stud Alcohol* 18:588–623, 1957.

79. Gorenstein EE: Cognitive–perceptual deficit in an alcoholism spectrum disorder. *J Stud Alcohol* 48:310–318, 1987.

80. Hesselbrock MN, Weidenman MA, Reed HB: Effect of age, sex, drinking history and antisocial personality on neuropsychology of alcoholics. *J Stud Alcohol* 46:313–320, 1985.

81. Malloy P, Noel N, Rogers S, *et al*: Risk factors for neuropsychological impairment in alcoholics: Antisocial personality, age, years of drinking, and gender. *J Stud Alcohol* 50:422–426, 1989.

82. Workman-Daniels KL, Hesselbrock VM: Childhood problem behavior and neuropsychological functioning in persons at risk for alcoholism. *J Stud Alcohol* 48:187–193, 1987.

83. Glenn SW, Nixon SJ: Investigation of Cloninger's subtypes in a male alcoholic sample: Applications and implications. *J Clin P* submitted.

84. Nathan P, Skinstad AH: Outcomes of treatment for alcohol problems: Current methods, problems and results. *J Consult Clin Psychol* 55:332–340, 1987.

85. Sokolow L, Welte J, Hynes G, Lyons J: Treatment-related differences between male and female alcoholics. *Focus Women* 1:42–56, 1980.

86. Annis HM: Treatment of alcoholic women, in Edwards G, Grant M (eds): *Alcoholism Treatment in Transition.* Baltimore, MD, University Park Press, 1980, pp 128–139.

87. Vannicellli M: Treatment outcome of alcoholic women: The state of the art in relation to sex bias and expectancy effects, in Wilsnack SC, Beckman LJ (eds): *Alcohol Problems in Women.* New York, Guilford, 1984, pp 369–412.

88. Kammeier ML, Conley JJ: Toward a system for prediction of posttreatment abstinence and adaptation, in Galanter M (ed): *Currents in Alcoholism.* New York, Grune & Stratton, 1979, vol 6, pp 111–119.

89. Blume SB: Researchers on women and alcohol, in *Alcoholism and Alcohol Abuse Among Women: Research Issues* (Research Monograph No. 1, U.S. Department of Health, Education and Public Welfare Publication No. ADM-80-835). Washington, DC, US Government Printing Office, 1980, pp 121–151.

90. Wilsnack SL: Alcohol abuse and alcoholism in women, in Pattison EM, Kaufman E (eds): *Encyclopedic Handbook of Alcoholism.* New York, Gardner, 1982, pp 718–735.

91. O'Connor PG, Horwitz RI, Gottlieb LD, *et al*: The impact of gender on clinical characteristics and outcome in alcohol withdrawal. *J Subst Abuse Treat* 10:59–61, 1993.

92. DeSoto CB, O'Donnell WE, DeSoto JL: Long-term recovery in alcoholics. *Alcohol Clin Exp Res* 13:693–697, 1989.

93. Weisner C, Schmidt L: Gender disparities in treatment for alcohol problems. *J Am Med Assoc* 268:1872–1876, 1992.

94. Rosenberg H: Prediction of controlled drinking by alcoholics and problem drinkers. *Psychol Bull* 113:129–139, 1993.
95. Davies DL: Normal drinking in recovered alcohol addicts. *Q J Stud Alcohol* 23:94–104, 1962.
96. Kendall RE: Normal drinking by former alcohol addicts. *Q J Stud Alcohol* 26:247–257, 1965.
97. Moos RH, Finney JW, Cronkite RC: *Alcoholism Treatment: Context, Process and Outcome.* New York, Oxford University Press, 1990.
98. Babor TF, Hoffman M, Del Boca FK, *et al:* Types of alcoholics. I. Evidence for an empirically derived typology based on indicators of vulnerability and severity. *Arch Gen Psychiatry* 49:599–608, 1992.
99. Glenn SW, Parsons OA: Prediction of resumption of drinking in posttreatment alcoholics. *Int J Addict* 26:237–254, 1991.
100. Fabian MS, Parsons OA: Differential improvement of cognitive functions in recovering alcoholic women. *J Abnorm Psychol* 92:87–95, 1983.
101. Parsons OA, Schaeffer KW, Glenn SW: Does neuropsychological test peformance predict resumption of drinking in posttreatment alcoholics? *Addict Behav* 15:297–307, 1990.
102. Glenn SW, Parsons OA, Sinha R: Assessment of recovery of electrophysiological and neuro-psychological functions in chronic alcoholics. *Biol Psychiatry* 36:443–452, 1994.
103. Ron MA: *The Alcoholic Brain: CT Scan and Psychological Findings.* Cambridge, Cambridge University Press, 1983 (Psychol Med monograph, Suppl 3).
104. Carlen PL, Wilkinson DA, Wortzman G, Holgate RC: Partially reversible cerebral atrophy and functional impairment in abstinent alcoholics. *Can J Neurol Sci* 11:441–446, 1984.
105. Cala LA, Jones B, Burns P, *et al:* Results of computerized tomography, psychometric studies, and dietary studies in social drinkers, with emphasis on reversibility after abstinence. *Med J Aust* 2:264–269, 1983.

The Emergence of Problem-Drinking Women as a Special Population in Need of Treatment

Laura Schmidt and Constance Weisner

Abstract. This chapter chronicles the development of advocacy for improvements in alcohol treatment services for women during the 1970s and 1980s, tracing its influence in terms of real change in treatment systems in the United States. We follow the development of a "women's alcoholism movement" from its inception in the late 1970s through its transition during the late 1980s into a broader movement focused on drug abuse and perinatal addiction. We describe the new governing images of problem-drinking women that advocates presented, their claims about the nature of substance abuse problems in women, and their recommendations for a more "gender-sensitive" treatment system. We also review increased federal involvement in this issue over the course of the 1980s, as pressure mounted on policymakers to respond to the crisis over drug-exposed infants by making treatment services more accessible to women. The chapter concludes by considering these developments from the perspective of national treatment system statistics, finding modest growth in specialized and women-only treatment units, as well as moderate increases in the representation of women in substance abuse treatment caseloads.

1. Introduction

Around the middle of the 1970s, constituents in the alcohol field began to advocate for the special treatment needs of "underserved" female problem drinkers in the US population. What followed was a familiar debate about numbers—one that seems to inevitably accompany the identification of a new

Laura Schmidt • Alcohol Research Group and Department of Sociology, University of California, Berkeley, California 94709. **Constance Weisner** • Alcohol Research Group and School of Public Health, University of California, Berkeley, California 94709.

Recent Developments in Alcoholism, Volume 12: Women and Alcoholism, edited by Marc Galanter. Plenum Press, New York, 1995.

social problem about which there is only inconclusive evidence. In this case, a loose coalition of women's advocates had begun to warn of a growing but "hidden epidemic" of alcohol problems in women; they argued that the traditional gap in rates of consumption by men and women had begun to narrow, while gender disparities in treatment access had not.[1-3] Meanwhile, a small but fairly continual stream of social scientists denied that there was evidence of a dramatic rise in women's alcohol consumption or convergence in male and female drinking patterns.[4,5] Some went on to suggest that claims of an "epidemic" were more indicative of a political tendency toward alcohol "problem inflation" than any real change in women's drinking patterns.[6]

Despite this skepticism, by the early 1980s, advocates for improving alcohol treatment services for women had organized a sizeable political coalition on the issue. This self-identified "women's alcoholism movement," however, did not grow out of organizations in the feminist movement, as did other activist groups focused on women's health issues that organized at the time. Rather, it largely drew from the ranks of traditional alcoholism constituencies, most notably the National Council on Alcoholism (NCA).* It used the time-honored techniques of lobbying members of Congress sensitive to alcohol issues, offering testimony in public hearings, and launching public education campaigns about alcohol problems. These were the same techniques that had successfully advanced important alcohol policies in the past, such as the "Hughes Act," which had created a National Institute on Alcohol Abuse and Alcoholism (NIAAA) in 1970.[7,8]

Fortuitously, the women's alcoholism movement was able to draw support from two other developments occurring inside the national alcoholism arena of the 1980s. First, controversy over women's substance abuse and "fetal rights" proved a consistent theme throughout the decade; the 1980s began with debates over fetal alcohol syndrome babies and closed with a crisis over drug-exposed infants.[9] Though initially advocates for improving women's treatment focused almost exclusively on alcohol issues, in the late-1980s they would broaden their agenda to include what had become higher-profile issues involving drug treatment for women and mothers. Second, there was a general expansion and diversification of substance abuse treatment systems over the course of the decade, evident in a doubling of national bed capacity and significant broadening in types of treatment modalities.[10,11] While growing controversy over maternal substance abuse provided a strong political rationale for improving women's access to treatment, the

---

* NCA is a voluntary association organized in 1944 by three women including Marty Mann, one of the first women to join Alcoholics Anonymous. Its program has emphasized educating the public about the basic facts of alcoholism as a disease and encouraging medical and public health responsibility for the problem. NCA has proved influential as a political lobby at the national level and has developed an expansive network of 190 state and local chapters, as well as effective strategies for influencing public opinion and policy on alcoholism. In the late 1980s, NCA renamed itself the National Council on Alcohol and Drug Dependency to reflect the inclusion of drug problems in its agenda.

general expansion in treatment systems created an organizational environment richer in resources for founding specialized women's programs.

By the mid-1980s, these developments and a vigorous political campaign had led to some tangible changes in national policy on substance abuse and women. As the treatment system expanded and diversified, new federal legislation in 1984 required that each state devote 5% of its federal funding allocations to specialized women's alcohol and drug services.[12] Meanwhile, a growing private sector of alcoholism treatment adopted new marketing policies designed to attract women into treatment. The federal government had also convened special conferences on the issue by the mid-1980s and had made research on women's drinking a national priority in the scientific grant-reviewing process. By the late 1980s, it would earmark sizeable portions of its national "drug war" allocations for the treatment of pregnant women[13] and would institute a "Women's Health Research and Services Work Group" to coordinate ongoing appraisal of research needs and to develop regular "Action Plans."[14] While these public and private sector policy developments are notable, it is yet to be determined whether they actually gave rise to significant changes in treatment services for women.

Our purpose in this chapter is to chronicle the development of advocacy for improvements in women's alcohol treatment during the 1970s and 1980s and as clearly as possible to trace its influence in terms of real change in the US substance abuse treatment system. First, we examine the type of coalition that formed around the issue of treatment for women and the particular claims it made about the problem. Second, we discuss the federal response to political pressure to improve treatment services for women, including how this response changed over the course of the 1980s as concerns about maternal substance abuse intensified. Last, we study change in the organization of services for women using national statistics on trends in substance abuse treatment units between 1982 and 1992.* In particular, we are interested in examining the development of substance abuse programs that serve exclusively women and whether change in treatment systems has proved consistent with the goals of political advocates.

2. A "Women's Alcoholism Movement"

The idea of a special population—or a group that is both "underserved" and requires a specialized treatment approach[15]—has been a leading principle in US alcohol policy, that is, at least since the inception of NIAAA in 1970. During its first years of operation, NIAAA provided special grants to state

* We rely on survey data from the National Drug and Alcohol Treatment Utilization Survey (NDATUS), the only available national database on substance abuse treatment units, to analyze trends involving women in treatment systems. Methodological limitations in the NDATUS surveys make it important to interpret findings cautiously; these issues are discussed in the Appendix (Section 6) and at points in the text where appropriate.

chapters of the NCA to support local grass roots commissions on women and ethnic minority issues. Whether intentional or not, drawing advocates of special populations into the alcohol arena has helped to broaden the political base of support for alcohol policies and to deepen public demand for services and research.[8] Over the years, a growing emphasis on special populations can be detected in NIAAA's regular reports to Congress, where the sheer number of groups identified as "underserved" has grown significantly.[10] It is also evident in the institute's ongoing promotion of "treatment matching"; since the 1970s, clinicians and researchers have been encouraged to develop ways of pairing specialized treatment modalities with particular special populations.[16] Finally, Table I suggests that sustained political interest in this area has influenced the shape of substance abuse treatment systems in the United States. The NDATUS survey shows significant growth between 1982 and 1992 in the proportion of treatment units that provide services designed for special populations such as ethnic minority populations and youth, as well as a decline in units offering no specialized services.

Advocates for improving alcohol treatment for women have been one of the more enduring coalitions devoted to a special population. Their general success is suggested in Table I, where it is shown that the number of treatment units offering specialized services for women has more than doubled since 1982 and that growth in women's services has held pace with that of other "special populations."* The strength of this particular coalition is largely due to the early involvement of NCA, an organization that views itself as having "led the field" in advocacy for women.[1] As noted above, early grass roots coalition building through state task forces on women took place under the auspices of the NCA during the 1970s. At this time, NCA's national leaders also began to lobby Congress and to hold public symposiums on issues such as fetal alcohol syndrome and women's access to treatment.[3,17] By the mid-1980s, NCA leaders were key spokespeople in debates over earmarking federal funds for women's treatment[18] and had begun to sponsor a yearly "National Fetal Alcohol Syndrome Awareness Week."[19] And as the decade closed, they had become central voices in Congressional debates about the problem of drug-exposed infants; here they played a crucial role in redirecting a debate about jailing pregnant addicts toward one focused on women's access to treatment.[20] Throughout, the NCA's success in leadership has been accomplished largely through specialty groups that it has spawned—groups that have remained loosely coupled with the parent organization but still able

---

* It is important to note here that the NDATUS surveys have not been very clear as to what counts as a "specialized service for women." Thus, some treatment settings claiming to offer special services may simply have hired a female counselor, whereas others may offer a well-developed program or track of specialized therapy designed for women. It is also possible that reporting bias changed over the course of the decade, though it is impossible to ascertain the extent to which this occurred. For example, under growing political demands that programs do something identifiable for problem-drinking women, administrators may have grown more sensitive to the importance of reporting specialized services that they offered for women.

Table I. Proportion of US Substance Abuse Treatment Units[a] Offering Special Population Services: 1982, 1987, and 1992

	1982 (N = 5677)	1987 (N = 6866)	1992 (N = 9262)
Women	23	28	53
Blacks	9	7	37
Hispanics	10	11	32
Native Americans	NA[b]	5	17
Youth	24	31	38
Cocaine users	NA	12	45
Public inebriates	10	6	19
No special services	50	NA	18

[a]Includes alcohol-only, drug-only, and combined alcohol and drug treatment units.
[b]NA, Data not available.

to reach out to narrower constituencies focused on particular aspects of women and substance abuse. These have included the National Women's Congress on Alcohol and Drug Problems (founded 1980),[21] the National Association of Women in Alcoholism and Other Drug Dependencies (founded 1988),[22] and the Coalition on Alcohol and Drug Dependent Women and Their Children (founded 1988).[23]

Treatment-provider coalitions and mutual aid groups have been important stakeholders, working in tandem with the NCA to reform the treatment system for women. During the 1970s, a National Coalition for Women's Alcoholism Programs formed to secure support for specialized programs sponsored by the NIAAA.[7] By the early 1980s, treatment-provider groups were convening regular national symposiums on issues such as "Intervention and Outreach Strategies to Meet the Needs of the Hidden Female Alcoholic,"[24] and "The Emerging Female Alcoholic: The Patient of the '80s."[25] National conferences did not merely provide opportunities for training; they also offered contexts for political mobilizing, as was suggested by the comments of one NIAAA representative at the 1980 "Women in Crisis" conference:

> I hope that you as activist women will help change at least some segments of society's view of the alcohol-abusing woman so they can see her as a person in need of help and a person worthy of the best care available.[26]

Nation-wide mutual help organizations, such as Alcoholics Anonymous (AA) and Women for Sobriety (WFS) have provided additional constituencies, with the latter closely reflecting the spirit and objectives of the women's alcoholism movement. WFS was founded in 1976 as a program tailored to the special needs of female alcoholics, who were believed to be inadequately served by traditional mutual help groups such as AA.[27] However, it is clear that during the 1980s representation of women in AA increased, as did the number of women-only AA groups.[28] While AA did not itself act politically, it provided a potential recruiting ground for women activists.

The women's alcoholism movement therefore drew its support largely from the ranks of traditional alcoholism constituencies; conspicuously absent were representatives from organizations in the broader feminist and women's health movements. This was not due to a lack of interest in building alliances with feminists. Indeed, at a "Mobilizing Organized Change" conference in the mid-1970s, the then-director of the NCA made an appeal to "broaden the base" of the women's alcoholism movement by "shaping a new awareness" of alcohol problems among feminists:

> Women in the field of alcohol have not been making their concerns known to the women's community at large—to the women's organizations, women's groups and women leaders. Women in the alcohol field must interact with, and become part of, the big picture of women's issues in their communities, in their cities, and in their states. Alcohol concerns must be seen as a valid concern by the women's community in general.[3]

The movement's limited success in becoming part of the "big picture of women's issues" may be attributable to basic differences in philosophy. The broader women's movement generally adopted a "wet" perspective on alcohol issues, evident in its crusades to obtain access to all-male drinking establishments such as the "Men's Bar" in New York City's Biltmore Hotel[29] and in its protests against public warning signs in bars about drinking during pregnancy.[30] The women's alcoholism movement, however, took the opposing "dry" position and focused on improving services for women and on conducting health education campaigns to warn women of, among other things, the dangers of drinking while pregnant.[31] Its rejection of "wet" feminism was quite explicit:

> Widespread drinking among women is usually seen as a "symbol of liberation," tangible evidence of the social equality of men and women. But in fact, women's increased drinking, along with their greater freedom to smoke cigarettes, drive sports cars, and wear pants to work, is not so much a sign of actual equality as it is a cheap substitute for it.[2]

Given our present interest in treatment systems, it also is noteworthy that these ideological differences tended to reduce the possibilities for building organizational alliances between women's substance abuse programs and the growing network of women's health centers sponsored by feminists. Though the women's alcoholism movement sought to "educate" feminist health providers about substance abuse,[32] women's centers sometimes "actively resisted recognizing that some women had problems with alcohol or other drugs" because this tended to "pathologize and blame women."[33] Indeed, central concepts in the alcoholism perspective, such as "codependency" and "enabling," were likely to be viewed by women's health advocates as offensive, since they could be interpreted as reinforcing traditional stereotypes of female dependency on men. These tensions reflected a general problem for feminist advocates involved with behavioral health issues, including mental illness and drug and alcohol problems. "Wet" and "dry" feminists shared an interest in helping women to win access to the same choices as men. However, those fighting for equal access to alcoholism treatment faced the unique problem of having to cast their beneficiaries in a weak light, as victims of a stigmatizing condition.

Consequently, a primary objective was to educate the public in a more sympathetic view of problem-drinking women, in particular, one that characterized their condition as a medical as opposed to a moral problem. Here, the movement could draw upon the extensive experience of the alcoholism constituency groups to which it was closely tied:

> We must once and for all time break down the stigma that has held the female alcoholic back from treatment—we must shout out what Marty Mann, the founder of NCA, voiced 32 years ago: Alcoholism is a treatable disease, and no woman in our country today should be allowed to suffer or die from this disease fearing it as a moral weakness.[3]

These public information efforts focused on two new governing images of women's alcohol problems. The first image was that of the housewife-alcoholic who drank to relieve daily boredom and frustrated personal aspirations.[3,29] The second was that of the working woman who drank to relieve job stress, "role overload," and the abuses of job discrimination[34]; for the working woman, "drinking may blot out the reality of a despised work situation from which she sees few avenues of escape."[2] In both cases, the new characterizations suggested a more sympathetic view of the problem-drinking woman; for instance, both referred to women of the middle-class who at the very least had a better chance of eliciting sympathy than did the usual stereotypes of downwardly mobile male alcoholics. Moreover, both governing images conveyed an implicit theory of the etiology of alcoholism in women, one that emphasized her unenviable place in patriarchal society. Both implied that women's victimization by traditional gender roles was a key cause of alcoholism, though of the two, it was perhaps the housewife-alcoholic who could be considered the greater victim. As women moved into the workplace,

> . . . naturally they [would] take on the diseases of the working male— hypertension, alcoholism. Naturally the woman under pressure will be tense. But frustration is more likely to lead to alcoholism. Self-expression is not achieved in the house. The hidden housewife's only high comes out of a bottle.[3]

This implicit theory, which located the origins of female alcoholism in gender roles, was conveyed in its purest form by the "womanliness hypothesis."[35] This suggested that the female alcoholic drank to feel more feminine, and thus to suppress her inner conflicts about traditional female roles[36]: "Rather than repudiating [the feminine role], she opts for overidentifying with it; she becomes feminine with a vengeance."[2]

The policy recommendations implied by these governing images of the problem were twofold and related to deficiencies in both the quantity and quality of alcohol treatment for women. First, the image of the "hidden" housewife-alcoholic suggested that the problem was more prevalent than generally believed. Public education and outreach were required to improve the chances that "invisible" alcoholics would obtain treatment.[37] Their invisibility was mainly attributable to the "brutally harsh stigma" attached to problem drinking by women,[2] which led to denial of the problem among families, professionals, and women themselves. Families often formed a "silent conspiracy" to hide the substance-abusing woman; thus advocates should increase awareness by espousing slogans such as, "For every woman drug addict hiding in a closet, there are usually several family members leaning against the door."[38] Law enforcement officers, judges, and physicians tended to "protect" women from the shame of being alcoholic[39,40]; hence, professionals should be made wary of the "magnolia blossom syndrome," where a women's "manner may be suspiciously demure, with a soft voice, fluttery eyes, and a tendency toward being over-cooperative" in an effort to hide her drinking problem.[29]

Finally, denial could be "so powerful [as to] permeate the alcoholism field itself."[2] "Sex bias" among researchers led to undercounting women with alcohol problems in national health surveys, as well as to a paucity of general knowledge about women's drinking.[41-43] Alcohol treatment providers' stereotypes suggested that women might be harder to treat,[44,45] and gender bias resulted in a treatment system that offered few of the services needed by women, such as child care and vocational counseling.[46] To cut through these many layers of denial, new tactics were needed to directly reach out to the middle-class and "hidden" housewife-alcoholic:

> One counselor suggests this untraditional way to get a message inside the front door: Train Tupperware hostesses, Avon Ladies, and Welcome Wagon greeters in techniques of talking to a woman who drinks too much, then send them into homes with "soap, perfume, deodorants, and lots of literature." The approach would reach some "unaffiliated" women—those who don't even belong to the PTA.[29]

The movement's second type of policy recommendation focused on the quality of treatment offered to women, emphasizing that women required a specialized or "gender-sensitive" approach. Since clearly, "the answer to female alcoholism [was] not going to come by returning women to their former roles,"[3] treatment for women would likely involve some aspect of "feminist consciousness-raising."[2,29] Women-only treatment programs or, at minimum separate groups within coed programs, were justified on several grounds. Women's diminished status in sexist society, not to mention stigmatizing public attitudes toward female alcoholism, could lead them to internalize feelings of inferiority. Womens' unique problems with self-esteem were best treated within specialized programs focusing on women's "autonomy" and "authentic expression of self."[47] In all-women programs, clients could be exposed to "role models" who demonstrated more positive identities for women.[48,49] Conflicts over sexual identity, sex roles, and sexual abuse in problem-drinking women were also best explored in all-women treatment settings.[50,51] As a director of NCA's Office on Women described the situation:

> We get up, in group therapy, in front of a therapist who is male and we talk about our bad days, how wild and irresponsible we were, and we repent and put our virgin mary suits on again. . . . And they don't challenge it— they encourage it. . . . The message is don't disrupt, don't do anything that would make us men have to confront our feelings about who women really are.[2]

Finally, the traditional "confrontational approach" often used in alcoholism therapy had been designed to "break through men's tendencies to minimize their problems and [to] try to maintain control at all costs." Yet confrontation was "opposite to how most women relate to others" and for them proved not only "frightening and alienating"[36] but also counterproductive: "Since interaction in therapy tends to reflect social relationships in the larger society, there is also a tendency for men to 'take charge' in coed therapy groups, while women silently look on."[52]

Some of these arguments about alcohol problems in women and their appropriate treatment seem plausible. However, they were largely founded on a new liberal-feminist political awareness of the problem rather than on scientific evidence—as the available evidence was rather weak and inconclusive. We have already noted that the general question of rising prevalence— or a "hidden epidemic" of female alcoholism—has been a debated issue. It has, for instance, led to debates among researchers about whether the usual indicators of problem drinking are applicable to women or whether entirely new measures are needed.[53,54] Furthermore, while there is reliable evidence that women have been underrepresented in alcoholism treatment programs,[36] it is not entirely clear whether this is primarily due to a lack of access and a poorly educated public as women's advocates emphasized or due to the many other factors that can potentially influence treatment entry. For instance, some studies indicate that while women are less likely than men to seek alcoholism treatment, they are more likely to seek psychiatric help for a drinking problem.[55,56] This may be because problem-drinking women are more likely to perceive their symptoms as psychological in nature[57,58] or because they experience different patterns of alcoholism–mental illness comorbidity than men.[59,60]

Finally, while there are clear practical advantages to making women-only treatment settings an available option,[5,61,62] there is little hard evidence to support advocate's claims that specialized or women-only programs perform better for women therapeutically. From a practical standpoint, women-only facilities are more likely to offer the benefits of ancillary services needed by women such as child care and vocational services[63] and may attract populations that would otherwise not be seen,[64] such as women with dependent children, lesbians, and women who have suffered sexual abuse in childhood.[65] However, reviews of the treatment outcomes literature over the past decade[6,10,44,66] have pointed to the lack of evidence about the advantages of specialized treatment approaches for women. Ironically, this is largely attributable to the smaller numbers of women found in substance abuse programs, where clinical trial studies have had difficulty obtaining adequate sample sizes of women to draw statistically reliable conclusions. Thus, an Institute of Medicine review[67] and other scientific reviews[68] have pointed to the sample size problem as one of the main hindrances to gathering evidence on treatment outcomes in women with the same precision as those for men. The most recent generation of outcome studies comparing treatment effects for men and women has generally found that women respond the same or slightly better than men to alcohol treatment[69–72]; however, studies of specialized women's therapies are virtually nonexistent. It thus remains the case that there is little conclusive evidence to support the relative advantages of using women therapists, women's therapy groups, women-only treatment programs, or any other specialized approach for treating women. Conclusions reached by literature reviews conducted more than a decade ago still generally apply:

> Little of what passes as commonly accepted knowledge in this area is, in fact, founded on a sound empirical basis. . . . A major task facing the serious student of the woman alcoholic is that of distilling fact from fancy.[44]

3. The Federal Response

As we suggested earlier, the founding goals of the women's alcoholism movement were generally compatible with the NIAAA's emphasis on "special populations." Moreover, during the 1970s, the federal institute used a "categorical project grants" approach that made it bureaucratically possible to prioritize funding for special or "underserved" populations over "generic" ones.[10] Thus, conditions during the 1970s proved ripe for improvements in women's treatment. By 1976, the NIAAA had introduced into its grant review process a set of procedures that assured special consideration of treatment for women. And by the end of the decade, the institute had funded 41 new model programs designed for women.

In 1981, however, new federal commitments to cost containment, deregulation, and the decentralization of federal authority (or a "new federalism") led to the development of a new, bureaucratically streamlined approach to allocating funds for treatment.[11,73] This involved consolidating 80 categorical grants into 9 "block grants" awarded to the states with minimal spending regulations attached but an approximate 25% overall reduction in funds.[74] Philosophically, this signaled a move away from federal assurances to safeguard the coverage of "special population" needs. More practically, federal belt-tightening and deregulation meant that the states would become the locus for intensifying battles over funds. As treatment providers lamented, the new policies dealt a

> . . . severe blow to women and other underserved populations. The belief that local communities would adequately provide for these groups through the block grant has not proven to be true. Stigmatized groups as well, such as people of color, and people with disabilities, gays and lesbians, and the aging, are not given priority by local communities.[75]

Despite these concerns, it appears that the new federal policies did not completely unravel the achievements of the 1970s; most of the new model programs "kept their identities" as specialized women's centers, though some had to seek outside funding and raise client fees to keep afloat.[76] But the general flavor of the 1981 policy changes set the stage for a renewed effort by women's advocates, so that by the time Congress was ready to consider reauthorizing the block grants in 1983, they had mobilized an aggressive lobby supporting new categorical grants for women.[1] Though such proposals ultimately failed, the surrounding debate yielded a different kind of policy: an amendment to the block grant legislation that required each state to set aside 5% of its block grant allocation for new or expanded alcohol and drug abuse services for women. In real terms, the 1984 "women's set-aside" sequestered $63.5 million for women's services over a 3-year period. Attached to the rather loosely defined requirement was a lengthier list of "recommendations" that mirrored the objectives of the women's alcoholism movement: states were encouraged to spend set-aside dollars on developing women-only treatment units, programs offering special ancillary services for women such as vocational counseling and child care, and services for pregnant women.

The new policy met with mixed reviews from the varying coalitions of state alcoholism authorities, federal evaluators, and representatives of the women's alcoholism movement. Not unexpectedly, the national organization of state alcohol directors was lukewarm on the policy as it implied backsliding on the federal commitment to increasing state discretion; they argued that "as a concept, set-asides do not appear conducive to a block grant approach," and that it imposed control over "funds for specific programs and needs that many states had already identified."[77] More objectionable was the fact that, by "defining treatment priorities from Washington,"[18] the set-aside had the potential to "reduce services for other populations and . . . shift resources from other priorities for which state and local authorities had planned."[1] Indeed, some state directors complained that, in order to meet legislative requirements, large numbers of men had been placed on waiting lists for treatment.[78] Federal evaluators identified additional technical problems with the legislation, most notably weak federal monitoring of states' compliance. Thus, an evaluation found that fewer than half of the states examined had actually fulfilled the mandate of providing new or expanded services for women.[79]

Women's advocates generally supported the set-aside policy, though they acknowledged the variation in its implementation across states.[1,80] However, as needed, they used the policy's failures to justify further reforms. For instance, the NCA used the occasion of releasing its evaluation of the set-aside policy to issue additional recommendations to improve treatment for women.[81] Following suit, the Coalition on Alcohol and Drug Dependent Women and Their Children would later link the crisis over drug-exposed infants to the failures of the set-aside policy:

> Presumably, if states had complied with the spirit and the letter of federal law since 1984, we would have programs operating and would not be in our current crisis. . . . [States] have used this money to support existing services, they have channeled this money to support a "women's group" in an otherwise predominantly male oriented treatment setting, or in one case I am aware of, they simply told all service providers that they must serve 5% more women without any increase in funding.[82]

In sum, the set-aside approach of the early 1980s involved the redistribution of existing resources rather than the allocation of new ones; it thus held the potential to pit interest groups and "special populations" against one another, it appeared to be poorly implemented, and held potential to limit local responsiveness. The latter part of the decade, however, brought a significant shift in federal policy on women and substance abuse, one driven by deepening public concern over the problem of drug-exposed infants and a national "war on drugs." By 1988, the problem of drug-exposed infants seemed a national preoccupation, and one that carried with it intensified scrutiny over womens' drinking during pregnancy. A new sense of urgency was evident in a sharp rise in federal hearings on the drug-exposed infants,[83–85] growing media attention,[86] and in the comments of Senators who called upon government "to stop the surveys and budget the funds needed to help thousands of infants born in this country exposed to drugs and alcohol."[87]

At this juncture, it appears that many in the women's alcoholism movement began to direct their efforts to the larger issue of maternal substance use. This brought a new tone to the movement, as well as new challenges in its campaign to soften the stigma associated with substance abuse in women. In the debate over drug-exposed infants, women's advocates played a characteristic role, one that built on more than a decade of efforts to alter governing images of female alcoholism. Emphasizing that women who abused drugs had a medical problem, they attempted to redirect the debate away from the more punitive approaches that seemed to prevail in policy discussions of perinatal addiction, such as proposals for jailing women who used drugs during their pregnancies[88] or cutting off their welfare entitlements.[89] Advocates sent

> . . . a clear message that the enhancement and coordination of services is the appropriate response to pregnant addicts and affected children. The flurry of prosecutions of pregnant addicts and the enactment of punitive

laws in a number of states flies in the face of an assessment of alcoholism
and other drug dependence as treatable illnesses.[20]

Predictably, the pregnant addict's case was based on her "invisibleness" from
the treatment system; it was thus argued that over half of the drug treatment
programs in New York City discriminated against women by routinely excluding those who were pregnant,[90] and that the best solution would be to secure
"expanded and priority access" for women.[91] As before, advocates drew support from treatment provider coalitions who used conferences to draft recommendations for a more therapeutic approach[92] and who issued formal statements opposing criminal sanctions in cases of maternal substance abuse.[93]

These arguments were generally welcomed with bipartisan interest in
Congress, even among those members who had favored legislating a more
punitive approach to the pregnant addict[94]; after all, a criminal justice response to the problem only seemed legitimate in a context where treatment
first had been made available. They enacted an assortment of new funding
projects specifically targeted to pre- and postpartum women, which began in
1988 by doubling the "women's set-aside" and clearly specifying that the
funds be spent on services designed "especially for pregnant women and
women with dependent children." Thus, between 1988 and 1990, the "wom-
en's set-aside" grew from $24.4 to $119.3 million, or by nearly 500%. However, in an atmosphere of crisis, increasing the set-aside allocation was believed to be insufficient.[80] Thus Congress passed a host of other bills that
released additional millions, including: $85 million in demonstration grants
for prenatal and infant care services through the Medicaid program[95]; $4.5
million for model programs for drug-using pregnant and postpartum women
through the national Office on Substance Abuse Prevention (OSAP)[96]; a year
later, $45 million for expanding of the OSAP model programs; and finally, $50
million under a Child Abuse Prevention and Treatment Act for services to
maternal addicts and their children.[96]

In sum, the latter 1980s brought an important shift in the federal response to female substance abuse, a shift from emphasizing the redistribution
of existing funds to the allocation of entirely new and generous ones. Surely,
this development was welcomed by many women's advocates after years of
political lobbying. Though for some, the victory would be tainted by a realiza-
tion that it had not been won by generating sympathy for women alone:

> Tragically, it is only when a woman's ability to bear healthy children is
> threatened by the consequences of alcoholism and drug addiction that we,
> as a society, are willing to take notice. We take notice not because we care
> about women, but, because we allege to care about children.[83]

4. Women in Treatment Systems

Since the founding of the women's alcoholism movement, the evolution
of treatment systems for women has tended to follow two separate courses.

Table II. Proportion of Women[a] Treated in US Alcoholism, Drug Abuse, and Combined Alcohol-Drug Treatment Units: 1982, 1987, and 1992

	1982	1987	1992
Alcohol-only units	30	21	22
Drug-only units	21	35	36
Combined units	26	27	29
Overall percentage	25	28	29
Number of women	113,407	164,495	213,101

[a]Based on point prevalence data.

This has first involved growth in the proportion of alcohol and drug treatment units providing specialized women's services. Today, a little more than half of all public and private units in the United States offer some sort of women's services (see Table I). This has been accompanied by a modest increase in the proportion of women in the treatment system. Using a point prevalence approach, the NDATUS surveys found that while women comprised 25% of the caseload in 1982, they comprised 29% in 1992 (Table II). This increase in point prevalence, however, should be interpreted in light of the fact that women tend to be treated in outpatient programs more often than in residential programs.[67] Because the former have slower rates of turnover, point prevalence estimates of the overall proportion of women in the treatment system could be artificially inflated. Table II also indicates that over the past decade the trend has been toward providing treatment for women in drug abuse units; this may be one reflection of the growing national emphasis on controlling drug abuse in women and mothers, especially pertaining to cocaine. This trend is particularly noteworthy since elsewhere in the treatment system there was a quite dramatic trend toward providing care in combined alcohol and drug abuse programs.[97] For instance, over the course of the decade, the proportion of combined units in the national treatment system more than tripled, while there were significant declines in the proportion of treatment units providing drug- or alcohol-only services.[74]*

A second, though less widespread trend in treatment services for women has involved the growth of women-only alcohol and drug units. The NDATUS survey suggests that since the early days of the women's alcoholism movement, these programs have represented a small but growing segment of the treatment industry. In 1982, the survey found that women-only units comprised 3% of substance abuse treatment units in the country, whereas by 1992, they comprised 6%. It is important to consider these proportionate changes in the context of overall expansion of treatment systems during the

* Here, it is important to note potential bias in NDATUS results for 1992. Due to its particular liscensure requirements, the rather large state of New York reported no combined alcohol and drug treatment units, but instead classified all of its units as alcohol- or drug-only units.

1980s. Though women-only units remain a small segment of the treatment industry, their actual numbers have tripled since 1982, increasing from 186 to 537 units in 1992. It is within this small sector of the national treatment system that we are most likely to find that the women's alcoholism movement has been influential. Descriptions of women-only programs in the early 1980s suggested that they did not just serve an exclusively female population, but that they also tended to be "staffed almost entirely by women, and [to] deal with alcohol problems in the context of a woman's total experience in society."[32]

The NDATUS survey provides some indication that women-only units are unique from others in the national treatment system and that their development has been informed by the ideology of the women's alcoholism movement. These programs tend to emphasize ancillary services combined with intensive, often live-in alcoholism treatment services. Therapeutically, they tend to deemphasize the medical approach and to focus on meeting broader types of needs. These characteristics are generally consistent with advocates' view that alcohol problems should be treated "in the context of a woman's total experience," and that treatment should assist women to establish independence as well as to obtain more fulfilling life and work situations. Tables III and IV provide general information on the types of services offered by women-only units for the most recent years that these figures are available. The first shows that while units elsewhere in the national treatment system emphasize ambulatory outpatient services, women-only units emphasize longer-term and more intensive services, such as those offered in halfway houses and designed to assist clients in major life transitions. Table IV indicates that women-only units are more likely than others to offer child care as

Table III. Distribution of Bed Capacity across Treatment Modalities in Women-Only Sector,[a] 1992 (in Percents)[b]

	Women-only sector	Other units
Detoxification-hospital	1	1
Detoxification-residential	1	1
Rehabilitation-residential hospital	*	1
Rehabilitation-residential short-term	3	2
Rehabilitation-residential long-term	39	7
Ambulatory-outpatient	40	80
Ambulatory-intensive outpatient	17	7
Ambulatory-detoxification	*	1
Total	100	100
	(14,271)	(927,391)

[a]Treatment units include alcohol-only, drug-only and combined alcohol and drug programs.
[b]N of bed capacity for each column in parentheses.
*Less than 0.5%

Table IV. Proportion of Substance Abuse Treatment Units[a] in the US Offering Selected Services: Women-Only and Other Units, 1992

	Women-only units (N = 537)	Other units (N = 8369)
Individual therapy	96	96
Group therapy	96	94
Self-help	78	56
Medical care	27	32
HIV risk prevention	80	66
Medications	20	34
Child care	33	6
Transportation	52	25
Employment counseling	45	26
Vocational services	35	20
Housing assistance	39	17
Financial counseling	36	18
Academic services	29	15
Legal services	9	5
Dual diagnosis[b]	22	39

[a]Includes alcohol-only, drug-only, and combined alcohol and drug treatment units.
[b]Combined substance abuse and psychiatric services.

well as other types of ancillary services that can facilitate personal and career development, such as vocational services, housing assistance, financial counseling, academic services, and legal services.

There are reasons to believe that women may especially benefit from adjunct medical services: for example, research indicates that women are more responsive to some medically oriented alcoholism therapies than are men,[98] and that they are more likely to experience some types of alcoholism–mental illness comorbidities.[59,60,99] However, as suggested by Table IV, units in the women-only treatment sector appear committed to a more "social model" orientation emphasizing self-help and tend to deemphasize medical services such as medications and dual diagnosis treatment. Table V corroborates this by showing that over time the institutional development of the women-only treatment sector has occurred disproportionately outside of medical treatment settings. Since its inception, the women-only sector has been made up largely of freestanding, community-based facilities.

The NDATUS surveys also suggest that women-only treatment units were established on a somewhat different ownership and funding base than the rest of the substance abuse treatment system; over time, however, they have been subjected to broad changes also affecting other parts of the system. Table VI shows that, as compared with other types of programs at the beginning of the 1980s, women-only units were more likely to have a voluntary or private nonprofit status. While the vast majority of these units have remained non-

Table V. Institutional Location of Women-Only Substance Abuse Treatment Units[a] in the US: 1982, 1987, and 1992 (in Percents)[b]

	1982		1987		1992	
	Women-only	Other	Women-only	Other	Women-only	Other
Community mental health center	3	20	1	14	3	15
General hospital	3	11	4	13	4	10
Other hospital	1	5	2	6	*	4
Correctional facility	5	2	2	1	3	2
Freestanding/ community-based	74	47	90	60	88	66
Other	14	16	3	7	2	3
Total[c]	100	101	102	101	100	100
	(186)	(5446)	(261)	(6535)	(537)	(8369)

[a]Includes alcohol-only, drug-only, and combined alcohol and drug treatment units.
[b]N of treatment units for each column in parentheses.
[c]Columns may not total to 100% due to rounding error.
*Less than 0.5%.

profit, there has been a modest trend toward privatization in ownership over the years; currently 7% of women's programs have private for-profit status. The growth of for-profit women's programs probably reflects a larger trend toward privatization in treatment systems during the late 1970s and 1980s, attributable to the expansion of private insurance coverage and changing market incentives in the for-profit treatment industry.[74,100,101] Also, throughout this period, women-only programs have maintained a stable presence in the public sector (Table VI). This departs from the trend toward declining

Table VI. Funding Status of Units in Women-Only Substance Abuse Treatment[a] Sector, 1982, 1987, and 1992 (in Percents)[b]

	1982		1987		1992	
	Women-only	Other	Women-only	Other	Women-only	Other
Private for-profit	2	6	4	15	7	19
Private nonprofit	87	66	91	65	81	63
Public[c]	11	29	5	21	12	18
Tribal government	NA[d]	NA	NA	NA	*	1
Total[e]	100	101	100	101	100	101
	(186)	(5446)	(261)	(6536)	(537)	(8369)

[a]Includes alcohol-only, drug-only, and combined alcohol and drug treatment units.
[b]N of treatment units for each column in parentheses.
[c]Includes units funded by federal, state, and local governments.
[d]NA, Data not available.
[e]Columns may not total 100% due to rounding error.
*Less than 0.5%.

Table VII. Funding Sources of Substance Abuse Units[a] in the Women-Only Treatment Sector, 1982, 1987, and 1992 (in Percents)

	1982		1987		1992	
	Women-only	Other	Women-only	Other	Women-only	Other
Federal government	9	11	4	5	10	6
Public welfare	3	2	7	3	3	3
State/local government[b]	54	45	52	37	65	46
Public third-party[c]	2	9	NA[d]	NA	8	13
Private third-party	8	20	11	35	2	15
Client fees	12	9	12	15	6	11
Private donations	12	3	10	2	5	11
Other sources	1	1	4	2	2	2
Total[e]	101	100	100	4	101	4
	($21,783)	($1,596,382)	($44,078)	101	101	100
				($2,683,031)	($147,772)	($3,439,977)

[a]Includes alcohol-only, drug-only, and combined alcohol and drug treatment units.
[b]Includes, e.g., block grants, state, and local fees.
[c]Includes, e.g., Medicare, Medicaid.
[d]NA, Data not available.
[e]Columns may not total to 100% due to rounding error. Total dollars (in thousands) for each column in parentheses.

public sector ownership noted elsewhere in the treatment system[74] and is a reflection of the federal government's increased support of maternal drug use services in the late 1980s.

Finally, Table VII shows that, over the course of the decade, there has been disproportionate growth in the amount of government support for women-only treatment programs. At the same time, the proportion of their budgets drawn from less stable voluntary sources, such as private donations and client fees, has been reduced. This trend may reflect improvements in the access of these units to block grant funds achieved through mechanisms such as the women's set-aside and special grants for maternal substance abuse. Again, the most substantial increases in public funding for women-only units occurred between 1987 and 1992, as the government increased funding in response to the crisis over drug-exposed infants as part of its "war on drugs." For instance, the proportion of funding to women's programs from state and local government sources increased from 52 to 65% between 1987 and 1992, following slight declines in the earlier part of the decade.

5. Conclusion

In America, public attention to social problems and to the needs of "special populations" tends to rise and fall over time in what may seem an ever-replenishing stream of new "drug epidemics," "crime waves," and social crises of other sorts.[102] Public issues tend to have short life spans because it requires considerable resources to maintain their prominence on the national policy agenda, especially as more novel, competing issues unfold. The government's response can be equally fleeting as it tries to adjudicate among the competing claims of groups. As the case of problem-drinking women demonstrates, the federal response to the claims of special populations is often piecemeal, involving new demonstration grants, "seed money," categorical grants, and funding set-asides. Piecemeal funding provides special populations with the political recognition they deserve, while requiring only a limited or temporary public investment. Of course, one consequence of the incremental funding approach can be chronic fragmentation in health care systems, as their parts expand and contract with fluctuating budget limits.[103]

Having chronicled more than a decade of its ongoing political and public education activities, we can conclude that the women's alcoholism movement has been relatively effective in keeping the issue of women and substance abuse alive in the public arena. Within a context of limited federal spending, it has also achieved some measurable success in improving women's access and in making specialized women's services more available. The NDATUS surveys suggest that since 1982, there has been a modest, disproportionate increase in the point prevalence of women found in the treatment system. Over time, the proportion of treatment programs in the nation providing specialized women's services has expanded, as has the small sector within the treatment system devoted to women-only programs. Today, women-only units operate on a more solid funding base of public sector resources than they did a decade ago and are a little less likely to rely on voluntary sources such as private donations. Finally, it appears that the ideology of the women's alcoholism movement has been institutionalized in treatment programs of the women-only sector. These programs, for instance, tend to combine intensive alcoholism treatment with vocational, child-care, legal, and housing assistance that can support women in achieving independence and in making career and life transitions.

In part, the political successes of women's advocates are attributable to the fact that they built their movement on an enduring base of support in traditional alcoholism constituencies, such as the NCA, treatment provider coalitions, and mutual aid groups. The common ground shared by these groups brought unity and cohesion to the women's alcoholism movement, though this meant that it shared less with groups outside the alcohol arena, most notably those in the mainline feminist movement. Nowhere were the philosophical differences between these two movements more clear than in their radically different positions on the issue of alcohol and drug-exposed infants. While the women's alcoholism movement embraced the perinatal addiction issue as a rationale for improving public education and treatment, the broader feminist movement tended to see it as a symbol of the state's encroachment on women's privacy and reproductive freedom.

A second source of success and endurance has been the movement's ability to shape its own agenda to the changing political commitments of the federal government. In the early days, the women's alcoholism movement especially benefited from the NIAAA's commitment to "underserved" or special populations. Later, advocates found that greater strides could be made when the claims of children and "fetal rights" were combined with those of women. When, in the late 1980s, they positioned women's treatment needs within the context of the crisis over drug-exposed infants, it appears that advocates achieved their greatest success; this was evident in an assortment of new multimillion dollar federal projects to improve women's access to treatment and also in the growth of public sector women's programs, as demonstrated in the NDATUS surveys. It remains unclear, however, whether the original population for whom they served as advocates—namely, problem-drinking women—were as well served by the new policies as those women whose drug problems directly threatened their offspring.

A final aspect of the movement's success lay in its ability to institutionalize a new perspective on women and alcoholism—one that drew authority both from liberal feminism and from the ideology of traditional alcoholism constituencies. Though never fully succeeding in building strong alliances with "wet" feminists, advocates for problem-drinking women still drew upon a feminist "politics of recognition."[104] This emphasized that in a sexist society, lack of recognition and frustrated aspirations could lead women to internalize a sense of inferiority, which in turn could serve as a unique causal agent in alcoholism. Like most feminists, advocates' arguments emphasized both the importance of equal opportunities for men and women and the uniqueness of women's experience. Arguing from a feminist "politics of universal equality," the women's alcoholism movement demanded gender parity in access to treatment; as they put it, "alcoholism is an equal-opportunity disease, and we're asking for equal opportunity to recover."[33] At the same time, they argued from a "politics of difference" for recognition of the distinctiveness of alcohol problems in women and, hence, for the importance of women-only programs and "gender-sensitive" treatment modalities.

However, while liberal feminism may have provided a general logic to advocates' political claims, it was traditional alcoholism ideology that contributed to their substance. As we have emphasized, the movement's close ties to established constituencies in the alcohol arena influenced its central goals, which included public education in more sympathetic governing images of problem-drinking women and political lobbying for improvements in treatment and research. Though we have emphasized the direct linkages between the ideology of the women's alcoholism movement and contemporary groups such as the NCA, we should note in closing that in a larger sense the movement drew ideas and political momentum from an older tradition of "dry feminism" in the alcohol arena—one developed within the temperance movement of the 19th and early 20th centuries, in organizations such as the Women's Christian Temperance Union and by powerful dry feminists such as Frances Willard, Elizabeth Cady Stanton, and Susan B. Anthony.[105] At no point was the influence of this legacy more clear than in the 1976 Senate hearings on women and alcohol. It was there that Susan B. Anthony Jr., great-grandniece and namesake of the original, gave public testimony of her own recovery from alcoholism and her subsequent involvement in the women's alcoholism movement:

> More than half a century ago, women attained their greatest unity in fighting for and winning the radical social change of voting rights. Today, women are uniting once more, not only for their own social and economic liberation, but simultaneously for radical personal change in themselves and their children. My goal, as I celebrate my 30th anniversary as a recovered woman alcoholic, is to use the time that is left to help make our society one in which sobriety is not only possible, but also is desirable. . . . I, therefore, want to add to my one-day-at-a-time goal of sobriety, the one-day-at-a-time goal of becoming a socially concerned contemplative. . . . And then perhaps I can say, with my sister alcoholics, as Aunt Susan said in her last public speech: "Failure is impossible!"[3]

6. Appendix: Methodology and Limitations of the NDATUS Survey

This chapter relies on data from the National Drug and Alcohol Treatment Utilization Survey (NDATUS). The NDATUS is the only ongoing survey of the national treatment system in the United States, involving a census of private, public, and nonprofit sector alcohol and drug treatment units. It emphasizes the collection of point prevalence data on characteristics such as unit structure, types of services provided, and caseload characteristics, by way of a self-administered questionnaire completed by administrators of treatment units. The National Institute on Drug Abuse and the National Institute on Alcohol Abuse and Alcoholism jointly sponsored the surveys between 1979 and 1993, and the responsibility has since been transferred to the Office of Applied Studies, Substance Abuse and Mental Health Services Administration.

Methodological limitations in the survey make it important to interpret findings cautiously; specific biasing factors are noted as they arise in the text's description of findings. In general, readers should first be reminded that because of the surveys' reliance on point prevalence data, findings cannot readily be generalized to the level of, for instance, annual utilization rates of treatment units. Also, point prevalence data on caseload characteristics may be biased by the fact that the surveys cannot guarantee lack of duplication of individual clients across treatment units, though there is no duplication within individual treatment settings. Second, because the surveys collect data at the unit level, as opposed to the level of the individual client, disaggregated analyses of client populations are not possible. Furthermore, over the years the targeted level of organizations (i.e., administrative vs. individual unit) has been loosely defined and appears to have been interpreted differently by different unit administrators. Third, coverage of the NDATUS census listing is incomplete. Because listings are obtained in cooperation with state alcohol and drug administrations, coverage of public sector units is more complete than coverage of private sector units that are not under state jurisdiction. Response rates are poorer among private sector programs as well. However, there is no indication so far of systematic bias due to lack of coverage. Finally, particularly because questionnaires are self-administered by treatment unit administrators, there is potential for inconsistencies to arise in the interpretation of questions in the survey instruments, though a glossary of terms is provided to respondents.

ACKNOWLEDGMENTS. Preparation of this manuscript was supported by a National Alcohol Research Center Grant (# AA05595) awarded to the Alcohol Research Group by the National Institute on Alcohol Abuse and Alcoholism. We are indebted to Beatrice Rouse, Substance Abuse and Mental Health Service Administration, US Department of Health and Human Services, for her generous assistance and advice on the NDATUS analysis. This study also benefited from library assistance by Andrea Mitchell, and draws on materials obtained through the library at Alcohol Research Group. Jessica Warner provided help with archival research. Robin Room provided a valuable and timely critique of the manuscript.

References

1. National Council on Alcoholism: *A Federal Response to a Hidden Epidemic: Alcohol and Other Drug Problems among Women.* Washington, DC: National Council on Alcoholism, 1987.

2. Sandmaier M: *The Invisible Alcoholics: Women and Alcohol Abuse in America*. New York, McGraw-Hill, 1980.

3. United States Senate, Subcommittee on Alcoholism and Narcotics of the Committee on Labor and Public Welfare: *Alcohol Abuse among Women: Special Problems and Unmet Needs*. Washington, DC, US Government Printing Office, 1976.

4. Ferrence RG: Sex differences in the prevalence of problem drinking, in Kalant OJ (ed): *Alcohol and Drug Problems in Women: Research Advances in Alcohol and Drug Problems*. New York, Plenum Press, 1980, vol 5, pp 125–201.

5. Roman P: *Women and Alcohol Use: A Review of the Research Literature*. Washington, DC, US Department of Health and Human Services, 1988.

6. Fillmore KM: "When angels fall": Women's drinking as cultural preoccupation and as reality, in Wilsnack CC, Beckman LJ (eds): *Alcohol Problems in Women*. New York, Guildford, 1984, pp 7–36.

7. Wiener C: *The Politics of Alcoholism: Building an Arena Around a Social Problem*. New Brunswick, NJ: Transaction Books, 1981.

8. Lewis J: Congressional rites of passage for the rights of alcoholics. *Alcohol Health Res World* 12:240–251, 1988.

9. Noble AL: *Law, Medicine and Women's Bodies: The Social Control of Pregnant Drug Users*. PhD dissertation, Department of Sociology, University of California, Davis, 1993.

10. Institute of Medicine: *Broadening the Base of Treatment for Alcohol Problems*. Washington, DC, National Academy Press, 1990.

11. Schmidt L, Weisner C: Developments in alcoholism treatment: A ten-year review, in Galanter M (ed), *Recent Developments in Alcoholism*. New York, Plenum, 1993, vol 11, pp 369–396.

12. United States General Accounting Office: *Block Grants: Federal Set-Asides for Substance Abuse and Mental Health Services*. Rockville, MD, US General Accounting Office, 1987.

13. OSAP youth and pregnant women grant applications. *Alcohol Drug Abuse Week* 1:6, April 1989.

14. United States Alcohol, Drug and Mental Health Administration: *Assessing Future Research Needs: Mental and Addictive Disorders in Women*. Washington, DC, ADAMHA News Supplement, July–August 1991.

15. Gomberg EL: Special populations, in Gomberg EL, Whilte HR, Carpenter JA (eds): *Alcohol, Science and Society Revisited*. Ann Arbor, University of Michigan Press, 1982, pp 337–354.

16. Lewis J: Washington report. *J Stud Alcohol* 37:1383–1392, 1976.

17. An illustrated booklet . . . *Alcohol Rep* 8:10, May 1980.

18. NCA says women's set-aside a success, urges extension. *Alcohol Rep* 15:2–3, April 1987.

19. The first fetal alcohol syndrome awareness week proclaimed. *Alcohol Rep* 8:7, February 1980.

20. Field groups backing Kohl bill for drug/alcohol programs for women and children. *Alcohol Drug Abuse Week* 2:2–3, May 1990.

21. A national women's congress on alcohol and drug problems was formed. *Alcohol Rep* 8:9, May 1980.

22. NAWAODD focuses on women's issues. *Alcohol Rep* 8:8, May 1980.

23. Drive begins to allow medicaid to pay for pregnant addicts' residential treatment. *Alcohol Drug Abuse Week* 9:2, 2–3, August 1990.

24. The Second Annual Women in Crisis Conference, with "Women and Alcohol" as one of the four major themes. *Alcohol Rep* 8:8, April 1980.

25. The emerging female alcoholic. *Alcohol Rep* 9:7, February 1981.

26. The woman who has a problem with alcohol. *Alcohol Rep* 8:9, November 1980.

27. Kaskutas L: Women for sobriety: A qualitative analysis. *Contemp Drug Problems* vol 16, pp 177–199, 1989.

28. Beckman LJ: Alcoholics anonymous and gender issues, in McCrady BS, Miller WR (eds): *Research on Alcoholics Anonymous: Opportunities and Alternatives*. New Brunswick, NJ, Rutgers Center of Alcohol Studies, 1993, pp 233–248.

29. Youcha G: *A Dangerous Pleasure: Alcohol from the Woman's Perspective—Its Effect on Body, Mind and Relationships*. New York, Hawthorn Books, 1978.

30. A bill to require retail vendors of alcoholic beverages. *Alcohol Rep* 13:7, November 1985.

31. Morrissey ER: Contradictions inhering in liberal feminist ideology: Promotion and control of women's drinking. *Contemp Drug Problems* 13:65–88, 1986.
32. Sandmaier M: Women helping women: Opening the door to treatment. *Alcohol Health Res World* 2:17–23, 1977.
33. Reed BG: Linkages: Battering, sexual assault, incest, child sexual abuse, teen pregnancy, dropping out of school and the alcohol and drug connection, in Roth P (ed): *Alcohol and Drugs Are Women's Issues.* Metuchen, NJ, Women's Action Alliance and Scarecrow Press, 1991, vol 1, pp 130–149.
34. Gomberg EL: *Alcohol and Women.* New Brunswick, NJ, Rutgers University Center of Alcohol Studies, 1989.
35. Wilsnack SC: The needs of the female drinker: Dependency, power or what? in Chafetz, Morris E (ed): *Proceedings of the Second Annual Alcoholism Conference of the National Institute on Alcohol Abuse and Alcoholism.* Washington, DC, US Department of Health, Education and Welfare, 1972, pp 65–83.
36. Wilsnack SC: Femininity by the bottle, in Eddy CC, Ford JL (eds): *Alcoholism in Women.* Dubuque, IA, Kendall/Hunt, 1980, pp 16–39.
37. Van Den Bergh N: Having bitten the apple: A feminist perspective on addictions, in Van Den Bergh N (ed): *Feminist Perspectives on Addictions.* New York, Springer Publishing, 1991, pp 3–30.
38. Peluso E, Peluso LS: *Women and Drugs: Getting Hooked and Getting Clean.* Minneapolis, MN, CompCare Publications, 1988.
39. Senseman LA: The housewife's secret illness: How to recognize the female alcoholic. *R I Med J* 49:4–42, 1966.
40. Celentano DD, McQueen DV, Chee E: Substance abuse by women: A review of the epidemiologic literature. *J Chron Dis* 33:383–394, 1980.
41. Forth-Finegan JL: Sugar and spice and everything nice: Gender socialization and women's addiction—a literature review, in Bepko C (ed): *Feminism and Addiction.* New York, Haworth Press, 1991, pp 19–48.
42. United States National Institute on Alcohol Abuse and Alcoholism: *Proceedings from First National Alcohol Conference.* Washington, DC, US Department of Health, Education and Welfare, 1973.
43. Gomberg ESL: Alcoholism in women: Social and psychological concomitants. *Q J Stud Alcohol* 18:588–623, December 1957.
44. Vanicelli M: Treatment outcome of alcoholic women: The state of the art in relation to sex bias and expectancy effects, in Beckman LJ, Wilsnack SC (eds): *Alcohol Problems in Women,* 2nd ed. New York, Guilford Press, 1984, pp 369–412.
45. Annis HM: Treatment of alcoholic women, in Edwards G, Grant M (eds): *Alcoholism Treatment in Transition.* London, Croom Helm, 1980, pp 128–139.
46. Beckman LJ, Kocel KM: The treatment-delivery system and alcohol abuse in women: Social policy implications. *J Soc Issues* 38:139–151, 1982.
47. Nol J: Selfobject search: The role of addictions in a patriarchal culture, in Van Den Bergh N (ed): *Feminist Perspectives on Addictions.* New York, Springer Publishing, 1991, pp 31–44.
48. Glover-Reed B: Drug misuse and dependency in women: The meaning and implications of being considered a special population or minority group. *Int J Addict* 20:13–62, 1985.
49. United States National Institute on Alcohol Abuse and Alcoholism: *Advances in Alcoholism Treatment Services for Women.* Rockville, MD, US Department of Health and Human Services, 1982.
50. Dowin C: Sex role setups and alcoholism, in Van Den Bergh N (ed): *Feminist Perspectives on Addictions.* New York, Springer Publishing, 1991, pp 47–60.
51. Smith C: Healing the feminine: A feminist residential model for treating chemical dependency, in Van Den Bergh N (ed): *Feminist Perspectives on Addictions.* New York, Springer Publishing, 1991, pp 115–124.
52. Sandmaier M: *Alcohol Programs for Women: Issues, Strategies and Resources,* Washington DC, National Clearinghouse for Alcohol Information, National Institute on Alcohol Abuse and Alcoholism, 1977.

53. Wilsnack SC, Klassen AD, Schur BE, Wilsnack RW: Predicting onset and chronicity of women's problem drinking: A five-year longitudinal analysis. *Am J Public Health* 81:305–318, 1991.
54. Ames G, Schmidt C, Klee L, Saltz R: *Indicators of Women's Drinking Problems: A Report of Research Findings.* Sacramento, CA, California State Department of Alcohol and Drug Problems, 1988, Contract A-0010-6.
55. Weisner C, Schmidt L: Gender disparities in treatment for alcohol problems. *J Am Med Assoc* 268:1872–1876, 1992.
56. Beckman LJ, Amaro H: Patterns of women's use of alcohol treatment agencies, in Wilsnack SC, Beckman LJ (eds): *Alcohol Problems in Women.* New York, Plenum Press, 1984, pp 319–348.
57. Thom B: Sex differences in help-seeking for alcohol problems—1. The barriers to help-seeking. *Br J Addict* 81:777–788, 1986.
58. Thom B: Sex differences in help-seeking for alcohol problems—2. Entry into treatment. *Br J Addict* 82:989–997, 1987.
59. Schuckit MA, Pitts FN, Reich T, Winokur GL: Alcoholism. I. Two types of alcoholism in women. *Arch Gen Psychiatry* 20:301–306, 1969.
60. Schuckit MA, Rimmer J, Reich T, Winkour G: The bender alcoholic. *Br J Psychiatry* 119:672–678, 1979.
61. Blume SB: The female alcoholic: Is she different? *Physicians' Alcohol Newsletter* 22:4, 1974.
62. Bissell L: Testimony, in *Alcohol Abuse Among Women: Special Problems and Unmet Needs.* Washington, DC, Government Printing Office, 1976, pp 47–55.
63. Survey finds barriers to women's alcoholism treatment. *Alcohol Rep* 16:6, October 1988.
64. Reed BG, Leibson E: Women clients in special women's demonstration programs compared with women entering co-sex programs. *Int J Addict* 16:1425–1466, 1981.
65. Copeland J, Hall W: A comparison of women seeking drug and alcohol treatment in a specialist women's and two traditional mixed-sex treatment services. *Br J Addict* 87:1293–1302, 1992.
66. Annis HM, Liban CB: Alcoholism in women: Treatment modalities and outcomes, in Kalant OJ (ed): *Alcohol and Drug Problems in Women.* Research Advances in Alcohol and Drug Problems. New York, Plenum Press, 1980, vol 5, pp 385–422.
67. Institute of Medicine: *Report of Conference on Assessing Future Research Needs: Mental and Addictive Disorders in Women.* Washington, DC, National Academy of Sciences, 1990.
68. Dawson DA, Grant BF: Gender effects in diagnosing alcohol abuse and dependence. *J Clin Psychol* 49:298–307, 1993.
69. Duckert F: Predictive factors for outcome of treatment for alcohol problems. *J Subst Abuse* 5:31–44, 1993.
70. Jarvis TTJ: Implications of gender for alcohol treatment research: A quantitative and qualitative review. *Br J Addict* 87:1249–1261, 1991.
71. O'Connor PG, Horwitz RI, Gottlieb LD, *et al:* The impact of gender on clinical characteristics and outcome in alcohol withdrawal. *J Subst Abuse Treat* 10:59–62, 1993.
72. Sanchez-Craig M, Spivak K, and Davila R: Superior outcome of females over males after brief treatment for the reduction of heavy drinking: Replication and report of therapist effects. *Br J Addict* 86:867–876, 1991.
73. United States General Accounting Office: *Block Grants: Overview of Experiences to Date and Emerging Issues.* Washington, DC, US General Accounting Office, 1985.
74. The March Reagan budget, in *Alcohol and Drug Abuse Report.* Washington, DC, National Association of State Alcohol and Drug Abuse Directors, Dec–Jan, 1982, p 2.
75. Women's program director cites lack of insurance as barrier to treatment. *Alcohol Rep* 16:2–3, June 1988.
76. The majority of women's alcoholism treatment programs survived the initiation of the block grant. *Alcohol Rep* 11:7, May 1983.
77. NCA urges continuation of women's set-aside. *Drug Abuse Rep* 2:2–3, April 1987.
78. United States National Institute on Drug Abuse Subgroup on Access and Utilization: Planning Meeting 1 of Health Services. Washington, DC, January 27–28, 1994.

79. United States General Accounting Office: *ADMS Block Grant: Women's Set-Aside Does Not Assure Drug Treatment for Pregnant Women.* Washington, DC, US General Accounting Office, 1991.

80. NCA study says women's set-aside effective. *Alcohol Rep* 15:6, August 1987.

81. National Council on Alcoholism: *Recommendations for the Improvement of Prevention and Treatment Efforts for Women with Alcohol and Other Drug Related Problems.* Washington, DC, National Council on Alcoholism, 1987.

82. House told states show little commitment to helping addicted women. *Alcohol Rep* 18:3–4, May 1990.

83. United States General Accounting Office: *Drug Exposed Infants: A Generation at Risk.* Washington, DC, US General Accounting Office, 1990.

84. United States Department of Health and Human Services: *Report of Hearings: Born Hooked: Confronting the Impact of Perinatal Substance Abuse.* Washington, DC, US Government Printing Office, 1989.

85. United States House of Representatives: *No Place to Call Home: Discarded Children in America.* Washington, DC, US Government Printing Office, 1991.

86. Reeves JL, Campbell R: *Cracked Coverage: Television News, the Anti-Cocaine Crusade and the Reagan Legacy.* Duke University Press, 1994.

87. Hearings for federal policy on pregnant women and infants held. *Alcohol Drug Abuse Week* 1:7, August 1989.

88. Maternal cocaine use raising criminal issues. *Alcohol Drug Abuse Week* 1:7, May 1989.

89. Bills proposed for pregnant addicts, mothers, families and prisoners. *Alcohol Drug Abuse Week* 2:1, May 1990.

90. Chavkin W: Drug addiction and pregnancy: Policy crossroads. *Am J Public Health* 80:483–487, 1990.

91. Crack babies overwhelming child welfare system, panel told. *Alcohol Drug Abuse Week* 2:4–5, March 1990.

92. Participants at a conference on policy. *Alcohol Rep* 15:6–7, 1986.

93. ASAM takes stance against criminal sanctions for pregnant addicts. *Alcohol Drug Abuse Week* 1:10, November 1989.

94. New ADAMHA program for pregnant addicts authorized. *Alcohol Drug Abuse Week* 1:5, October 1989.

95. Cocaine babies new worry for treatment centers. *Drug Abuse Rep* 3:4, February 1988.

96. OSAP youth and pregnant women grant applications available. *Alcohol Drug Abuse Week* 1:6–7, April 1989.

97. Weisner C: The merging of alcohol and drug treatment: A policy review. *J Public Health Policy* 13:66–80, 1992.

98. Sokolow L, Welte J, Hynes G, Lyons J: Treatment-related differences between female and male alcoholics. *J Addict Health* 1:42–56, 1980.

99. Blume SB: Women and alcohol: A Review, *J Am Med Assoc* 256:1467–1470, 1986.

100. Yahr H: A national comparison of public- and private-sector alcoholism treatment delivery system characteristics. *J Stud Alcohol* 49:233–239, 1988.

101. Weisner C, Room R: Financing and ideology in alcohol treatment. *Soc Problems* 32:167–184, 1984.

102. Bosk CL: The rise and fall of social problems: A public arenas model. *Am J Sociol* 94:53–78, 1988.

103. Alford AR: *Health Care Politics: Ideological and Interest Group Barriers to Reform.* Chicago, IL, University of Chicago Press, 1975.

104. Taylor C: The politics of recognition, in Taylor C, Gutmann A (eds): *Multiculturalism and "the Politics of Recognition."* Princeton, NJ, Princeton University Press, 1992, pp 25–73.

105. Levine H: Temperance and women in the 19th-century United States, in Kalant OJ (ed): *Alcohol and Drug Problems in Women: Research Advances in Alcohol and Drug Problems.* New York, Plenum Press, 1980, vol. 5, 25–67.

IV

Social and Cultural Issues

Edward Gottheil and Ellen F. Gottheil,
Section Editors

Overview

Edward Gottheil and Ellen F. Gottheil

Previous chapters in this volume have addressed gender differences in substance use and misuse, such as how males and females differ in amounts, patterns, and styles of use, and what differences there are, for example, in metabolism, interpersonal relationships, and outcome. In this section we are concerned with questions about the extent to which such gender differences differ across societies and cultures. Is the extent to which men drink more heavily more often than women in Philadelphia, for example, the same in Salt Lake City; the same for Japanese living in Seattle or for Japanese living in Tokyo?

More and more, books on substance abuse now contain sections on "special populations," which include women, ethnic minorities, adolescents, prison inmates, the elderly, the homeless, and so forth. While it is difficult to conceive of Asians as a minority and women outnumber men, what makes these groups and the elderly and the homeless "special" is that in the United States these groups have been understudied in terms of research and underserved in terms of treatment. They have needed and continue to need "special" attention. Over the past few decades these problems at least have been recognized and some progress has been made. For example, federal regulations mandated a set-aside of funds for the expansion or development of new treatment programs for women and now require that women and minorities be represented in all research grant applications. Information on these groups is growing and recent reviews demonstrate the surprising extent to which the knowledge base has increased.[1-3]

To examine gender differences in substance use/misuse across cultures in

Edward Gottheil • Department of Psychiatry and Human Behavior, Thomas Jefferson University, Philadelphia, Pennsylvania 19107. **Ellen F. Gottheil** • Department of Psychiatry and Behaviorial Sciences, University of Washington Medical School, Seattle, Washington 98195.

Recent Developments in Alcoholism, Volume 12: Women and Alcoholism, edited by Marc Galanter. Plenum Press, New York, 1995

a systematic fashion one might conceive of a matrix with the rows representing characteristics (e.g., parental use of opiates, cirrhosis, marital status, AA attendance) and the columns representing ethnic/racial groups (e.g., African-Americans, Hispanic-Americans, Native Americans, Asian-Americans, and "whites"). A cell in the matrix located in the Native-American column and the frequency of intoxication row, then, would provide data regarding the frequency with which Native-American males and females become intoxicated.

The first problem with the conceptualized matrix is that more of the cells would be empty than full; but that is only the beginning. Asians, of course, include Indians who differ from Chinese and Japanese and each other. Navajos differ from Apaches and other Navajos. African-Americans and Hispanic-Americans are also anything but homogeneous. The leftover miscellaneous group, most commonly referred to as white, Anglo, or Caucasian, is rather difficult to characterize since it is not differentiated by language, color, or continent of origin. We could perhaps increase the number of columns in the matrix to include separate columns for groups such as Cubans, Navajos, and Pacific Islanders. Similarly, there are problems regarding the number, importance, and definitions of the rows representing characteristics. For example, the same amount of alcohol is likely to have a different effect if consumed by a fourth-generation Irish male in New York or a newly arrived Korean female in Minnesota. Many definitions have been offered that have varied across time and place and from study to study. As we increase the numbers of columns and rows of the matrix, however, the number of empty cells multiplies, and it becomes apparent why this section is not titled cross-cultural comparisons but, more modestly, social and cultural issues.

Undaunted, the contributors to this section have provided us with important ideas, data, and insights into these complex sociocultural issues. The chapter by Rouse, Carter, and Rodriguez-Andrews includes 120 references and provides an excellent review of treatment-related issues. They suggest that a very practical reason for being concerned with the treatment needs of what are now ethnic minorities derives from estimated population shifts. It is expected that by the year 2050, the US population will have grown from 255 to 383 million. During this time, the Anglo-American population will increase by about 6% from 191 to 202 million, while the African-, Hispanic-, and Asian-American populations will about triple from 65 to 184 million and will then constitute 47% of the population. The implications for planning, training, prevention, and treatment are apparent.

After describing some special issues affecting women in general (e.g., child-care demands, criminalization of pregnant drug users), Rouse and her co-workers draw on African-American, Hispanic-American, and Native-American studies to note differences (physiological responses to drugs and pharmacological agents, cultural backgrounds, economic status, and opportunities) that may differentially affect risk for substance abuse, interest in treatment, and type of treatment needed. They discuss treatment utilization (including, for example, underutilization by minorities even when they have insurance), the need for reliable and standardized assessment and survey instruments, psychosocial and cultural barriers to treatment, and treatment outcome. They conclude with recommendations for providing services that are relevant and sensitive to the needs of women, minorities, and minority women, ending with the caveat, however, that these have not been evaluated in carefully controlled studies.

If the social and cultural issues relating to gender, ethnicity, and substance use and their interactions do not seem sufficiently complex, Edwards, Thurman, and Beauvais add the factor of adolescence to the analytic mix. In the first half of their chapter, they describe the findings of national studies which indicate that alcohol use rates are highest for whites and then decrease in order for Hispanics, blacks, and Asians, with American Indians falling somewhere in between. For adolescents the use rates follow the same order as for adults with the notable exception, however, that Indian youths have higher rates of use than any of the other groups including the whites. Females have lower rates of use than males across all of the above age and ethnic categories. They also report that, in contrast to the white majority culture where peers exert more influence than families on adolescent substance use patterns, peers appear to have less influence on minority group individuals who belong to families that are highly invested in maintaining and defending their own way of life. Over time, with acculturation, minority individuals tend to become more like the larger group and drink more. Females, however, are more resistant than males to change and slower to adopt the practices of the new culture. Such differential age and gender effects are then described more specifically as they occur within each of the different ethnic groups.

In the second half of their chapter, Edwards, Thurman, and Beauvais examine a new set of data that was obtained using the same instrumentation and methodology from white, Hispanic, African-American, Asian-American, and American Indian male and female adolescents attending 8th and 12th grade classes in 150 communities across the United States. One example of their interesting findings was that the prevalence of use by males and females was very similar at the 8th grade level across the ethnic groups, but that by the time they reached the 12th grade there were generally wide gaps, with males using more than females. Another example concerned a question about whether friends would be likely to try to stop them from getting drunk. Responses indicated that peer sanctions weakened for all groups and both genders between the 8th and 12th grades, but there was a differential gender effect with more influence exerted on the female adolescents, across all ethnic groups and both grades, not to get drunk.

Barthwell's chapter focuses primarily on sociocultural factors that influence drinking and alcoholism among African-American women. In addition to the effects of age, education, country of origin, and acculturation which may have different effects on African-American males and females, she notes differences in employability and socioeconomic status. She also discusses differential consequences over time of immigration status (nonvoluntary or voluntary), migratory patterns, and personal struggles to blend African and American cultural influences into an African-American experience and identity.

While sociocultural studies usually involve comparisons between cultural groups and subgroups, Barthwell concentrates on differences within groups and especially on the interactive effects of different cultures within specific individuals such as the biracial, triracial, or multiracial issues of transcultural marriages. She illustrates with a case example of a child, Betsy, born to an African-American female and a man of German–English descent, and traces the family background of her mother back through six generations and spanning 100 years. A majority of the ancestors were African-Americans but they also included Native-Americans, Caucasians, Creoles, French, and Spanish, differing also in their religious affiliations. Included were many alcoholics, male and female, and a few using other drugs.

How, then, would one attempt to begin to categorize the cultural background and influences on Betsy and hazard a prediction of her likelihood of becoming an alcoholic? Barthwell observes that in acknowledging the extent of diversity that occurs within groups we limit the generalizability of the results of our studies. On the other hand, in recognizing this diversity we also tend to restrain or counteract the propensity for stereotyping.

The power of bringing together data from ten studies conducted in five countries over a 19-year period and examining them with sophisticated, meta-analytic statistical strategies is beautifully exemplified in the chapter by Fillmore and her associates. The first issue they address is the relative risks of men and women for alcohol-related problems when controlling for age and alcohol consumption. One might expect such a comparison to reveal that women would be at higher risk because the same amount of alcohol would result in higher blood alcohol concentrations (biological hypothesis) or, conversely, that men would be at higher risk because of their societal norms and roles (sociocultural hypothesis). Apart from the overall results based on pooled data across the studies, the finding of heterogeneous results among the studies would suggest the operation of sociocultural factors.

To account for variations from study to study in relative male–female risks for alcohol-related behaviors such as belligerence or symptomatic drinking, Fillmore and co-workers test hypotheses regarding the effects of two societal dimensions: traditionality–modernity (operationalized as the number of women in the workplace) and societal stress (operationalized as female suicide rates). They then proceed to conduct a series of logical, systematic analyses testing their theoretically based hypotheses, culminating with hypotheses about the combined effects of societal stress and modernity that could be additive or could cancel each other out and equalize risks for men and women.

Despite some limitations of the study which are recognized and discussed by the authors, there are a number of very interesting and often surprising results, such as finding no differences in male–female risks, when age and intake are controlled, for general health problems or for a past history of treatment for alcoholism. The results are best summarized in the authors' own words in their chapter but it is difficult to restrain from quoting one other finding, i.e., the quotable

> Therefore, we conclude that in the context of the family, the school, and the job, and also with regard to financial matters, ladies, even when drinking, are more likely to continue to act like ladies, whereas gentlemen are less likely to continue to act like gentlemen.

These chapters on sociocultural issues in substance use demonstrate that a great deal of significant information has been and is still being gathered about women and ethnic minorities and also to some extent about variations in gender differences across sociocultural subgroups. They also serve to illustrate the multidimensionality and heterogeneity of the findings and the many and varied knowledge gaps remaining to be filled by further research. This research is of importance not only to social scientists and substance use theorists but to clinicians, service delivery administrators, and economists. For example, Rouse and co-workers report that at present there is no evidence that programs designed for women and minorities have been shown to be more effective than mainstreaming. Clearly, it will be necessary to continue to fill in our knowledge gaps through the kind of creative and systematic research described in these chapters if we are to develop more effective services that are relevant and sensitive to the needs of women and minorities.

References

1. Institute of Medicine: Broadening the base of treatment for alcohol problems, in *Special Populations in Treatment*. Washington, DC, National Academy Press, 1990, Section IV, pp 354–406
2. Lex BW: Alcohol problems in special populations, in Mendelson JH, Mello NK (eds): *Medical Diagnosis and Treatment of Alcoholism*. New York, McGraw-Hill, 1992, pp 71–155.
3. Lowinson JH, Ruiz P, Millman RB, Langrod JG (eds): Special populations, in *Substance Abuse: A comprehensive Textbook*, ed 2. Baltimore, 1992, part VIII, pp 794–910.

18

Race/Ethnicity and Other Sociocultural Influences on Alcoholism Treatment for Women

Beatrice A. Rouse, James H. Carter, and Sylvia Rodriguez-Andrew

Abstract. This chapter discusses sociocultural influences on the availability, access, diagnosis, and treatment of alcoholism for women, particularly those in minority groups. Race/ethnicity and other sociocultural influences are presented in terms of the societal context and the counselor–client relationship. The latest data on heavy drinking, alcohol-induced mortality, and alcoholism treatment utilization are presented on African-American, Hispanic, and white women. Data also are presented on the ability to pay for treatment through insurance or earnings. Information on Native Americans and Asian/Pacific Islanders is included whenever possible.

Introduction

Women needing treatment for alcohol and other substance abuse have a variety of special issues to be addressed to increase their treatment success. These include child-care responsibilities, history of incest and domestic violence, the criminalization of pregnant drug abusers, and a variety of gynecological/obstetric and other medical conditions. Women of minority ra-

The views expressed in this chapter are those of the authors and are not meant to represent the official positions of their respective organizations.

Beatrice A. Rouse • Office of Applied Studies, Substance Abuse and Mental Health Services Administration, Rockville, Maryland 20857.   **James H. Carter** • Department of Psychiatry, Duke University Medical Center, Durham, North Carolina 27710.   **Sylvia Rodriguez-Andrew** • College of Social Work, San Jose State University, San Jose, California 95192.

Recent Developments in Alcoholism, Volume 12: Women and Alcoholism, edited by Marc Galanter. Plenum Press, New York, 1995

cial/ethnic groups present additional needs to ensure treatment availability, access, and effectiveness. This chapter examines sociocultural influences on alcoholism prevalence, access to care, and treatment effectiveness among different racial/ethnic groups of women.

In 1977, in response to Congress and various federal agencies, the Office of Management and Budget (OMB) developed the standards currently used to report federal statistics on race and ethnicity.[1] According to OMB's Directive 15, all federal agencies were to use the following five categories to report racial and ethnic data: (1) American Indian/Alaskan Native, (2) Asian/Pacific Islander, (3) black, (4) Hispanic, and (5) white. OMB added "Hispanic" because Congress passed Public Law 94-311 in the prior year. This law mandated the collection of statistics on the health of Americans of Spanish origin or descent. Agencies could collect data on more specific categories if the data could be aggregated into the five designated racial/ethnic groups. The Census Bureau used these five groups in the 1980 census and in following years. This chapter will use these five groups to report on federal data systems.

According to the Bureau of Census,[2] as of Spring 1991, blacks comprised 12% and Hispanics comprised 9% of the total U.S. population. Between 1980 and 1988, the white population in the U.S. increased 6%, the black population increased 13%, the Asian/Pacific Islanders increased 70%, and the American Indian, Eskimo, and Aleut populations increased 19%.[3] The Census Bureau projects a significant population shift by the year 2050 due to increases in the black, Hispanic, and Asian populations.[4] Currently, whites comprise 75% of the nation's population; the Census Bureau estimates that by the year 2050, whites will comprise only 53%.

Race and ethnicity are important in alcohol addiction because of potential physiological differences in metabolic rates and response to pharmacological treatment regimens. Researchers have found gender, race, and ethnic differences in alcohol and other drug metabolism and physiological responses.[5–12] These differences may account for differential alcoholism and drug abuse rates and may be important when using medications in treatment regimens. For example, Rudorfer's[9] research with antipsychotic drugs supports the belief that racial groups display genetically determined differences in drug metabolism, affecting both the pharmacokinetic and pharmacodynamic actions of several psychotropic drugs. The body eliminates antipsychotic drugs, excluding lithium carbonate, primarily by the liver biotransformation process rather than through kidney excretion. Research has shown that there are distinct phenotypes for hepatic metabolism involving the cytochrome P-450 system. Therefore, such compounds as the beta-adrenoreceptor blocking drug, i.e., propranolol, should be used with caution in African-American populations who are occasionally noted to have a deficient cytochrome P-450 system.[13,14]

Some racial/ethnic groups experience adverse physiological reactions to alcohol, but social factors can override the physical discomfort felt.[15] This chapter examines only sociocultural influences on alcoholism and treatment.

Researchers use various terms interchangeably to denote sociocultural influences. Cultural factors include nationality, language, cultural heritage, ethnicity, and religion. These are often meshed with such socioeconomic factors as education, occupation, and income level. We propose that sociocultural factors are relevant not only to the explanation of the causes of alcoholism but also to its conceptualization, measurement, and treatment.

1.1. Heterogeneity of Minority Racial/Ethnic Groups and Their Socioeconomic Characteristics

Most of the Hispanics in the United States are of Mexican origin (62.6%), followed by Puerto Ricans (11.6%), Cubans (5.3%), Central and South Americans (12.7%), and other Hispanics (7.8%). As a group, Hispanics are young and diverse. Although they reside in every state, nearly 90% live in ten states.[16] Most (70%) Hispanics are under the age of 35. The median age for Hispanics is 26 versus 34 years for non-Hispanics. The majority of Hispanics (63%) have children under the age of 18 living with them. The number of Hispanic families maintained by a single woman has increased. In 1970, 15% of Hispanic families had women head-of-householders; by 1990, it had increased to 22%. Unlike their non-Hispanic counterparts, Hispanic women are more likely to be employed as operators, fabricators, and laborers or in service occupations.[17]

Most Mexican-Americans (80%), the largest Hispanic group, live in either California or Texas. The median education for Mexican-Americans (age 25 and over) is 10.8 years of schooling completed versus 12.7 for non-Hispanic whites. Mexican-American women (6.0%) are less likely than Mexican-American men to graduate from college (8.1%). Mexican-American women also have the highest fertility rate of any group: 26.6 live births per 1000 population compared with 14.2 for white Americans, 22.9 for African-Americans, and 23.5 for all Hispanic-Americans.

Approximately 23 million Puerto Ricans reside in the US mainland. About 10% graduate from college compared with 21% of white Americans. The median number of school years completed for Puerto Ricans is 12.0 years, one year less than white Americans. Women head 65.3% of Puerto Rican families living below the poverty level.

Cuban-Americans, the third largest subgroup, are older than Mexican-Americans, Puerto Ricans, and the general US population. The median age of Cubans is 38.7 years and their median education is 12.4 years.

Blacks are also a young and diverse group.[18] Blacks include US-born African-Americans and immigrants from such areas as the Caribbean, Africa, or Europe. Also, there are regional differences among African-Americans. The median age for blacks in 1991 was 28.0 years. A greater proportion completed high school in 1991 (82%) than in 1980 (75%). About 12% black men and women completed four or more years of college.

Native Americans, like most other primary minority groups, are younger than the general population, with 34% younger than 15 years of age. The Indian Health Service (IHS) recognizes over 550 American Indian and Alaska Native tribes.[19] Tribal sizes range from 30 to 250,000 members and their land sizes range from a few acres to the Navaho's four-state area. The largest percent served by the IHS lives in the Oklahoma City area (21%) and the Navaho area (15%). The smallest percent live in the Tucson, Arizona area (2%). The IHS serviced approximately 1.33 million Native Americans in fiscal year 1994. Additional numbers of Native Americans have undergone various degrees of acculturation and live throughout the United States.

Data on the different Asian and Pacific Islander groups are not routinely presented by the Bureau of Census. The Asian/Pacific Islander group varies widely. It includes Chinese, Japanese, Filipinos, Hawaiians, Koreans, Vietnamese, Cambodians, Laotians, and persons from other Asian countries and Pacific Islands. The Bureau of Census estimates that this is the most rapidly growing population group in the United States. Currently there are 8.5 million in the United States.[4]

1.2. Other Sociocultural Factors

Bales[20] presented three ways that sociocultural factors impact alcoholism rates. Sociocultural groups can differ in: (1) rates of inner tension and anxiety and need for tension reduction, (2) substitute relief for inner tension and anxiety, and (3) attitudes toward drinking. Research has found significant gender differences on these factors. Women alcoholics experience more anxiety,[21] more depression,[22] and more opposition to treatment[23] than do the men. Also, women alcoholics are more likely to be in a relationship with an alcoholic or drug-abusing significant other than men alcoholics.[24–26]

Racial/ethnic and other sociocultural groups also differ on these factors. Many minority racial/ethnic groups experience a disproportionately greater number of social and economic problems that increase tension and anxiety and reduce resources for dealing effectively with their problems. These factors contribute to problems associated with alcohol use among those who drink. There is great variation among the racial/ethnic groups in their attitudes toward drinking, the relative rates of alcohol use, and drinking by women.

Both macro- and microlevel factors have increased the stress levels for various racial/ethnic groups. For example, stress for American Indians and how they cope may vary with their level of acculturation. Those living on reservations have different sources of stress from those in urban areas. Immigrants have different sources and levels of stress prior to leaving their homeland and afterward coping with a new environment.[27] The sociopsychopathology of alcohol addiction in many African-American, Hispanic, and other minority women is inextricably intertwined with issues of racisim, sexism, unemployment, poverty, and substandard housing and child-care services.[28] For example, more women are becoming solely responsible for child care and development with increasingly fewer resources. The percentage of children living with both parents has declined for both blacks and whites.[18] Black women heading families without a husband are more likely than their white counterparts to be never married (41% black vs. 17% white).[18] These family responsibilities present complex psychosocial stressors.

African-American women must contend with the harsh reality that their households are more likely to be victimized by a serious violent crime than white households. These include rape, robbery, and aggravated assault.[29,30] Besides rape, another sex-related stressor for African-American women is HIV/AIDS. As of June 1994, among women age 13 or over, there were more cases of AIDS among black women (27,681) than among white (12,554) or Hispanic women (10,519).[31] Most women acquired HIV/AIDS because of their own or their partner's intravenous drug use.

There are countless minority women who not only must survive in a caldron of mounting crime, but must cope without skilled and decent-paying jobs. Opportunities are increasing. Still, too few African-American and other minority women have the choice of deciding whether to stay at home or to attempt to climb the corporate ladder, earning their equal share of wealth and prestige. Some lack the appropriate mentorship, career guidance, and education. Others have low self-esteem and are self-conscious about skin tone, hair texture, and social acceptance, reflecting the bias of a nation with different standards of beauty from their culture. Fortunately, there has been some progress. Dolls with African-American features are available. Successful women with African-American, Hispanic, and Asian features and fashions provide public role models in a variety of businesses and professions.

2. Alcoholism Treatment Need and Utilization

2.1. Rates of Alcohol Use and Abuse

Few national data were available on the extent of alcohol and other drug use among blacks and Hispanics before the mid-1980s. Even fewer data were available on drinking and related problems among black and Hispanic women. Most of the available literature aggregates the various minority ethnic/racial groups into one broad category, does not distinguish between the various Hispanic cultural groups, has small samples, and deals with limited geographic locations. Also, research does not consistently report findings based on both gender and race/ethnicity.

The National Alcohol Survey, funded by the National Institute on Alcohol Abuse and Alcoholism (NIAAA) in 1984, was an early effort to examine alcohol use among Hispanics. The survey, which contained a probability sample of 1453 Hispanics, found a high abstention rate among women (47%) and a high rate of "heavy" drinking among men (36%). Men in the general population tended to decrease their alcohol consumption between ages of 20 and 40. Hispanic men, however, continued to experience high levels of alcohol use and alcohol-related problems until their 40s. Interestingly, while women and men in the same age group reported similar rates of alcohol-related problems, the men's rate of heavy drinking was eight times higher.

The various Hispanic cultural groups differed in their drinking patterns. Among Hispanics in the NIAAA study, Mexican-Americans had the highest rates of both abstention and heavy drinking. Hispanics born in the United States were more likely to be heavy drinkers than foreign-born Hispanic drinkers. Mexican-American men reported the highest abstention rates *and* a high rate of heavy drinking compared with Cubans, Puerto Ricans, and Hispanics from other Latin American countries. Similarly, Mexican-American women drank more heavily than their other Hispanic counterparts but Mexican-American women also reported high rates of abstention. Puerto Rican women tended to be primarily moderate drinkers, with low rates of abstention and few heavy drinkers.

More recent data on drinking among both blacks and Hispanics were available from the National Household Survey on Drug Abuse (NHSDA), a national probability survey conducted periodically since 1971.[32] Currently, the Substance Abuse and Mental Health Services Administration (SAMHSA) conducts the NHSDA annually. The NHSDA sample represents respondents from the civilian noninstitutionalized population aged 12 and older. Since 1985, the survey contains an oversample of blacks and Hispanics to provide reliable estimates of alcohol and drug abuse in these groups. Since 1991, the NHSDA sample has included Alaska and Hawaii, civilians living on military bases, and persons living in noninstitutional group quarters. These group quarters included college dormitories, rooming houses, and homeless shelters.

In 1993, the total NHSDA sample contained 26,489 respondents. Of these, 12,478 were whites, 6183 were blacks, 6894 were Hispanic, and 934 were in other racial/ethnic groups. Table I shows data by under or at legal age of drinking (i.e., age 12–20 years and age 21 years and older). For both genders, blacks under legal age for drinking were the least likely to report any drinking or heavy drinking. Both men and women had comparable rates of any drinking when between 12–20 years old, but men were more likely to drink heavily. For women under legal age for drinking, heavy drinking rates were higher for whites, but the difference was not statistically significant. The difference between groups was also not statistically significant for the women of legal age for drinking.

Socioeconomic factors account for some racial/ethnic differences in alcohol and other drug use. Flewelling et al.[33] adjusted for demographic background, socioeconomic status, and social variables for drug use among respondents aged 18 to 49 in the 1991 NHSDA. The demographic variables included gender, age, region, and metropolitan status of residence. The socioeconomic variables included educational attainment, occupation of chief household wage earner, and household income. Social variables included marital status, employment and number of jobs and residential moves in the past 5 years. Without the adjustment for these variables, blacks were four times more likely than whites to use crack cocaine. After the adjustment, the

Table I. Alcohol Use in the Past Month by Age Group, Race/Ethnicity, and Gender[a]

| Race/gender | Age 12–20 years | | Age 21 and older | |
	Any use	Heavy use[b]	Any use	Heavy use
Total	28.6%	4.2%	53.4%	5.5%
Whites	30.9%	4.9%	56.2%	5.8%
Blacks	21.7%	0.9%	41.7%	5.1%
Hispanics	26.5%	4.8%	50.8%	5.2%
Men[c]	29.8%	6.5%	62.9%	9.9%
White	31.6%	7.7%	64.7%	10.4%
Black	24.8%	1.4%	53.0%	9.8%
Hispanic	31.4%	8.0%	65.9%	9.5%
Women[c]	27.3%	1.6%	45.0%	1.5%
White	30.1%	1.9%	48.6%	1.6%
Black	18.5%	0.3%	33.0%	1.5%
Hispanic	21.3%	1.3%	36.0%	1.0%

[a]From SAMHSA National Household Survey on Drug Abuse, 1993.
[b]Heavy drinking is defined as drinking five or more drinks per occasion on 5 or more days in the past 30 days.
 An occasion is defined as "at one sitting" or within a couple of hours.
[c]Total rates for men and women include other race/ethnicities in addition to white, black, and Hispanic.

differences between the races were no longer significant. Similarly, without the adjustment, Hispanics were twice as likely as whites to use cocaine in any form frequently. After the adjustment, the difference between whites' and Hispanics' cocaine use was no longer significant. Blacks and Hispanics were less likely to drink heavily even with the adjustment for the various sociodemographic variables.

Also, rates of alcohol and other drug use within racial/ethnic groups may vary. This hetereogeneity may be due to a variety of socioeconomic factors as well as differences in family history, heritage, tribal customs, immigrant status, or acculturation. Caetano[34] considered some of these factors in his analysis of alcohol consumption among Hispanics. Among the foreign born, Latin American women largely from South and Central America had the highest rates of abstention (74%), followed by Mexican (71%), Cuban (48%), and Puerto Rican women (45%). US-born Hispanic women reported the lowest rate of abstention. Immigrant men, on the other hand, reported a different pattern of alcohol consumption. Their drinking tended to be low frequency but high quantity. After they immigrated, their drinking changed to both high frequency and high quantity.[35]

2.2. Alcohol-Induced Mortality Rates

Black women had higher mortality rates than white women for a variety of conditions and for total mortality from natural causes.[36] The age-adjusted rate of deaths for 100,000 resident population for natural causes in 1991 was

538.4 for black women compared with 341.1 for white women. While under-reporting of deaths attributed to alcohol and other drugs is likely, the rates for blacks are still higher than for whites. For alcohol-induced deaths, the rates were 6.8 per 100,000 for black women compared with 2.7 for white women. For other drug-induced deaths, the rates were 3.9 per 100,000 compared with 2.6 for white women.

Data by gender were not available for Native Americans. The age-adjusted mortality rates for alcoholism among American Indians and Alaska Natives in the IHS areas remain much higher than that for US whites.[19] In 1988, the Native American rate was 6.3 times higher; this represents an improvement over 1980 when it was 8.4 times higher.

2.3. Alcohol and Other Drug Treatment Utilization

Some credit the reduction in alcohol-induced mortality among Native Americans to enhanced treatment efforts. Native American alcoholism treatment programs have increased their emphasis on prevention and outreach activities. Tribal governments are also increasingly providing and participating in alcoholism treatment programs. They emphasize the understanding and identification of Native American culture and traditions, but also tailor their programs to their clients' special needs. American Indians, for example, may have different ideas of what it means to be an American Indian depending on their level of acculturation and where they live. The types of alcoholism programs for Native Americans followed the same progression as those in the general population. Early programs focused on men and adolescents. Later, programs made provisions for women and some became family-oriented. Finally, programs provided facilities for the children of women in treatment for substance abuse.

Two national data systems provide data on the availability and utilization of services by racial/ethnic groups. These are the National Drug and Alcoholism Treatment Unit Survey (NDATUS) and the national Client Data System (CDS). SAMHSA conducts both surveys.

NDATUS assesses the nature and extent of treatment services for alcoholism and other drug abuse. SAMHSA contacted all identified substance abuse treatment units in the United States to provide data that described their programs and client count on a designated day. The point prevalence date for the most recent available survey was September 30, 1992. The overall response rate was 84.4%. Both private and public sector alcohol and other drug treatment facilities participated; but coverage and participation were greatest for publicly funded providers. In 1992, 9483 treatment units provided data.

NDATUS providers indicated whether they had staff that were specially trained or assigned to treat special population groups. For 1992, only 18% reported no such specialized programs. About a third (37%) reported that they had special programs for blacks, 32% for Hispanics, and 17% for American Indians/Alaskan Natives. Over half (53%) reported that they had special programs for women and 29% for pregnant users. Information was not available on the number of clients treated in such population-specific programs, the characteristics of the specialized staff, or the programs' effectiveness.

In the NDATUS, the ratio of men to women clients in treatment for alcoholism or drug abuse on September 30, 1992 was 2.4 to 1 (71% to 29%). Women were less likely than men to be in treatment for alcoholism only (29% vs. 41%) and more likely to be in treatment for drug abuse only (31% vs. 23%). NDATUS permits analysis by either race/ethnicity or gender but not both simultaneously. Such analysis is possible with SAMHSA's national CDS.

The Department of Health and Human Services developed the CDS to meet the reporting requirements of Public Law 100-690 in 1988. The CDS contains a minimum set of 19 items reported by all states on all admissions to substance abuse treatment programs that receive public funds. These items include basic characteristics of the provider, the client, and the substances used. Some states reported an optional additional 15 items that provide more details on the clients, their diagnoses, and their source of payment. The states phased in their reporting so that as of fiscal year 1992, CDS had consistent 12 months of reporting for 42 jurisdictions. Forty states, the District of Columbia, and Puerto Rico reported the complete minimum data set. The fiscal year 1992 data set does not contain Arizona, Georgia, Idaho, Kansas, Kentucky, Mississippi, Nebraska, Nevada, Washington, and Wyoming. Because many states do not use unique client identifiers, the data were not necessarily unduplicated client counts. The following data are initial admissions and do not include transfer admissions from one facility or service to another.

Alcohol was the primary substance for 59% of the 1.3 million admissions reported to the CDS in fiscal year 1992. On admission, Native Americans (84%), non-Hispanic whites (70%), and Mexican-Americans (49%) were most likely to report "alcohol only" as their primary substance. Blacks (43%) and Cubans (35%) were more likely to report cocaine and Puerto Ricans (41%) were more likely to report heroin as their primary substance.

Women accounted for 28% of the admissions. Of the 172,870 women admissions for alcohol treatment, 100,215 were for only alcohol and 72,655 for alcohol with other drugs. Women comprised about 40% of the 166,944 admissions for smoked cocaine, over half the admissions for sedatives and tranquilizers, and 45% for stimulants. Smoked cocaine was the primary substance for 13% of the total admissions, while together the stimulants, sedatives, and tranquilizers accounted for only 2%.

Table II shows that Native American men and women and white men in the CDS were the most likely to be in substance abuse treatment for alcohol only. Black, Puerto Rican, and Mexican-American women were more likely to have other drug abuse. Women aged 45 and older were more likely to be in treatment for alcohol abuse, while younger women were in treatment for other drugs.

While research suggests that minorities tend to underutilize the health

Table II. Admissions to National Client Data System by Race/Ethnicity, Gender, and Primary Substance of Abuse[a] (October 1991–September 1992)

| | Total number admissions | Primary substance of abuse | | | |
		Alcohol only	Alcohol and other drug	Other drugs	Total
Men					
White	544,361	48%	26%	26%	100%
Black	231,381	23%	21%	56%	100%
Puerto Rican	32,727	20%	16%	64%	100%
Mexican	47,422	39%	15%	46%	100%
Native American	17,035	60%	26%	13%	100%
Other	44,139	39%	16%	45%	100%
Women					
White	198,605	38%	23%	39%	100%
Black	111,987	12%	16%	72%	100%
Puerto Rican	10,351	10%	13%	77%	100%
Mexican	13,124	17%	12%	70%	100%
Native American	6,886	50%	27%	23%	100%
Other	12,291	25%	18%	57%	100%

[a]From SAMHSA, National Client Data System, 1992; 40 states, District of Columbia, and Puerto Rico reporting.

and social service systems, this may not apply to alcohol and drug treatment services. In 1987, for example, Hispanics accounted for 5.5% of the clients in alcoholism treatment programs and 9.8% of clients in drug treatment programs. Few data exist on source of referral by racial/ethnic group. Since states generally aggregate all Hispanic subgroups into the general category of "Hispanic," it is difficult to determine exactly who seeks treatment and under what circumstances. However, it appears that Hispanics are more likely to access treatment as involuntary rather than voluntary clients.[37]

Various factors may influence whether minority women are likely to be involuntary referrals to substance abuse treatment. Researchers examined rates of drug treatment referral for pregnant women in a Florida study. The black and white pregnant women had comparable rates of combined alcohol and drug use based on toxicological tests. Yet, the black women were ten times more likely than whites to be reported to public health authorities.[38] Also, poor women were more likely to be reported. It is not clear whether the differences were due to the type of drugs abused or to racial/ethnic group. For example, the examining physicians may have considered cocaine use during pregnancy more damaging than alcohol or marijuana. Yet, research consistently has found a wide range of detrimental effects of alcohol use, including fetal alcohol syndrome (FAS). The estimated incidence of FAS varies between 1.7 and 5.9 per 1000 live births.[39] Professionals have developed effective programs to train health care personnel to both identify and treat alcohol-abusing pregnant women.[40]

Several researchers have examined the treatment programs available for minorities. Some found services to be inadequate for minority groups.[41] A 1980 survey documented the underutilization of available services by Hispanics in Arizona, Illinois, California, Texas, New Mexico, Colorado, and Nevada.[42] In contrast, Flores[43] studied an East Los Angeles mental health service agency, predominately staffed by bilingual and bicultural service providers. Mexican-Americans' use of services was higher than anticipated. Flores suggested that the availability and accessibility of bilingual and bicultural staff contributed to the higher utilization rate.

A survey of substance abuse treatment services by Reed and Sanchez[44] in 1984 identified a total of 602 specialized treatment programs for Hispanics (9% of the treatment programs in the United States). The treatment field needs guidelines to determine whether specialized programs are also culturally relevant for their target populations. It also needs appropriate, timely data to evaluate what works best for whom and under what circumstances.

3. Screening and Assessment Instruments

Rates of alcoholism and alcohol abuse among women in general and in various sociocultural groups depend on both the definition of these conditions and the diagnostic instrumentation used.[45] Historically, the definition of alcoholism has had various changing emphasis placed on the physiological compared with the behavioral aspects.[46] The assessment of impaired control over drinking, denial of excessive drinking and its effects, mood changes, defense mechanisms, and difficulties in family functioning all depend on the cultural understandings of both the diagnostician and the client. Rogler[47] points out the impact of culture on the assessment, severity, and configuring of symptoms into disorders. Cervantes and Arroyo[48] are working to include culturally relevant, reliable, and valid criteria into the *Diagnostic and Statistical Manual of Mental Disorders*, Fourth Edition (DSM-IV). The interpersonal situation in which people conduct the diagnostic interview influences the validity and reliability of the diagnosis. Cultural distance due to differences in the backgrounds of the clinician and client in such areas as language, cognitive styles, and child-rearing practices can lead to diagnostic errors.

Screening and diagnostic assessment instruments should be valid, reliable, brief, and clinically relevant. Their clinical utility depends on the practitioner having established some type of rapport before administering the instrument. There are a variety of valid and highly reliable screening instruments for alcoholism. Some more widely used instruments include the four-item CAGE questionnaire,[49] the Michigan Alcoholism Screening Test (MAST),[50] the Alcohol Use Disorders Identification Test (AUDIT),[51] and the 52-item true/false Substance Abuse Subtle Screening Inventory (SASSI).[52] The MAST includes two shorter versions, the 13-item short MAST (SMAST)[53] and the 10-item Brief MAST.[54]

None of the tests directly addresses the specific concerns of minority women. The World Health Organization developed the AUDIT primarily for health care providers.[55] The ten-item AUDIT asks three questions on the quantity and frequency of use, three items on alcohol dependence, and four items on problems resulting from alcohol use. Both the MAST and the SASSI contain one item that pertains to neglect of family obligations because of drinking. The SASSI provides guidelines for identifying whether an individual fits the profile of a chemically dependent person. It includes separate profiles for scoring results based on gender. The widely used Addiction Severity Index (ASI) contains only one question that pertains to the impact of alcohol and other drugs on a woman's children and family.[56] An earlier study on the ASI found that patient age, gender, and race did not impact the interrater reliabilities for the severity scores.[57]

The number of alcohol and other drug abuse screening and diagnostic assessment instruments has proliferated in the past decade. Yet, the relevance of these instruments for gender and race/ethnicity needs further examination.[58,59] The Diagnostic Interview Schedule (DIS) and the Composite International Diagnostic Interview (CIDI) are among the few substance abuse assessment instruments adapted to other cultures.[60-62] Researchers have translated the section on alcohol and other drugs into Spanish. The CIDI provides a description of the specific withdrawal symptoms and the course and severity of addiction by drug class. The expanded alcohol and drug module of the CIDI is especially useful because it assesses age and recency of symptoms. Since both the DIS and CIDI include assessments of substance abuse and mental disorders, they permit making diagnoses of co-occurring conditions. Researchers have used the CIDI and DIS for epidemiological psychiatric research in Europe, South American, and Asia.

Clinicians and researchers usually screen for alcohol and other drug problems in a wide array of settings. Usually, these settings include correctional facilities, substance abuse treatment programs, and mental health facilities. People do not routinely screen for alcohol and other drug problems in settings typically considered outside the "substance abuse field." Minority women can be found in these settings, such as child protective services and hospital emergency rooms.

Most diagnostic assessment instruments were developed for research rather than for clinical applications. Even those instruments used primarily in clinical situations often do not have appropriate norms for various racial/ethnic groups. Thus, screening and assessment instruments often have little clinical utility with diverse racial/ethnic groups. Other reasons for their lack of clinical utility include the use of items that are inappropriate or irrelevant to the sociocultural group, emphasis on dissimilar values from the minority culture, and language difficulties. Colloquialisms, inadequate translations, and reading level can all cause language difficulties.

Assessments conducted in Spanish with Hispanics have resulted in both higher[63] and lower[64-66] levels of psychiatric pathology. Most substance abuse and mental health assessment instruments have not been adapted for Hispanics. This lack of cultural adaptation may account for part of the mixed results. Rogler *et al.*[67] suggest that most assessments are at best only translations in Spanish of the instrument. They suggest that the translations should attain equivalent meanings for symptoms.

4. Access to Treatment

Regier *et al.*[68] estimate that only 25% of the general population that meet diagnostic criteria for an addictive disorder receive care at any specialist, general, or voluntary care system. Rouse and Steigerwald[69] studied the referral sources of a national sample of clients discharged from substance abuse treatment. Adults were more likely to refer themselves for substance abuse treatment. The criminal justice system (34%) and the social agencies (31%) were the primary referral sources for persons under age 18.

In general, although minority groups may have similar or higher rates of health problems, they use health services less than whites even when insured.[70,71] Padgett *et al.*[72] examined the role of race/ethnicity in the use of outpatient mental health services by the insured. They analyzed the insurance claims data for 1.2 million federal employees and their dependents insured by Blue Cross/Blue Shield. Age, education, and having the high-option plan all predicted having an outpatient visit for mental health care. After adjusting for the various sociodemographic predictors, whites still were 1.7 more likely than blacks and Hispanics to use an outpatient facility. There are a variety of possible explanations for minorities using fewer services. These include less availability and acceptability of services, reluctance to use a treatment system dominated by English-speaking whites, difficulty finding facilities within available transportation, and a variety of cultural and attitudinal factors.

Recently, substance abuse programs have mounted special outreach and other efforts to get minority groups into treatment. Community health centers and neighborhood community centers can play an important role as "ports of entry" both to treatment and related services. Service providers increase their effectiveness by working collaboratively with local social services. Natural self-help groups, such as the church and other local institutions, can help women to access needed services. Such collaboration helps to link women, especially minority women, to alcoholism treatment and related services. The local Spanish-speaking media that typically offer short segments on local services and resources also can facilitate access to treatment for Hispanic women.

4.1. Psychosocial and Cultural Barriers

Efforts have increased to identify and eliminate barriers that prevent black, Hispanic, and other minority women from accessing treatment services. Allen[73] provided a comprehensive list of various types of treatment obstacles for women, classified into three domains. Characteristics of treatment programs, individuals, and the socioeconomic environment may prevent women from accessing and receiving effective treatment. She also developed the Allen Barriers to Treatment Instrument[74] to provide a standarized, objective, and valid means of assessing barriers faced by women.

The barriers that keep various minority women from entering treatment are similar to those of their white counterparts. There is a strong cultural mandate that intoxication or the appearance of alcohol-related problems is not acceptable behavior for women. Thus, women face additional stigma and rejection from their families compared with men when seeking treatment. Caetano[75] found gender differences in the medical and social consequences of alcohol dependence. More women than men alcoholics reported medical problems, which suggests that women may have delayed entry to treatment until their conditions were very severe. Also, he found that ethnicity significantly predicted the number of social consequences for women only. Other barriers include the inability to pay for treatment, the threat of legal intervention, fear of losing custody of children, lack of programs for women with children, and unresponsive service providers. Minority women, however, are likely to experience these barriers to a greater extent.

Harper[76] examined barriers to access and successful alcoholism treatment for blacks in the 1970s. A major obstacle to seeking treatment was their fear of the criminal and social consequences of being labeled an alcoholic. In a more recent review of barriers, Harper[77] concluded:

> Other cultural concerns include black language usage that can impede effective communication with therapists of other cultural backgrounds;[76,78] negative reactions and discriminatory actions of treatment personnel and law enforcers toward black alcoholics;[79–81] and suspicious reactions of black alcoholics to white counselors, middle-class black counselors, and traditional AA programs.[82] (p.73)

Therapists also need to consider differences in the client's ability to comply with treatment due to socioeconomic influences. Clients may break appointments because they lack transportation or other resources not because they lack a commitment to their treatment. For example, according to the 1990 census, 94% of the total population had a telephone in their household compared with only 77% of the Puerto Rican and 83% of the Mexican households.[2] Also, clients, especially women, may be ashamed to admit they do not have clean clothes or are homeless. Lack of sanitation facilities may cause embarrassment. Minority women are more likely to begin childbearing at younger ages and have sole responsibility for child care. Thus, they are more likely to have difficulties making appointments even when they want to participate in the treatment process. The lack of social supports may impose additional responsibilities without fallback arrangements.

4.2. Ability to Pay for Treatment

Access to treatment depends on the ability to have that treatment reimbursed. Clients can pay by earning sufficient income, having health insurance, or qualifying for public assistance. In 1990, as in earlier years, men were more likely to earn more money than women; the median earning for working men was $21,538 compared with $12,239 for working women.[2] Whites were more likely to earn more than blacks.[18] The median income in 1990 after adjusting for inflation was $36,920 for white families and $21,420 for black families. White and black women had comparable rates of annual average labor force participation for 1991 (57.4% vs. 57%), but more black women worked full-time. The median earning in 1990 was $12,280 for white women and $11,850 for black women. While the median earning for non-Hispanic women was higher ($12,438) than for Hispanic women ($10,099), there were significant differences among the Hispanic groups. The median income for Cuban women ($12,904) exceeded not only all other Hispanic women but also that for non-Hispanic women. The median income for Puerto Rican women ($11,702) also exceeded other Hispanic women.[2]

Women (86.9%) were slightly more likely than men (83.6%) to be covered by some form of health insurance during all or part of 1992.[83] This was due in part to the greater proportion of women covered by Medicaid (12.9% women vs. 94% men) and by Medicare (14.9% women vs. 11.6% men). Whites (86.4%) were more likely than blacks (79.9%) or Hispanics (67.4%) to have health insurance coverage. For income levels below the federal poverty level (FPL), more blacks (77.4%) than whites (69%) or Hispanics (58.8%) had some form of health insurance coverage, either private or public insurance.

In 1990, the poverty rate for families with women head of households with no husband present was 48% for blacks versus 27% for whites. Among families with related children under 18 years of age, those with black women as the head of householders (64%) were more likely to qualify as poor than those headed by white women (38%).[18] By 1992, the percentage of persons below the FPL was 33% for blacks, 29% for Hispanics, 13% for Asian/Pacific Islanders, 12% for whites, and 17% for others.[83] While Medicaid is often the payment source of last resource for those with substance abuse, Medicaid does not cover all poor. Only 42% of those in poverty and 75% of those in extreme poverty (below 25% of the FPL) have Medicaid coverage.[84]

Table III shows the rates of heavy drinking reported in the 1993 NHSDA by FPL, race/ethnicity, and gender. Among men and women below the poverty level, whites were most likely to report heavy drinking. Among women above poverty level, heavy drinking among the racial/ethnic groups did not differ significantly.

4.3. Language and Communication Difficulties

Minority women face additional obstacles and barriers due to communication difficulties. Not feeling understood and appreciated can prevent them from accessing treatment, staying in treatment, or continuing to participate in aftercare or relapse prevention programs. For example, the client and the counselor may differ in their meanings of the symptoms, ways of expressing distress or help-seeking behavior, and acceptance of assertive communication.

Table III. Heavy Drinking in the Past Month by Federal
Poverty Level, Race/Ethnicity, and Gender[a-c]

Race/gender	Below poverty level	Above poverty level
Men		
White	14.7%	9.5%
Black	8.2%	7.8%
Hispanic	14.0%	7.5%
Women		
White	2.8%	1.4%
Black	1.3%	1.3%
Hispanic	0.8%	1.2%

[a]From SAMHSA National Household Survey on Drug Abuse, 1993.
[b]Heavy drinking is defined as drinking five or more drinks per occasion
on 5 or more days in the past 30 days. An occasion is defined as "at one
sitting" or within a couple of hours.
[c]For definitions of Federal Poverty Level by income and family size and
composition, see: US Department of Commerce, Bureau of the Census:
Poverty in the United States: 1991. Current Populations Reports, Consumer Income, Series P-60, No. 181. Washington DC, US Government Printing Office, 1992.

Some verbal and nonverbal behavior in the client's culture may be a sign
of respect or acknowledgment of social status. Yet the clinician may interpret
such behavior as weakness or evasion. Marin[85] points out that the concept of
simpatia leads traditional Hispanics to appear to agree out of politeness and
respect. *Simpatia* would lead them to agree even when they do not intend to
comply or do not understand the message. Minority groups are not the only
people who display this "agreeableness." The phenomenon is well known to
researchers who have to guard against inducing the socially desirable responses on their research instruments.

Direct questioning may not be the most culturally appropriate way of
eliciting some information from minority groups. For some, a direct question
may be interpreted as threatening or disrespectful. Others may see the questions as more complex than intended. For example, if asked whether they
have difficulty making decisions, they would want to know what type of
decision and during what time period.[86] *Platica,* or "friendly conversation,"
may be more effective in determining the desired mental health status or
clinical condition.[87] *Platica* may be another way of emphasizing the importance of providing the client an acceptable environment for not agreeing and
for honest communication.

5. Treatment Effectiveness

There is continuing debate on what constitutes successful treatment.
Some studies of gender-related treatment outcomes suggest that recovery

rates for men and women are similar.[88] Vannicelli[89] conducted an early review of treatment outcome studies that reported gender-outcomes. Eighteen reported no difference in outcomes, four reported better outcomes for women, and one reported better outcomes for men. Scientific clinical studies to determine treatment outcomes for different racial/ethnic groups by gender are notably absent.

Any conceptualization of alcoholism and drug treatment effectiveness needs to consider the chronic, relapsing nature of the disease. Alcohol and other drug treatment providers have long held that aftercare is a critical component in the continuum of treatment services. It is especially important not to penalize clients if they experience a lapse. Only recently, clinicians and researchers have addressed factors associated with the likelihood of relapse among women. They also need to examine the factors affecting relapse in minority groups.

Finkelstein's[90] guiding principles of care for pregnant women are equally important for all women, regardless of pregnancy status or race/ethnicity. To increase substance abuse treatment effectiveness for culturally diverse clients, the services should be: (1) family-oriented, (2) promote competency building and empowerment, (3) community-based, (4) multidisciplinary, comprehensive, and coordinated, (5) address multiple problems and needs of alcohol- and drug-dependent mothers and their children, (6) individually tailored, and (7) long term.

5.1. Coexisting Conditions

As with women in the general population, minority women present other coexisting conditions as they enter alcoholism treatment. Often, women enter treatment with a history of failed and often abusive relationships that include rape and incest. Minority women are likely to have a variety of medical and other coexisting conditions that impair or delay treatment effectiveness. Researchers reviewed the medical records of 252 African-American women admitted to an inpatient drug rehabilitation program between July 1989 and July 1991.[91] Many women had problems related to lifestyles, such as sexually transmitted diseases, anemia, and dental diseases. They also had significant medical conditions, such as heart disease, abdominal surgical conditions, and breast masses. Such high rates of disease are compatible with the report of the Secretary's Task Force on Black and Minority Health.[92] Only 58% of those women referred to specialists kept their initial appointment. All but 0.7% of the patients were on general relief, Medicare, Medicaid, or lacked payment source. These findings affirm the usefulness of comprehensive health care intervention with impoverished African-Americans and the need for the services of culturally competent health care professionals.[93] With the myriad of problems noted with women in general and minority women in particular, case management becomes extremely important.

5.2. Counselor and Client Relationship

5.2.1. Labeling. The therapist's perceptions of the client's motivation and treatment compliance are crucial to treatment success.[94,95] Moore[96] found that most therapists (72%) held the client responsible for negative treatment outcomes while only 11% acknowledged their role in the client's treatment outcomes. An experiment with randomly selected clients labeled as having a good prognosis showed the impact of perceptions on client treatment outcomes.[97] Not only did their therapists later rate these randomly labeled clients as highly motivated and successful but the clients themselves were less likely to be absent from treatment.

Labeling is a form of behavioral expectation. The greater the distant between the person doing the labeling and the person with the behavior being labeled, the more likely the behavior will be labeled deviant or pathological.[98] Thus, it is likely that minorities are more likely to be labeled deviant.

Levy[99] differentiates between intracultural labeling and cross-cultural labeling. Intracultural labeling problems occur when a specific cultural group and the dominant culture differ on their definitions of appropriate behaviors. This is particularly a problem when the treatment system and the client differ on the definition of illness. To deal with different cultural definitions of deviance and illness, he suggests that the health care delivery system must determine the beliefs, values, and attitudes of the other culture. After knowing how the other culture really works, prevention and treatment planners can develop programs that use these differences to increase effectiveness.

Cross-cultural labeling problems occur when it involves the labeling of minority persons to their detriment. Such labeling influences the minority group to behave in expected ways that generally engender their feelings of inadequacy and inferiority. The effects of cross-cultural labeling are often difficult to separate from the effects of malnutrition, inappropriate living conditions, and inadequate economic resources. Levy[99] suggests conducting appropriate research to remove the erroneous and negative perceptions and labeling now used in health programs. Prevention and treatment programs can then be adapted and designed to meet the real needs of culturally distinct groups.

The counselor should be sensitive to cultural differences. Cultural explanations, however, should not be used to avoid dealing with maladaptive, dangerous, or self-destructive behaviors. Clinicians attempting to be "culturally sensitive" may minimize symptoms or normalize dysfunctional behavior. Martinez[100] cautions family therapists:

> Culture cannot be used to explain all behavior nor can it be dismissed totally as a superfluous concept. It is the responsibility of the therapist to maintain an informed perspective that balances a broadly defined cultural sensitivity that includes an awareness about sociocultural and spiritual issues with sound clinical judgment based on well-founded family therapy principles. (p79)

Some people may not be able to distinguish between cultural sensitivity and cross-cultural labeling. There are many cultural myths and stereotypes. Machismo or "macho" behavior, for example, is often considered primarily a Hispanic concept of manhood when it actually is a widespread phenomenon.[101] There is some evidence that counselors understand the need for cultural sensitivity, but often appropriate training is not available or accessible to them.[102]

5.2.2. Race/Ethnicity of Counselor. Most alcohol and other drug treatment service providers agree that the counselor and client relationship is an important factor in keeping clients in treatment. Yet, few have conducted such research on racial/ethnic groups in general and minority women in particular. Results regarding the role of the race of the therapist and client are mixed. Some suggest that the racial identity of the client and therapist should be the same.[103–105] Others maintain that the therapist's ability to facilitate a therapeutic relationship is more important.[106,107] This also entails helping clients to identify and build on their own strengths and assets. Many agree that culturally sensitive and responsive therapists are generally more credible, trusted, and effective.[108–111] Bell and Evans[112] have delineated factors that inhibit the counseling of black clients by blacks. They have also dealt with those factors specific to counseling by whites. They present general guidelines for effectively counseling black clients regardless of the therapist's background. Carter[113] also addressed psychotherapy issues with African-Americans, based on his counseling experiences. Fleming[114] provided background information helpful in working with American Indians and Alaska Natives. Ponterotto and Casas[115] presented guidelines for counseling Hispanics and other minority groups. Background information is also available for various Asian groups, including Asian-Americans,[116] Indochinese refugees,[117] and Asian/Pacific Island-Americans.[118]

6. Summary and Recommendations

Women need similar types of services as men, such as detoxification, treatment of coexisting physical and psychiatric conditions, education/ vocational training and support, and active relapse prevention. However, because of women's socioeconomic and cultural conditions, they require more child-care, medical treatment, and supportive services. Barriers to effective treatment access, diagnosis, and services exist. Such barriers include stigmatizing and punitive attitudes, uncertainty regarding the medical management of pregnant women in substance abuse treatment, inability to pay, language, and communication style differences.

Some race/ethnicity differences in alcoholism rates and treatment effectiveness are due to socioeconomic factors. There is significant variability within as well as diversity between the ethnic/racial groups. Race and ethnicity are complex sociocultural phenomena. For example, an individual coming to the clinician may share African, Hispanic, Asian, and Native American heritages within herself or her family. Cultural modifications also are taking place due to acculturation and large scale social and economic forces.[119,120]

A comprehensive and effective treatment approach to women alcoholics must include attention to both their special needs as women and to those sociocultural influences that impact access, diagnosis, and treatment. Special needs arise from the cultural attitudes and behaviors toward women as well as their social roles and responsibilities and economic conditions. Therefore, effective treatment for women needs to combine culturally compatible and sensitive psychological, medical, and social services. Socioculturally responsive strategies are needed to increase access to treatment, prevent early termination or discharge, and to maintain follow-up and after care. Often this requires coordination between the services of the social service, health care, and substance abuse treatment systems.

The clinicians's knowledge of sociocultural factors, good listening skills, and ability to develop a trustworthy and respectful relationship with a client are even more important because of the complexity and diversity of clientele encountered. Clinicians need research to determine the extent that culturally different groups require different treatment and outreach strategies. They also need training opportunities to know which strategies are most effective for which sociocultural groups. Appropriate research and evaluation are needed to determine how well different sociocultural groups' needs are being served. Researchers can help by conducting treatment and communication research to evaluate the effectiveness of various approaches to different racial/ethnic groups. Guidelines for outcome research have been established.[121] There is a great need for large-scale, representative, culturally sensitive, and methodologically sound clinical and epidemiological research.

ACKNOWLEDGMENTS. We wish to thank Philip Archambault, Certified Senior Counselor, Native American Rehabilitation Association of the Northwest, Inc. Oregon, for valuable information concerning Native American treatment programs. From the Office of Applied Studies, SAMHSA, Dr. Richard Thoreson and Janet Greenblatt contributed important information, and Dr. Daniel Melnick, Acting Director, provided insightful comments on the manuscript.

References

1. US Office of Management and Budget: *Race and Ethnic Standards for Federal Statistics and Administrative Reporting.* Statistical Policy Directive No. 15 (43 FR 19260), Washington, DC, May 4, 1978.
2. US Department of Commerce, Bureau of the Census: The Hispanic Population in the United States: March 1991. Current Population Reports, Series P20-455. Washington, DC, US Government Printing Office, October 1991.
3. US Department of Commerce, Bureau of the Census. United States Population Estimates,

by Age, Sex, Race, and Hispanic Origin: 1980 to 1988. Current Population Reports, Population Estimates and Projections, Series P-25, No. 1045. Washington, DC, US Government Printing Office, January 1990.

4. US Department of Commerce, Bureau of the Census: Population Projections of the United States, by Age, Sex, Race, and Hispanic Origin: 1993 to 2050. Current Population Reports, Series P25-1104. Washington, DC, US Government Printing Office, November 1993.

5. Ewing JA, Rouse BA, Pellizzari ED: Alcohol sensitivity and ethnic background. *Am J Psychiatry* 131:206–210, 1974.

6. Fenna D, Mix L, Schaefer O, Gilbert JAL: Ethanol metabolism in various racial groups. *Can Med Assoc J* 150:472–475, 1971.

7. Harada S, Agarwal DP, Goedde HW: Aldehyde dehydrogenase deficiency as cause of facial flushing reaction to alcohol in Japanese. *Lancet* 1(8253):982, October 31, 1981.

8. Harada S, Agarwah DP, Goedde HW, Ishikawa B: Aldehyde dehydrogenase isozyme variation and alcoholism in Japan. *Pharmacol Biochem Behav* 18:151–153, 1983.

9. Rudorfer MV: Pharmacokinetics and psychotropic drugs in special populations. *J Clin Psychiatry* 54:50–54, 1993.

10. Wolff PH: Ethnic differences in alcohol sensitivity. *Science* 175:449–450, 1972.

11. Mizoi Y, Tatsuno Y, Adachi J, et al: Alcohol sensitivity related to polymorphism of alcohol-metabolizing enzymes in Japanese. *Pharmacol Biochem Behav* 18(Suppl 1):127–133, 1983.

12. Park JY, Huang YH, Nagoshi CT, et al: The flushing response to alcohol use among Koreans and Taiwanese. *J Stud Alcohol* 45:481–485, 1984.

13. Venten CD, Joubert PH, Strydom WJ: Comparative pharmacokinetics and intravenous propranolol in black and white volunteers. *J Cardiovasc Pharmacol* 7:409–410, 1985.

14. Venten CD, Joubert PH: Ethnic differences in response to beta-1 adrenoceptor blocker by propranolol. *J Cardiovasc Pharmacol* 6:361–364, 1984.

15. Yamamoto J: Genetic, cultural and family factors in alcohol use in Asians, in Sorel E (ed): *Family, Culture, and Psychobiology.* Brooklyn, NY, Legas, 1990, pp 91–110.

16. Macias RF: Language and ethnic classification of language minorities: Chicano and Latino students in the 1990s. *Hispanic J Behav Sci* 15(2):230–257, 1993.

17. US Department of Commerce, Bureau of the Census: Hispanic Americans Today: Current Population Reports. Population Characteristics P23-183. Washington, DC, US Government Printing Office, 1993.

18. US Department of Commerce, Bureau of the Census: The Black Population in the United States: March 1991. Current Population Reports, Series P20-464. Washington, DC, US Government Printing Office, September 1992.

19. US Department of Health and Human Services, Indian Health Service: Trends in Indian Health—1993. Rockville, MD, Indian Health Service, Division of Program Statistics, 1994.

20. Bales RJ: Cultural differences in rates of alcoholism. *Q J Stud Alcohol* 6:480–499, 1946.

21. McLachlan JFC, Walderman RL, Birchmore DF, Marsden LR: Self-evaluation, role satisfaction and anxiety in the woman alcoholic. *Int J Addict* 14(6):609–632, 1979.

22. Schuckit MA, Pitts FN, Reich T, et al: Two types of alcoholism in women. *Arch Gen Psychiatry* 20:301–306, 1969.

23. Beckman LJ, Amaro H: Personal and social difficulties faced by women and men entering alcoholism treatment. *J Stud Alcohol* 46(2):135–145, 1986.

24. Reed BG: Drug misuse and dependency in women: The meaning and implications of being considered a special population or minority group. *Int J Addict* 20(1):13–62, 1985.

25. Beckman LJ: Woman alcoholics: A review of social and psychological studies. *J Stud Alcohol* 36(7):797–824, 1975.

26. Estep R: The influence of the family on the use of alcohol and prescription depressants by women. *J Psychoactive Drugs* 19(2):171–179, 1982.

27. Vargas-Willis G, Cervantes RC: Consideration of psychosocial stress in the treatment of the Latina immigrant. *Hispanic J Behav Sci* 9(3):315–329, 1987.

28. Thornton CI, Carter JH: Treating the black female alcoholic: Clinical observations of black therapists. *J Natl Med Assoc* 80:644–647, 1988.

29. Rand MR: Crime and the nation's households. Bureau of Justice Statistics Bulletin. Washington, DC, US Department of Justice, 1992.
30. Wyatt GE: The sociocultural context of African-American and white American women's roles. *J Soc Issues* 48:77–91, 1992.
31. US Department of Health and Human Services, Centers for Disease Control and Prevention: HIV/AIDS Surveillance Report, US AIDS Cases Reported through June 1994. Atlanta, National Center for Infectious Diseases, 6(1):10 1994.
32. US Department of Health and Human Services, Substance Abuse and Mental Health Services Administration, National Household Survey on Drug Abuse Population Estimates, 1993. DHHS Publication No. (SMA) 94–3017. Washington DC, US Government Printing Office, 1994.
33. Flewelling R, Ennett ST, Rachal JV, Theisen AC: National Household Survey on Drug Abuse: Race, Socioeconomic Status, and Drug Abuse, 1991. DHHS Pub. No. (SMA)93-2062. Rockville, MD, Substance Abuse and Mental Health Services Administration, 1994.
34. Caetano R: Drinking patterns and alcohol problems in a national sample of U.S. Hispanics, in Spengler D, Tate DA, Aitkin S, Christian CM (eds): *Alcohol Use Among U.S. Ethnic Minorities*. National Institute on Alcohol Abuse and Alcoholism Research Monograph No. 18, DHHS Publication No. (ADM) 89–1435, Washington, DC, US Government Printing Office, 1989, pp 147–162.
35. Cervantes RC, Gilbert MJ, Salgado de Synder VN, Padilla AM: Psychosocial and cognitive correlates of alcohol use in younger adult immigrant and US born Hispanics. *Int J Addict* 25(5/6):689–710, 1990.
36. US Department of Health and Human Services, Centers for Disease Control and Prevention: Health United States 1993. DHHS Pub. No. (PHS)94-1232, Hyattsville, MD, National Center for Health Statistics, May 1994.
37. Gilbert MJ, Cervantes RC: Alcohol services for Mexican Americans: A review of utilization patterns, treatment considerations and prevention activities. *Hispanic J Behav Sci* 8(3):191–224, 1986.
38. Chasnoff IJ, Landress HJ, Barrett ME: The prevalence of illicit drug or alcohol use during pregnancy and discrepancies in mandatory reporting in Pinellas County, Florida. *N Engl J Med* 322:1202–1206, 1990.
39. Phillips DK, Henderson GI, Schenker S: Pathogenesis of fetal alcohol syndrome. *Alcohol Health Res World* 13(3):219–227, 1989.
40. Weiner L, Rosett HL, Mason EA: Training professionals to identify and treat pregnant women who drink heavily. *Alcohol Health Res World* 10(1):32–36, 1985.
41. Delgado M: Using Hispanic adolescents to access community needs. *Soc Casework* 62:607–613, 1981.
42. US Department of Health and Human Services. Hispanics in HHS Programs. A Needs and Service Delivery Assessment: Preliminary Findings. Washington, DC, 1980.
43. Flores JL: The utilization of a community mental health service by Mexican Americans. *Int J Soc Psychiatry* 24(4):271–275, 1978.
44. Reed PG, Sanchez DS: Characteristics of Alcoholism Services in the United States—1984. Rockville, MD, National Institute on Alcohol Abuse and Alcoholism, 1986.
45. Dawson DA, Archer L: Gender differences in alcohol consumption: Effects of Measurement. *Br J Addiction* 87:119–123, 1992.
46. Morse RM, Flavin DK: The definition of alcoholism. Joint Committee of the National Council on Alcoholism and Drug Dependence and the American Society of Addiction Medicine to study the definition and criteria for the diagnosis of alcoholism. *J Am Med Assoc* 268(8):1012–1014, August 26, 1992.
47. Rogler LH: Culturally sensitizing psychiatric diagnosis: A framework for research. *J Nerv Ment Dis* 181(7):401–408, 1993.
48. Cervantes RC, Arroyo W: DSM-IV: Implications for Hispanic children and adolescents. *Hispanic J Behav Sci* 16:8–27, 1994.
49. Ewing JA: Detecting alcoholism: The CAGE questionnaire. *J Am Med Assoc* 252:1905–1907, 1984.

50. Selzer ML: The Michigan Alcoholism Screening Test: The quest for a new diagnostic instrument. *Am J Psychiatry* 127:1653–1658, 1971.
51. Babor TF, de la Fuerte JR, Saunders J, Grant M: AUDIT: The Alcohol Use Disorders Identification Test, Guidelines for Use in Primary Health Care. Geneva, WHO, 1992.
52. Miller GA: The Substance Abuse Subtle Screening Inventory Manual. Bloomington, IN, The SASSI Institute, 1985.
53. Selzer ML, van Rooijen L: A self-administered short Michigan Alcoholism Screening Test (MAST). *J Stud Alcohol* 36(1):117–126, 1975.
54. Allex D, Pokorny BA, Kaplan HB: The Brief Mast: A shortened version of the Michigan Alcoholism Screening Test (MAST). *Am J Psychiatry* 129(3):342–345, 1972.
55. Babor TF, de la Fuerte JR, Saunders J, Grant M: AUDIT: The Alcohol Use Disorders Identification Test, Guidelines for Use in Primary Health Care. Geneva, WHO, 1992.
56. McLellan AT, Parikh G, Bragg A, *et al:* Addiction Severity Index Administration Manual, 5th ed. Philadelphia, Pennsylvania VA Center for Studies on Addiction, 1990.
57. McLellan AT, Luborsky L, Cacciola J, Griffith J: New data from the Addiction Severity Index: Reliability and validity in three centers. *J Nerv Ment Dis* 173(7):412–423, 1985.
58. Rounsaville BJ, Tims FM, Horton AM Jr, Sowder BJ (eds): *Diagnostic Source Book on Drug Abuse Research and Treatment.* National Institute on Drug Abuse, NIH Pub No. 93-3508. Washington, DC, US Government Printing Office, 1993.
59. Allen JP, Litten RZ: Psychometric and laboratory measures to assist in the treatment of alcoholism. *Clin Psychol Rev* 13:223–239, 1993.
60. Helzer JE: Psychiatric diagnosis, family psychiatric history, in Rounsaville BJ, Tims FM, Horton AM Jr, Sowder BJ (eds): *Diagnostic Source Book on Drug Abuse Research and Treatment.* National Institute on Drug Abuse, NIH Pub No. 93-3508. Washington, DC, US Government Printing Office, 1993.
61. Helzer JE, Canino G: *Alcoholism in North America, Europe, and Asia.* New York, Oxford University Press, 1991.
62. Canino G, Bird H, Shrout P, *et al:* The Spanish DIS reliability and concordance with clinical diagnosis in Puerto Rico. *Arch Gen Psychiatry* 44:120–126, 1987a.
63. Del Castillo J: The influence of language upon symptomatology in foreign-born patients. *Am J Psychiatry* 127:242–244, 1970.
64. Marcos LR, Alpert M, Urcuyo L, Kesselman M: The effect of interview language on the evaluation of psychopathology in Spanish-American schizophrenic patients. *Am J Psychiatry* 130:549–553, 1973.
65. Malgady RG, Rogler LH, Costantino G: Ethnocultural and linguistic bias in mental health evaluation of Hispanics. *Am Psychol* 42:228–234, 1987.
66. Price CS, Cuellar I: Effects of language and related variables on the expression of psychopathology in Mexican-American psychiatric patients. *Hispanic J Behav Sci* 3:145–160, 1981.
67. Rogler LH, Cortes DE, Malgady RG: Acculturation and mental health status among Hispanics: Convergence and new directions for research. *Am Psychol* 46(6):585–597, 1991.
68. Regier DA, Narrow WE, Rae DS, *et al:* The de facto US mental and addictive disorders service system. *Arch Gen Psychiatry* 50:85–94, 1993.
69. Rouse BA, Steigerwald CE: National survey of drug abuse treatment services: Implications for treatment referrals, in *Problems of Drug Dependence 1992: Proceedings of the 54th Annual Scientific Meeting.* National Institute on Drug Abuse Research Monograph Series 132. DHHS Publication No. (ADM)93-3505. Washington, DC, US Government Printing Office, 1993, p 133.
70. Hayward RA, Shapiro MF, Freeman HE, Corey CR: Inequities in health services among insured Americans. *N Engl J Med* 318:1507–12, 1988.
71. Wells KB, Golding JM, Hough RL, *et al:* Acculturation and the probability of use of health services by Mexican Americans. *Health Serv Res* 24:237–257, 1989.
72. Padgett DK, Patrick C, Burns BJ, Schlesinger HG: Ethnicity and the use of outpatient mental health services in a national insured population. *Am J Public Health* 84(2):222–226, 1994.
73. Allen K: Development of an instrument to identify barriers to treatment for addicted women, from their perspective. *Int J Addict* 29(4):429–444, 1994.

74. Allen K: Psychometric assessment of the Allen barriers to treatment instrument. *Int J Addict* 29(5):545–563, 1994.
75. Caetano R: The association between severity of DSM-III-R alcohol dependence and medical and social consequences. *Addict* 88:631–642, 1993.
76. Harper FD (ed): *Alcohol Abuse and Black America.* Alexandria, VA, Douglass Publishers, 1976.
77. Harper FD: Alcoholism treatment and Black Americans: A review and analysis, in Watts TD, Wright R Jr (eds): *Black Alcoholism: Toward a Comprehensive Understanding.* Springfield Ill: Charles C. Thomas Publisher, 1983, pp 71–84.
78. Higgins E, Warner R: Counseling blacks. *Personnel Guidance J* 53:382–386, 1975.
79. Halleck SL: *Psychiatry and the Dilemmas of Crime: A Study of Causes, Punishment, and Treatment.* New York, Harper & Row, 1967.
80. Larkins J: *Alcohol and the Negro: Explosive Issues.* Zebulon, NC, Record Publishing, 1965.
81. Lowe G, Hodge E: Race and the treatment of alcoholism in a southern state. *J Soc Problems* 17:240–252, 1972.
82. Davis F: Alcoholism among American blacks. *Addict* 3:8–16, 1974, p.73.
83. US Department of Commerce, Bureau of the Census: Poverty in the United States: 1992. Current Population Reports, Consumer Income, Series P60-185, September 1993.
84. US Bipartisan Commission on Comprehensive Health Care (Pepper Commission): A Call for Action: Final report of the commission. Senate Print 101-114. Washington, DC, US Government Printing Office, September 1990.
85. Marin BV: Hispanic drug abuse: Culturally appropriate prevention and treatment, in Watson RR (ed): *Drug and Alcohol Abuse Prevention.* Clifton, NJ, Humana Press, 1990, pp 151–165.
86. Zane N, Sasao T: Research on drug abuse among Asian Pacific Americans. Unpublished manuscript. Santa Barbara, University of California, 1990.
87. Marin G, Marin BV, Juarez R: Prevention of AIDS in the Latino Community: Cultural issues. Presented at the American Psychological Association annual meeting. Atlanta, GA, August 1988.
88. Yih-Ing Hser M, Anglin MD, Booth MW: Sex differences in addict careers. *Am J Drug Alcohol Abuse* 13(3):231–251, 1987.
89. Vanicelli M: Treatment outcomes of alcoholic women: The state of the art in relation to sex bias and expectancy effects, in Wilsnack SC, Beckman LJ (eds): *Alcohol Problems in Women.* New York, Guilford Press, 1984, pp 369–412.
90. Finkelstein N: Treatment programming for alcohol and drug-dependent pregnant women. *Int J Addict* 28(13):1275–1309, 1993.
91. Curtiss AM, Lenz KM, Frei NR: Medical evaluation of African-American women entering treatment. *J Addict Dis* 12:29–44, 1993.
92. US Department of Health and Human Services: Report of the Secretary's Task Force on Black Health. Washington, DC, 1985, vol 1.
93. Thornton CI, Carter JH: Treating the black female alcoholic: Clinical observations of black therapists. *J Natl Med Assoc* 80:644–647, 1988.
94. Miller WR: Motivation for treatment: A review with special emphasis on alcoholism. *Psychol Bull* 98:84–107, 1985.
95. Davies P: Expectations and therapeutic practices in outpatient clinics for alcohol problems. *Br J Addict* 76:159–173, 1981.
96. Moore RA: Alcoholism treatment in private psychiatric hospitals: A national survey. *Q J Stud Alcohol* 32:1083–1085, 1971.
97. Leake GJ, King AS: Effect of counselor expectations on alcoholic recovery. *Alcohol Health Res World* 11(3):16–22, 1977.
98. Horowitz AV: *Social Control of Mental Illness.* New York, Academic Press, 1982.
99. Levy JE: The effects of labeling on health behavior and treatment programs among North American Indians. Behavioral Health Issues Among American Indian and Alaska Natives. *Am Indian Alaska Native Ment Health Res Monogr* 1:211–243, 1988.
100. Martinez KJ: Cultural sensitivity in family therapy gone awry. *Hispanic J Behav Sci* 16(1):75–79, 1994.

101. Ramirez O, Arce CH: The contemporary Chicano family: An empirically based review, in Baron A (ed): *Explorations in Chicano Psychology.* New York, Praeger, 1981, pp 3–28.

102. Ramirez SZ, Wassef A, Paniagua FA, *et al:* Perceptions of mental health providers concerning cultural factors in the evaluation of Hispanic children and adolescents. *Hispanic J Behav Sci* 16(1):28–42, 1994.

103. Beverly C: Toward a model for counseling the black alcoholic. *J Non-White Concerns in Personnel Guidance* 3:169–176, 1975.

104. Smith E: *Counseling the Culturally Different Black Youth.* Columbus, OH, Charles E. Merrill, 1973.

105. Murphy S, Deblassie RR: Substance abuse and the Native American student. *J Drug Educ* 14(4):315–321, 1984.

106. Carkhuff R, Berenson B: *Beyond Counseling and Therapy.* New York, Holt, Rinehart and Winston, 1967.

107. Rogers C: *On Becoming a Person.* Boston, Houghton Mifflin, 1961.

108. Sue S, Zane N: The role of culture and cultural techniques in pychotherapy: A critique and reformulation. *Am Psychol* 41:37–45, 1987.

109. Clifford PR: Drug abusers and access to treatment issues among inner city minority populations. *J Health Hum Resources Admin* 10(3):278–287, 1988.

110. Gutierrez LM: Working with women of color: An empowerment perspective. *Soc Work* 149-153, 1990.

111. Watts TD, Wright R Jr (eds): *Black Alcoholism: Toward a Comprehensive Understanding.* Springfield IL, Charles C. Thomas, 1983.

112. Bell P, Evans J: *Counseling the Black Client: Alcohol Use and Abuse in Black America.* Center City, MN, Hazelden Educational Services, 1981.

113. Carter JH: Frequent mistakes made in psychotherapy with blacks. *J Natl Med Assoc* 71:1007–1009, 1979.

114. Fleming CM: American Indians and Alaska Natives: Changing societies past and present, in Orlandi MA, Weston R, Epstein LG (eds): *Cultural Competence for Evaluators.* OSAP Cultural Competence Series #1. DHHS Pub No. (ADM) 92-1884,Washington DC: US Government Printing Office 1992, pp. 147–171.

115. Ponterotto JG, Casas JM: *Handbook of Racial/Ethnic Minority Counseling Research.* Springfield, IL, Charles C. Thomas, 1991.

116. Kim S, McLeod JH, Shantzis C: Cultural competence for evaluators working with Asian-American communities: Some practical considerations, in Orlandi MA, Weston R, Epstein LG (eds): *Cultural Competence for Evaluators.* OSAP Cultural Competence Series #1. DHHS Pub No. (ADM)92-1884, Washington DC, US Government Printing Office 1992 pp 203–260.

117. Yee BWK, Thu ND: Correlates of drug use and abuse among Indochinese refugees: Mental health implications. *J Psychoactive Drugs* 19(1):77–83, 1987.

118. Yen S: Cultural competence for evaluators working with Asian/Pacific Island-American communities: Some common themes and important implications, in Orlandi MA, Weston R, Epstein LG (eds): *Cultural Competence for Evaluators.* OSAP Cultural Competence Series #1. DHHS Pub No. (ADM)92-1884, Washington DC: US Government Printing Office 1992, pp 261–291.

119. Padilla AM, Salgado de Snyder VN: Hispanics: What the culturally informed evaluator needs to know, in Orlandi MA, Weston R, Epstein LG (eds): *Cultural Competence for Evaluators.* OSAP Cultural Competence Series #1. DHHS Pub No. (ADM)92-1884, Washington DC: US Government Printing Office, 1992, pp 117–146.

120. Szapocznik J, Scopetta MA, Kurtines WM, Aranalde MA: Theory and measurement of acculturation. *Interam J Psychol* 12:113–130, 1978.

121. American Society of Addiction Medicine: Public policy statement on recommendations for design of treatment efficacy research with emphasis on outcome measures. *J Addict Dis* 13(1):119–124, 1994.

Patterns of Alcohol Use among Ethnic Minority Adolescent Women

Ruth W. Edwards, Pamela Jumper Thurman, and Fred Beauvais

Abstract. There is agreement in the literature that women of the major ethnic groups in the United States have lower rates of alcohol use and suffer fewer alcohol-related problems than men. In adolescence, the highest rates of alcohol use are generally found among American Indians, followed in decreasing order by whites, Hispanics, African-Americans, and Asian-Americans. The role of sociocultural factors in alcohol use as found in the literature is discussed, including level of acculturation, generational status, culturally specific values and beliefs and peer influence. Lifetime and last 30-day prevalence, age of first time drunk, and peer sanction data from the 1989–93 database of The American Drug and Alcohol Survey™ are presented by gender and ethnicity for 8th and 12th graders. These data show similar rates of alcohol use by males and females in the 8th grade but more use by males in the 12th grade for all ethnicities except American Indians who live on reservations.

1. Introduction

The discussion of patterns of behavior within nearly any specific group of people is attended by a number of difficulties. Once a group is defined in a way that distinguishes it from the general population, questions will be raised about the accuracy and meaning of that definition. Defining women as a special group of interest is fairly straightforward, but when this consideration includes ethnic minority status, problems arise. The myriad social, political, and personal agendas that attend discussion of subgroup behaviors make

Ruth W. Edwards, Pamela Jumper Thurman, and Fred Beauvais • Tri-Ethnic Center for Prevention Research, Department of Psychology, Colorado State University, Fort Collins, Colorado 80523.

Recent Developments in Alcoholism, Volume 12: Women and Alcoholism, edited by Marc Galanter. Plenum Press, New York, 1995

accurate descriptions even more difficult. Fillmore[1] illustrates these biases very clearly in her discussion of the convergence between male and female drinking rates and associated problems over the last few decades. There appears to be a host of reasons why some authors would like to see this convergence as real and why others would prefer to dismiss it as an artifact. One of the strongest influencing attitudes is that problem drinking somehow runs counter to a prevailing societal belief that women do, or at least should, represent a more virtuous position in society. Armed with this belief, one would be likely to take every opportunity to dismiss any evidence that women may be becoming more like men in their drinking behavior.

This chapter is divided into two parts. The first part will review what is known about female patterns of alcohol use in general and then discuss differences by ethnic group. The emphasis will be on female adolescents, although much of the discussion will include patterns of male drinking as a point of reference. The second part of the chapter will present new data on adolescent alcohol use for five ethnic groups: American Indians, Hispanic-Americans, African-Americans, Asian-Americans, and white or Anglo-Americans. These data will be presented by gender for both 8th- and 12th-grade youth so that differences across this critical developmental span can be discussed. It is hoped that these data, collected across all ethnic groups with the same methodology, will help clarify the patterns of alcohol use within and between these groups.

An important caveat is necessary in any discussion of ethnic differences in social behavior and this entails a recognition of the need for precision in the definition of what constitutes a particular ethnic group. The literature is very uneven in this regard; thus, many seemingly contradictory findings are reported and it is easy for one to reach untenable conclusions. Broad ethnic classifications such as "Hispanic," "Asian," or "American Indian" should be viewed very cautiously since they often aggregate very diverse groups of people. The most helpful literature makes it very clear which groups have been included in such classifications, and even more helpful are sources that disaggregate data by subpopulations. Kitano and Chi,[2] for instance, report separately on levels of alcohol use among Chinese, Japanese, Koreans, and Filipinos in the Los Angeles area.[3] A further caution is the need for some specification of the generational status of the minority sample under study. Cervantes et al.,[4] for example, report important differences in alcohol use patterns between immigrant and US-born Hispanics (from Mexico and Central America).[5,6]

2. Patterns of Use

2.1. Prevalence Rates

There is near-unanimous agreement among studies throughout this century that women have lower rates of alcohol use and suffer fewer alcohol related problems than men.[1] This relationship holds for the majority population as well as for all ethnic minority groups.[7] Sex role theory is the most compelling explanation for this discrepancy; Thompson and Wilsnack[8] concluded,

> Girls may gain some special protection against abusing alcohol by starting to drink at a later age than boys, by adhering to traditionally feminine values (such as caring about other people) and gender-specific drinking norms. (p 59)

As previously mentioned, there is good evidence from a number of sources that the gap between the prevalence of male and female use of alcohol appears to be narrowing.

When national studies of alcohol use rates are examined, using broad ethnic classifications, a consistent pattern emerges. The highest rates of alcohol use are found among whites, followed in order by Hispanics, blacks, and Asians; this relationship holds for both adult and adolescent populations.[9] The placement of American Indians in this ordering is less clear for adults since few data are available. May[10] concludes that there is great variability across tribes with some tribes showing higher adult alcohol use rates than average US rates and some tribes lower. Indian adolescents, on the other hand, do not appear to demonstrate such variability and in nearly all instances have much higher rates of alcohol use than adolescents nationally, including all other ethnic minority groups.[11]

Within these general relationships there are a number of variations that can be found when ethnic minority populations are considered. One principle that seems to hold with minority populations is that as individuals become more acculturated, their alcohol use tends to resemble that of the majority culture and, in most cases, this means an increase in alcohol use.[12–14] In an interesting reversal of this trend, Trotter[15] reports on a group of Anglo females who exhibited a lower rate of alcohol use than the general female Anglo population. The context of this finding is important; this was a group of students at Pan American University in Texas where the majority of the student population are Mexican-Americans, with fairly strong traditional values. Trotter hypothesized that the Anglo females, being in the minority, were conforming to the relatively conservative drinking standards for women in that part of the country. While the influence of acculturation holds generally for both genders, the acculturation process appears to operate somewhat differentially for males and females, with females less likely to change their drinking behavior as a result of contact and interchange with another culture.[16]

The literature describing the values and beliefs of ethnic minority groups is replete with discussion of the centrality of the family within black,[17] Hispanic,[18] Asian-American,[19] and American Indian[20] cultures. Although those of the majority culture would also espouse this value, the importance of the family comes into sharp relief among groups in the process of defending and maintaining a traditional way of life. It appears that, indeed, within ethnic minority communities the family does play a central role in shaping behaviors among its members, and, in this instance, there is evidence that alcohol use among ethnic minority children is strongly influenced by family values and beliefs. This is somewhat in contrast to what is found among the majority population. Oetting and Beauvais[21] have shown that for white youth "peer clusters" are the major determinant of adolescent substance use patterns and that the influence of peers on drug use outweighs that of the family (peer clusters are the small groups of closest friends and are the milieu in which attitudes toward drugs are determined and in which substance using behaviors are normed). Within white culture, family influences are more distal in the chain of influence than peer clusters. When path analytic models are examined for white youth, peer clusters account for 55% of the variance in drug use, but for Indian youth they account for only 18% of the variance.[22] Recent analyses for Mexican-American youth show that peers only account for 16% of the variance in drug use.[23] Additionally, in models for Indian youth, there is a direct negative path from parental sanctions against substance use to substance use, whereas for white youth the parental influence is mediated through peer influence.

There are no data to date to indicate whether family influence may differentially affect ethnic minority females and males, although there is some reason to believe it may. If sex roles among ethnic minorities do dictate that females have more family responsibility in terms of care of family members and maintaining cultural traditions, then it would be reasonable to assume that family values would be more powerful in determining behavior for females than for males (see Leland,[24] for an extended discussion).

2.2. Sociocultural Factors and Their Relationship to Alcohol Use

2.2.1. Hispanic Populations. While gender differences in alcohol use exist for all Hispanic subgroup populations,[25] they appear to be most pronounced among Mexican-Americans, with males reporting much higher rates of alcohol use and abuse and negative consequences of use than females.[5,26] The most common explanation given is that gender roles are very strong within the Mexican-American population. Men are expected to be providers for their family, but along with that responsibility comes a sense of independence in behavior and, perhaps, even a "right" to engage in male-oriented drinking events.[24,26] Belief in these "rights" and expectations can lead to higher levels of drinking. Women, on the other hand, are held to standards of "respect" and "virtue," both of which provide an atmosphere of protection and implicitly proscribe drinking behavior.[26,27] Goldberg and Botvin[28] found other gender differences among a sample of mixed Hispanic junior high students in New York that may also contribute to differential rates of use. Males and females differed on levels of assertiveness in varying social situations. Males, for instance, scored higher on "dating assertiveness," which in a previous study was associated with greater levels of intoxication.

There is strong evidence that over time these role expectations may be weakening, and as they do the rates of drinking and associated consequences for Hispanics are converging for Mexican-American males and females. Gilbert[13,26] discusses the strong relationship between increased drinking among both Mexican-American males and females as their generational status in the United States increases. The one exception to this is that alcohol use for immigrant females did not increase even with extended tenure in the United States. Gilbert attributed this finding to the very stringent restrictions against alcohol use by females that exist in Mexico and which apparently persist despite immigration. Despite higher levels of drinking for both genders with increasing generational status, however, the rates for females never reach those found for males. The convergence between male and female drinking rates may be particularly pronounced among adolescents since the acculturation process is strongest at this developmental stage.[29] Even this relationship, however, may not be straightforward. Chavez and Swaim,[5] for instance, found that the male/female disparity actually increased from the 8th to the 12th grade, a change mostly accounted for by more conservative drinking among females. This suggests that protective factors may increase in salience through this period. Gilbert and Cervantes,[30] on the other hand, found a clear association between higher levels of education (postsecondary) and increased alcohol use in a population of Mexican-American females. It is clear that the patterns of gender differences in drinking are very complex and will likely vary with the age of the population under consideration and the socioeconomic context.

Bolstering the notion that greater acculturation is related to increased drinking among Hispanic women are a number of studies showing lower rates of alcohol use among those women with lower educational attainment who were unemployed.[29,31] Gilbert[32] identified several arenas of influence and interaction that comprise the acculturation process and that help shape the changing beliefs and values regarding drinking; these include media exposure, informal interactions with friends and neighbors, workplace interactions, and, most importantly, the educational system.

In addition to role expectations, there are cognitive expectations about the positive value of alcohol use that relate to the differences in use rates between males and females.[4] Across a number of measures of expectations, Hispanic men held more positive views about the consequences of alcohol use than women. More importantly, these expectations became more positive along the acculturation continuum from immigrant to multiple US generation status and the level of expectation predicted the differential level of drinking between Hispanic men and women.

2.2.2. Asian Populations. A number of studies of Asian subpopulations have shown that, in general, all Asian groups have lower rates of alcohol use than Caucasians. Within Asian populations the highest rates are found for Native Hawaiians (which approached those of Caucasians), followed by Hapa-

Haoles (half Hawaiian, half Caucasian) and Japanese. It is difficult to rank other Asian groups since various studies find differing rates, although the Chinese appear to have the lowest rates of all groups across a number of studies.[33,34] Although the data are not as complete as they are for Hispanics, Asian groups also show a large disparity in alcohol use between genders, with women having lower rates.[3,33] This relationship holds for foreign-born, Hawaiian, and US mainland-born groups including adolescents.[35] In fact, Rachal et al.[36] found that heavy drinking was five times higher for Asian adolescent males compared with females—the highest ratio of all ethnic groups found in a national study. For both genders and across all Asian subgroups, the level of drinking and alcohol problems increase with increasing contact with Western values and norms.[3] While the evidence is not overwhelming among Asian groups, there is some indication that Asian males are more susceptible to increased alcohol use through acculturation than females.[37] Further implicating the role of norms in rates of alcohol consumption is a study by Danko et al.,[38] which showed a very high level of correspondence between perceived "normal" and "problem" drinking and levels of drinking among five Asian ethnic groups.

Asian culture differs from Western or Anglo cultures on a number of dimensions that appear to temper drinking behavior. These include "responsibility to others, interdependence, restraint, moderation and group achievement."[3] It is not known, however, to what degree these attributes have greater applicability to women than to men with respect to drinking behavior. One dimension common among Asian cultures that most likely leads to lower use of alcohol by women is the tendency to limit alcohol use to specifically defined situations, for example, family celebrations, or cultural ceremonies.[33,39] In most instances there are strong sanctions against alcohol use by women in these contexts.

A central area of controversy in considering alcohol use among Asian people is whether or not drinking rates are affected by the "flushing response." This response is marked by a reddening of the skin, other physiological changes (e.g., increased heart rate), and unpleasant subjective feelings; it is found most commonly in people of Oriental background. It has been hypothesized that the negative effect of this flushing response may account for the lower rates of alcohol use among Asian populations. Sue[3] and Johnson[40] have reviewed the research pertaining to this question and concluded that there are few data to support such a hypothesis and that sociocultural explanations are much more compelling. It is also unlikely that the flushing response would account for gender differences since it appears to be experienced equally by males and females.

2.2.3. African-American Populations. The pattern of alcohol use in African-American populations differs from that of others. Where surveys have been done among younger populations, mostly adolescents and college students, African-Americans show lower levels of alcohol use and problems than white youth and than most other ethnic minority groups. However, problems arising from alcohol increase in older segments of the population and rival or are greater than those for whites and others beginning in the middle adult years.[41-45] It has been suggested that the lower rate of drinking among African-American youth is primarily related to a later onset of drinking behavior.[46]

There also appears to be a strong bimodal distribution of attitudes regarding the acceptance of alcohol use among African-American populations. The temperance movement which peaked late in the last century, combined with the strong influence of fundamentalist religious values, has created a strong antialcohol sentiment that continues to influence attitudes toward alcohol among a large segment of the contemporary African-American population.[43,47] Alternately, there appears to be another group of African-Americans among which there is a wide acceptance of alcohol use. As might be expected, rates of use among these two portions of the population reflect the differing norms. In addressing the issues of norms in general, Herd[43] concludes, ". . . that internalized norms, such as religious beliefs and attitudes towards women's roles and conduct, may have comparatively more influence on black drinking patterns than socioeconomic factors" (p.25). In contrast, there is a study by Taylor and Jackson[48] indicating that life events (i.e., socioeconomic stress) were among the highest predictors of alcohol use among African-American women.

A further pattern distinguishing African-Americans from other ethnic groups is the smaller discrepancy in drinking rates between males and females, at least among younger populations.[46] Furthermore, Harford and Lowman[46] found that rates of recent drinking did not increase for African-Americans (both male and female) between the 10th and 12th grade as they do for the majority population youth. To the extent that discrepancies do exist between African-American males and females, they may be attributable to differences in peer and parental influences. Having reviewed what data do exist on these factors, Prendergast et al.[47] conclude,

> Most evidence seems to indicate that parental influences are more important than peer influences in explaining alcohol and other drug use among black youth, although the influence of peers might be more salient in certain instances, for example, in accounting for heavy drinking behavior. Also, boys and girls may respond differently to these influences. (p 10)

A later study by Beck and Zannis[17] reached similar conclusions.

2.2.4. American Indian Populations. When national, comparative studies are done across ethnic minority groups, American Indian adolescents are found to have the highest rates of alcohol use.[11,41] Although there is some variation across reservations and tribes, alcohol use appears to be a universal problem for American Indian adolescents in the United States. This is in contrast to what May[10] concluded about alcohol use among adult American

Indian populations; apparently some set of factors begin to operate after adolescence that lead to differential rates of adult alcohol use among different tribes.

Gender comparison studies of reservation American Indian, nonreservation American Indian, and Anglo youth conducted by Beauvais[11] indicate that there is a slight tendency toward higher use among males for all three groups. He emphasizes, however, that though this pattern is consistent, the differences are not large. A higher use rate for males is evident for reservation American Indian 8th graders, but rates are nearly comparable for both males and females in the nonreservation group at the 8th-grade level. This pattern of a small, or nonexistent, gender discrepancy in alcohol use rates is quite unusual among ethnic minority as well as majority youth. In an earlier study, Oetting and Beauvais[49] found significant gender differences at the elementary school level but the discrepancy all but disappeared during high school. They concluded, ". . . something important happens among the females during their junior high years; whatever factors protected them from alcohol when they were younger are no longer effective" (p 243). This homogeneity among American Indian adolescent males and females is underscored in a study by King et al.[50] They were trying to determine if males and females made differential use of social support systems when confronted with drug use behavior. Contrary to studies with other ethnic minorities, no male–female differences were found.

Among adult American Indian populations the gender difference may be supported by Heath,[51] who notes that women constitute only 20% of the clients in American Indian alcoholism treatment programs. There are growing indications, however, that this proportion may be increasing,[52] and this may present a particularly serious problem for American Indian communities given the already high rates of fetal alcohol syndrome in some locations.[53] Demonstrating the variability of differing American Indian populations, Weibel-Orlando[54] found some groups where adult American Indian women had higher levels of alcohol use than the men.

Several factors have been cited in discussions of the high rates of American Indian drinking and drug use. Beauvais[11] suggests that involvement with alcohol and drugs may be related to the lack of opportunity on reservations. Often there are very few chances for decent and well-paying jobs and unemployment on or near some reservations can be as high as 80%. There are also few chances to obtain higher education. Even though some scholarships are available through tribal services, family support for educational pursuits may not be strong for various reasons. Further, returning to the reservation or tribal area following completion of a degree may still hold limited opportunities for employment. There is no evidence to suggest that these socioeconomic factors may have differential gender effects, although this is a question that needs attention.

It has been suggested that the impact of acculturation, more specifically acculturation stress, leads to higher levels of alcohol use among American

Indian youth. Yet, as seen above, Mexican-American immigrants actually have lower rates of alcohol use than Mexican-Americans whose families have been in the United States for more than one generation. Furthermore, Oetting and Beauvais[55] found that level of cultural identification, including biculturality, among American Indian youth was not predictive of drug use. If acculturation level does account for alcohol use, it must operate in a very subtle manner and, as Oetting and Beauvais observed, it is probably mediated by more powerful factors, not the least of which is the influence of peers. Acculturation may also operate differentially between genders, an effect that to date has been obscured by the lack of studies addressing gender specific patterns. The scarcity of such studies on American Indian populations is actually more general than just addressing acculturation issues, and what is available is usually tribally specific.[56,57]

2.3. Summary

The literature reveals a number of consistent findings about alcohol use among ethnic minority women including lower rates than for men, later onset of use, the differential effects of acculturation between men and women, and the impact of sex-role expectation on levels of use. The remainder of this chapter will examine a new set of data in light of the previous findings and hopefully will confirm what has been found previously and perhaps provide some new insights. The primary value of this new data set is that the instrumentation and methodology are identical across ethnic groups.

3. Method

The American Drug and Alcohol Survey™ (ADAS)[59] is a survey service that provides communities with data on drug use of youth who are attending school. Approximately 150 communities across the United States use the survey each year to assess and monitor substance use levels of their in-school youth. These communities represent a sample of convenience and while the predominant ethnicity is white, their populations also include significant numbers of Hispanic, African-American, Asian-American, and American Indian students. For purposes of this chapter, the databases from 1989–90 through 1992–93 have been combined to increase the numbers of ethnic minority students included, so that when the data are further broken down by gender, the numbers of students will be sufficient such that meaningful comparisons may be made. In interpreting these data, however, it is important to consider that inner-city youth are underrepresented in this sample. Data from an ongoing study of the epidemiology of substance use among reservation-based American Indian youth[11] are also presented to illustrate the different patterns of substance use that may occur within different subpopulations of the same ethnic group. This study utilizes the same instrumentation and data collection techniques in collecting substance use prevalence information as for those included in The American Drug and Alcohol Survey™ database, and the data were collected over the same time span.

4. Results and Discussion

Table I shows lifetime and last 30-day prevalence of alcohol use by ethnicity, grade, and gender. Parallel questions on incidence of having "gotten drunk" are also included as a better indication of problematic alcohol use.

4.1. Gender and Grade

Data from both 8th graders and 12th graders are presented because there are some important differences in patterns to be noted by comparing the two age levels. For all five ethnic groups presented, the prevalence of alcohol use by males and females at the 8th grade level is very similar. However, by the 12th grade there is generally a wide gap, with males reporting significantly more alcohol use than females, a finding that is congruent with previous studies. One possible explanation of this is that there are differential dropout rates for alcohol-using males and females, with those females using alcohol in the 8th grade dropping out more frequently than their male counterparts. Previous studies have shown, however, that dropout rates do not alter the differential rates of alcohol use found in school-based surveys, at least for African-American students.[47] A more likely explanation is sex-role related. Early use of alcohol is generally seen as indicative of serious problem behavior. Given the equal rates of alcohol use for both genders at the 8th grade level (including being drunk in the past month), it could be concluded that this problem behavior occurs equally for both males and females. The greater proportion of males initiating use after the 8th grade may be reflecting a pattern of "normative" behavior wherein there is a greater permissiveness for male drinking but less for female drinking as these youth get older.

4.2. Ethnicity and Grade

Overall, at both the 8th and 12th grade levels, the Asian-Americans in this sample report by far the lowest alcohol use, with African-Americans the next lowest. American Indian youth, both those living on and off reservations, report higher rates of alcohol use and of having gotten drunk than the youth of other ethnic groups. Hispanic and white youth fall in between. These findings generally mirror past studies. While this pattern is generally apparent at both the 8th and 12th grades of both genders, there is a shift in the pattern for Hispanics and whites. While approximately two in five Hispanic 8th graders have gotten drunk compared with only one in four white 8th graders, by the 12th grade, this difference between the two groups has

Table I. Lifetime and Last 30-Day Prevalence of Alcohol Use by Gender and Ethnicity

	Asian-American				African-American				Hispanic			
	8th grade		12th grade		8th grade		12th grade		8th grade		12th grade	
	Males $n = 765$	Females $n = 704$	Males $n = 802$	Females $n = 784$	Males $n = 2948$	Females $n = 2993$	Males $n = 2274$	Females $n = 2652$	Males $n = 2987$	Females $n = 3216$	Males $n = 1803$	Females $n = 1903$
Ever tried alcohol	56.1%	54.3%	81.7%	79.1%	68.5%	68.4%	87.4%	84.5%	76.4%	74.1%	91.8%	89.6%
Ever gotten drunk	12.2%	12.8%	47.5%	42.1%	27.7%	23.6%	60.7%	47.4%	38.9%	36.6%	74.5%	64.1%
Used alcohol in last month	15.3%	17.2%	43.9%	36.3%	25.7%	25.8%	52.1%	36.5%	34.3%	36.2%	64.2%	53.2%
Drunk in last month	2.1%	3.3%	21.9%	15.8%	10.1%	8.2%	31.9%	14.2%	15.1%	15.4%	42.0%	28.0%

	American Indians (nonreservation)				American Indians (reservation)				White			
	8th grade		12th grade		8th grade		12th grade		8th grade		12th grade	
	Males $n = 1498$	Females $n = 1534$	Males $n = 680$	Females $n = 576$	Males $n = 870$	Females $n = 890$	Males $n = 382$	Females $n = 413$	Males $n = 38,745$	Females $n = 40,024$	Males $n = 35,190$	Females $n = 35,990$
Ever tried alcohol	77.8%	77.4%	93.5%	90.5%	64.5%	60.6%	94.2%	92.0%	72.7%	69.5%	92.3%	92.1%
Ever gotten drunk	41.2%	41.8%	83.2%	71.1%	44.9%	40.2%	87.8%	84.1%	26.3%	24.0%	74.6%	69.8%
Used alcohol in last month	32.1%	36.7%	63.9%	54.6%	31.1%	30.2%	55.8%	54.3%	27.0%	26.4%	60.7%	55.3%
Drunk in last month	15.6%	16.8%	43.8%	32.1%	19.5%	17.7%	44.1%	37.9%	8.3%	8.0%	41.0%	32.4%

virtually disappeared. Further, although lifetime prevalence rates for Hispanic and white 8th graders are comparable, the indicators of ongoing use are higher for Hispanics of this age group (e.g., about 37% "ever drunk" vs. 26% for whites, and 15% "drunk in past month" vs. 8%). A similar pattern of earlier, heavy drinking is also evident for the American Indian 8th graders, both male and female.

4.3. Age of First Involvement with Alcohol by Gender and Ethnicity

A useful way of looking at exposure to alcohol use by different groups is through utilization of what Oetting and Beauvais[59] have termed the "drug acquisition curve." The drug acquisition curve is a chart of the cumulative percentage of a group that has exhibited a given behavior, such as having gotten drunk, by a given age. Figure 1 shows drug acquisition curves for responses by 12th graders by gender for each ethnicity under consideration in this study to the question, "How old were you the first time you got drunk?"

Oetting and Beauvais[59] interpret the point at which the curves start accelerating rapidly upward as the "age of exposure," the point at which children begin to be exposed to a drug at a higher rate. For young American Indian males, this acceleration of the curve for getting drunk the first time is between ages 9 and 10. For young American Indian females, it is between the ages of 10 and 11 but increases sharply at age 11. The cumulative percentage of American Indian females living on reservations who have gotten drunk is at least as great as that for their male counterparts by age 13, and continues to equal that of males throughout adolescence. This is not true for nonreservation American Indians or for African-Americans, Asian-Americans, Hispanics, or whites. For these groups, the cumulative percentage of females who have gotten drunk is lower at all ages than their male counterparts.

Based on the data presented in the previous section, one would expect that the age of exposure to alcohol for Hispanics would be much earlier than for whites. The acquisition curves, however, do not reflect this. At age 13, for instance, if male and female rates for both groups are averaged, the curves for Hispanics and whites are nearly identical. This pattern suggests that school dropout may be a factor in the equality of these rates. Recall that the acquisition curve is based on reported "first time drunk" for *12th graders*—i.e., those who remain in school. It is quite possible that since the Hispanic dropout rate is higher than that for whites and since dropouts have been found to use alcohol at a higher rate,[60] the heavier and earlier drinking youth are not still in school by the 12th grade, and hence are not included in the curves.

4.4. Peer Influence on Alcohol Use by Gender and Ethnicity

Other studies have demonstrated that social relationships differ for males and females and that these differences may have an impact on levels of drug use. The American Drug and Alcohol Survey™ contains a number of items

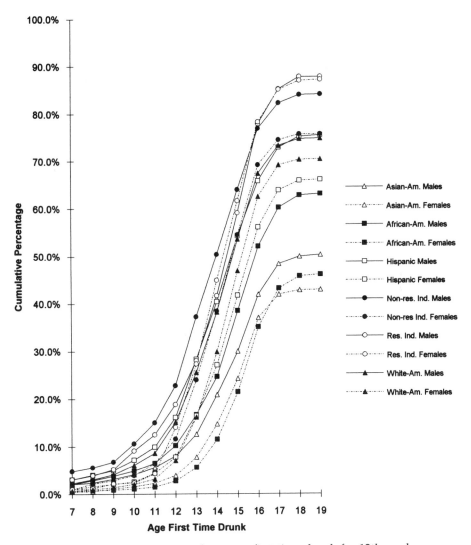

Figure 1. Acquisition curve for age at first time drunk for 12th graders.

asking about peer relationships and alcohol use. Figure 2 shows the percentage of youth who indicated that their friends would try to stop them from getting drunk "a lot," by grade, gender, and ethnicity. It is clear that peer sanctions are stronger at the 8th grade level for all groups and both genders; this accounts, in part, for the lower 8th grade alcohol use rates. For both 8th and 12th graders of all ethnic groups, there is more peer influence *not* to get drunk for females than for males; again, a partial explanation for the gender discrepancy in youth. At the 8th grade level, this discrepancy between males and females in peer influence to "not get drunk" is most pronounced for

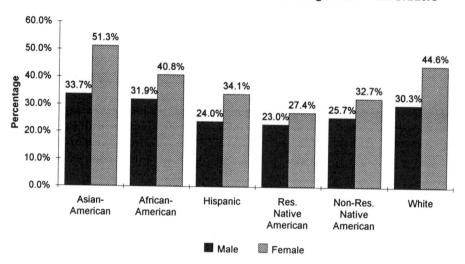

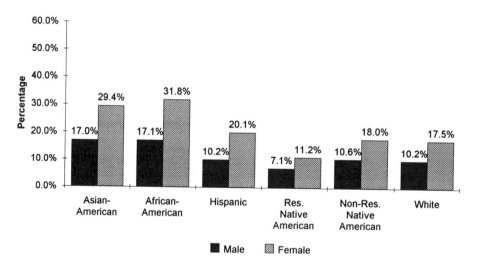

Figure 2. (A) Friends try a lot to stop you from drinking—8th graders. (B) Friends try a lot to stop you from drinking—12th graders.

Asian-Americans and white Americans. by 12th grade, the difference between males and females has dropped off for whites but has increased for African-Americans, with a third of African-American females indicating their friends would try "a lot" to stop them from getting drunk versus almost half that for African-American males. A final demonstration of the strong relationship between peer influence and levels of use is the relative lack of sanctions among American Indians, a group that has been consistently shown to have the highest levels of alcohol use. The gender discrepancy in sanctions against alcohol use is the smallest of any of the ethnic groups for American Indians, where rates of alcohol use for males and females are nearly the same.

5. Conclusion

Previous research, as well as the present study, confirm that there are robust patterns of gender and ethnic differences in alcohol use. Correlational data strongly suggest that these patterns are influenced by a variety of social and cultural factors that operate differentially across gender and ethnic minority status. These findings present a couple of major challenges. First, the relationships will require a considerable amount of additional inquiry to fully understand the causative pathways. Second, it will take a great deal of creativity to design prevention strategies that capitalize on the protective influences of sociocultural factors, particularly gender-specific factors. This variability in the alcohol use patterns across genders and across minority populations must be taken into consideration to maximize effectiveness and efficiency of prevention programs.

References

1. Fillmore K: "When angels fall": Women's drinking as a cultural preoccupation and as reality, in Wilsnack S, Beckman L (eds): *Alcohol Problems in Women: Antecedents, Consequences and Intervention.* New York, Guilford Press, 1984, pp 7–36.
2. Kitano H, Chi I: Asian Americans and alcohol: The Chinese, Japanese, Koreans and Filipinos in Los Angeles, in Spiegler D, Tate D, Aitken S, Christian C (eds): *Alcohol Use among US Ethnic Minorities.*NIAAA Research Monograph 18. Rockville, MD, National Institute on Alcohol Abuse and Alcoholism, 1989, pp 373–382.
3. Sue D: Use and abuse of alcohol by Asian Americans. *J Psychoactive Drugs* 19:57–66, 1987.
4. Cervantes R, Gilbert M, Salgado de Snyder N, Padilla A: Psychosocial and cognitive correlates of alcohol use in younger adult immigrant and US born Hispanics. *Int J Addict* 25:687–708, 1990–91.
5. Chavez E, Swaim R: Hispanic substance abuse: Problems in epidemiology. *Drugs Society* 6:211–230, 1992.
6. Gordon A: State of the art review: Caribbean Hispanics and their alcohol use, in Spiegler D, Tate D, Aitken S, Christian C (eds): *Alcohol Use among US Ethnic Minorities.* Research Monograph 18. Rockville, MD, National Institute on Alcohol Abuse and Alcoholism 1989, pp 135–146.

7. Spiegler D, Tate D, Aitken S, Christian C: Research highlights, in Spiegler D, Tate D, Aitken S, Christian C (eds): *Alcohol Use among US Ethnic Minorities.* Research Monograph 18. Rockville, MD, National Institute on Alcohol Abuse and Alcoholism, 1989, pp xv–xxiv.
8. Thompson K, Wilsnack R: Drinking and drinking problems among female adolescents: Patterns and influences, in Wilsnack S, Beckman L (eds): *Alcohol Problems in Women: Antecedents, Consequences and Intervention.* New York, Guilford Press, 1984, pp 37–65.
9. Rebach H: Alcohol and drug use among American minorities, in Trimble J, Bolek C, Niemcryk S (eds): *Ethnic and Multicultural Drug Abuse: Perspectives on Current Research.* New York, Haworth Press, 1992, pp 23–57.
10. May P: Substance abuse and American Indians: Prevalence and susceptibility. *Int J Addict* 17:1185–1209, 1982.
11. Beauvais F: Trends in Indian adolescent drug and alcohol use. *J Natl Center Am Indian Alaska Native Ment Health Res* 5(1):1–12, 1992.
12. Caetano R: Alcoholism and drinking patterns among US Hispanics. *Br J Addict* 82:789–799, 1987.
13. Gilbert M: Mexican-Americans in California: Intracultural variations in attitudes and behavior related to alcohol, in Bennett L, Ames G (eds): *The American Experience with Alcohol: Contemporary Cultural Perspectives.* New York, Plenum Press, 1985, pp 255–277.
14. Cheung, Y: Ethnicity and alcohol/drug use revisited: A framework for future research. *Int J Addict* 25:581–605, 1990–91.
15. Trotter R: Ethnic and sexual patterns of alcohol use: Anglo and Mexican-American college students. *Adolescence* 17:305–325, 1982.
16. Corbett K, Mora J, Ames G: Drinking patterns and drinking related problems of Mexican-American husbands and wives. *J Stud Alcohol* 52:215–223, 1991.
17. Beck K, Zanis M: Patterns of alcohol consumption among suburban adolescent black high school students. *J Alcohol Drug Educ* 37:1–13, 1992.
18. Galan F: Alcoholism prevention and Hispanic youth, in Wright R, Watts T (eds): *Alcohol Problems of Minority Youth in America.* New York, Edwin Mellon Press, 1989, pp 81–95.
19. Zane N, Sasao T: Research on drug abuse among Asian Pacific Americans, in Trimble J, Bolek C, Niemcryk S (eds): *Ethnic and Multicultural Drug Abuse: Perspectives on Current Research.* New York, Haworth Press, 1992, pp 181–210.
20. Beauvais F, Laboueff S: Drug and alcohol abuse intervention in American Indian communities. *Int J Addict* 20:139–171, 1985.
21. Oetting ER, Beauvais F: Peer cluster theory: Drugs and the adolescent. *J Counsel Dev* 65(1):17–22, 1986.
22. Swaim RC, Thurman PJ, Beauvais F, Oetting ER, Wayman J: American Indian adolescent substance use as a function of number of risk factors, submitted.
23. Swaim RC: Personal communication, February 1994.
24. Leland J: Alcohol use and abuse in ethnic minority women, in Wilsnack S, Beckman L (eds): *Alcohol Problems in Women: Antecedents, Consequences and Intervention.* New York, Guilford Press, 1984, pp 66–96.
25. Austin M, Gilbert M: Substance abuse among Latino youth. Prevention Research Update No. 3, Portland, OR, Northwest Regional Educational Laboratory, Spring 1989.
26. Gilbert M: Current information on drinking behavior among Hispanic youth, in Wright R, Watts T (eds): *Alcohol Problems of Minority Youth in America.* New York, Edwin Mellon Press, 1989, pp 53–79.
27. Trotter R: Mexican American experience with alcohol: South Texas example, in Bennett L, Ames G (eds): *The American Experience with Alcohol.* New York, Plenum Press, 1985, pp 279–296.
28. Goldberg C, Botvin G: Assertiveness in Hispanic adolescents: Relationship to alcohol use and abuse. *Psych Rep* 73:227–238, 1993.
29. Holck S, Warren C, Smith J, Rochat R: Alcohol consumption among Mexican American and Anglo women: Results of a survey along the U.S.-Mexican border. *J Stud Alcohol* 45:149–154, 1984.

30. Gilbert M, Cervantes R: Patterns and practices of alcohol use among Mexican-Americans: A comprehensive review. *Hispanic J Behav Sci* 8:1–60, 1986.
31. Caetano R: Drinking patterns and alcohol problems in a national sample of US Hispanics, in Spiegler D, Tate D, Aitken S, Christian C (eds): *Alcohol Use among US Ethnic Minorities.* Research Monograph 18. Rockville, MD, National Institute on Alcohol Abuse and Alcoholism, 1989, pp 147–162.
32. Gilbert M: Alcohol consumption patterns in immigrant and later generation Mexican-American women. *Hispanic J Behav Sci* 9:299–313, 1987.
33. Austin G, Prendergast M, Lee J: Substance use among Asian-American youth. Prevention Research Update, 5. Portland, OR, Northwest Regional Laboratories, 1989.
34. Murakami S: An epidemiological survey of alcohol, drug and mental problems in Hawaii: A comparison of four ethnic groups, in Spiegler D, Tate D, Aitken S, Christian C (eds): *Alcohol Use among US Ethnic Minorities.* Research Monograph 18. Rockville, MD, National Institute on Alcohol Abuse and Alcoholism, 1989, pp 343–353.
35. Welte J, Barnes G: Alcohol use among adolescent minority groups. *J Stud Alcohol* 48:329–336, 1987.
36. Rachal J, Maisto S, Guess L, Hubbard L: Alcohol use among youth, in *Alcohol and Health Monograph 1.* Rockville, MD, National Clearinghouse for Alcohol Information, RPO 483, 1982.
37. Akutsu P, Sue S, Zane N, Nakamura C: Ethnic differences in alcohol consumption among Asians and Caucasians in the United States: An investigation of culture and physiological factors. *J Stud Alcohol* 50:261–267, 1989.
38. Danko G, Johnson R, Nagoshi C, *et al:* Judgments of "normal" and "problem" alcohol use as related to reported alcohol consumption. *Alcohol Clin Exp Res* 12:760–767, 1988.
39. Yu E, Liu W, Xia Z, Zhang M: Alcohol use, abuse and alcoholism among Chinese Americans: A review of the epidemiologic data, in Spiegler D, Tate D, Aitken S, Christian C (eds): *Alcohol Use among US Ethnic Minorites.* Research Monograph 18. Rockville, MD, National Institute on Alcohol Abuse and Alcoholism, 1989, pp 329–342.
40. Johnson R: The flushing response and alcohol use, in Spiegler D, Tate D, Aitken S, Christian C (eds): *Alcohol Use among US Ethnic Minorities.* Research Monograph 18. Rockville, MD, National Institute on Alcohol Abuse and Alcoholism, 1989, pp 383–396.
41. Bachman J, Wallace J, O'Malley P, *et al:* Racial/ethnic differences in smoking, drinking, and illicit drug use among American high school seniors, 1976–89. *Am J Public Health* 81:372–377, 1991.
42. Caetano R: Ethnicity and drinking in northern California: A comparison between whites, blacks and Hispanics. *Alcohol Alcohol* 19:31–44, 1984.
43. Herd D: The epidemiology of drinking patterns and alcohol related problems among US blacks, in Spiegler D, Tate D, Aitken S, Christian C (eds): *Alcohol Use among US Ethnic Minorities.* Research Monograph 18, Rockville, MD, National Institute on Alcohol Abuse and Alcoholism, 1989, pp 3–50.
44. Robbins L: Alcohol abuse in blacks and whites as indicated in the epidemiological catchment area program, in spiegler D, Tate D, Aitken S, Christian C (eds): *Alcohol Use among US Ethnic Minorities.* Research Monograph 18. Rockville, MD, National Institute on Alcohol Abuse and Alcoholism, 1989, pp 63–73.
45. Lillie-Blanton M, MacKenzie E, Anthony J: Black–white differences in alcohol use by women: Baltimore survey findings. *Public Health Rep* 106:124–133, 1991.
46. Harford T, Lowman C: Alcohol use among black and white teenagers, in Spiegler D, Tate D, Aitken S, Christian C (eds): *Alcohol Use among US Ethnic Minorities.* Research Monograph 18. Rockville, MD, National Institute on Alcohol Abuse and Alcoholism 1989, pp 51–62.
47. Prendergast M, Austin G, Maton K, Baker R: Substance abuse among black youth. Prevention Research Update No. 4. Portland, OR, Northwest Regional Educational Laboratory, 1989.
48. Taylor J, Jackson B: Factors affecting alcohol consumption in black women. *Int J Addict* 25(12):1415–1427, 1990.

49. Oetting ER, Beauvais F: Epidemiology and correlates of alcohol use among Indian adolescents living on reservations, in Spiegler D, Tate D, Aitken S, Christian C (eds): *Alcohol Use among US Ethnic Minorities*. Research Monograph 18. Rockville, MD, National Institute on Alcohol Abuse and Alcoholism, 1989, pp 239–267.

50. King J, Beals J, Manson S, Trimble J: A structural equation model of factors relating to substance use among American Indian adolescents. *Drugs Society* 6:253–268, 1992.

51. Heath DB: American Indians and alcohol: Epidemiological and sociocultural correlates, in spiegler D, Tate D, Aitken S, Christian C (eds): *Alcohol Use among US Ethnic Minorities*. Research Monograph 18. Rockville, MD, National Institute on Alcohol Abuse and Alcoholism, 1989, pp 207–222.

52. Vanderwagon C, Mason RD, Owan TC: IHS Alcoholism/Substance Abuse Prevention Initiative: Background, Plenary Session, and Action Plan. Washington, DC, Department of Health and Human Services (no date).

53. May PA, Hymbaugh KH: A pilot project on fetal alcohol syndrome among American Indians. *Alcohol Health Res World* 7(2):3–9, 1982/83.

54. Weibel-Orlando JC: Women and alcohol: Special populations and cross-cultural variations, in National Institute on Alcohol Abuse and Alcoholism (ed): *Women and Alcohol: Health-Related Issues*. Research Monograph 16, DHHS Pub. No. (ADM) 86-1139. Washington, DC, US Government Printing Office, 1986, pp 161–87.

55. Oetting ER, Beauvais F: Orthogonal cultural identification theory: The cultural identification of minority adolescents. *Int J Addict* 25(5A & 6A):655–685, 1990.

56. Forslund MA: Drinking problems of Native American and white youth. *J Drug Educ* 9:21–27, 1979.

57. Hurlburt G, Gade E: Personality differences between Native American and Caucasian women alcoholics: Implications for alcoholism counseling. *White Cloud J* 3(2):35–39, 1984.

58. Oetting ER, Beauvais F, Edwards RW: *The American Drug and Alcohol Survey™*. Ft. Collins, CO, Rocky Mountain Behavioral Science Institute, 1985.

59. Oetting ER, Beauvais F: The drug acquisition curve: A method for analysis and prediction of drug epidemiology. *Int J Addict* 18(8):1115–1129, 1983.

60. Chavez EL, Edwards R, Oetting ER: Mexican-American and white American school dropouts' drug use, health status, and involvement in violence. *Public Health Rep* 104(6):594–604, 1989.

Alcoholism in the Family
A Multicultural Exploration

Andrea G. Barthwell

Abstract. The initial focus is on defining race, culture, and ethnicity, followed by a review of the extent of alcohol and alcohol use consequences among African-Americans and Native Americans. Cultural specificity in an historical context is provided. A brief overview of gaps in the incident and prevalence data is presented. The biosociocultural context of drinking among African-American women with specific emphasis on cultural disruption, socialization, and social class is explored. A triracial infant girl (African-American/Native American/German–Irish-American), whose family genogram documents, by the case study method, six generations back to slavery, is presented. The alcohol use patterns within this family are somewhat illustrative of historical patterns and of racial and ethnic import. An absence of religiosity/spirituality is noted. The family genogram is followed by a discussion of the limitations of the case study method of family genograms. The final section relates the findings of the family genogram back to the extant data and the gaps in the collection of data regarding the epidemiology of alcoholism across groups. It highlights the recent findings and questions raised by those findings from cross-cultural and racial studies of alcoholism among women of color.

1. Introduction

Alcoholism can be viewed as a disorder that results from the interaction of multiple causal factors—biophysical, psychological, and sociocultural—over time. Women differ from men in rates of alcohol use initiation, consequences of use (with same duration and frequency of use), maintenance of use patterns, and attempts to stop and success at cessation. Thus, alcoholism in women is a multidimensional disorder that can be influenced by biological and sociocultural interaction which combine processes to produce alcoholics

Andrea G. Barthwell • Interventions, Chicago, Illinois 60605.

Recent Developments in Alcoholism, Volume 12: Women and Alcoholism, edited by Marc Galanter. Plenum Press, New York, 1995.

among African-American women (as persons or as a group). What is clear from a review of the literature is that how African-American women drink and the consequences of that drinking are culturally (and gender) linked. This chapter examines the sociocultural factors that influence alcoholism among African-American women and applies this knowledge to a case study of a family of African-American women with triracial (African, European, Native American) involvement over six generations.

2. Basic Assumptions and Definitions

2.1. Ethnicity and Culture

The distinctions between ethnic and cultural differences are important to define. Ethnic differences refer to variations in personal or social characteristics. Ethnicity involves group membership and implies cultural differences that may or may not exist. Cultural differences constitute a host of socio-psychological variables which are in turn linked to lifestyles and perspectives. Therefore, cultural differences constitue more proximal determinants of alcoholism and imply certain differences in attitudes, values, and perceptual constructs as a result of different culturally based experiences.

Culture is defined as the advanced structure of language, behavior, customs, knowledge, symbols, ideas, values, matter, and mind that provides a people with a general design for living and patterns for interpreting their reality. An ethnic group is a group that is socially distinguishable or set apart by others and/or itself primarily on the basis of cultural or nationality characteristics. A racial group is not something that is naturally generated as a part of the self-evident order of the universe, but is a social group that persons inside or outside of the group have decided it is important to single out as inferior or superior, typically on the basis of real or alleged physical characteristics objectively selected.[1]

Culture is defined as customs, beliefs, values, knowledge, and skills that guide a people's behavior along shared paths, and social norms are shared rules that specify appropriate and inappropriate behavior. Social mores are norms that people consider vital to their well-being and to their most cherished values. Sanctions are those socially imposed rewards and punishments that compel people to comply with norms. Shared values, norms, mores, traditions, customs, art, history, folklore, and institutions define a group of people. Groups are bound together by the intangible nonmaterial elements of culture.

While many researchers acknowledge that the heterogeneity among minority populations exists, only recently has it been acknowledged in descriptions of study samples and incorporated in research designs. The heterogeneity within ethnic groups derives from socioeconomic status, education, acculturation, gender, age, country of origin, and racial makeup, variables that may interact.

If diversity within groups is acknowledged, it can limit the ability to generalize results while serving to negate stereotypes. African-Americans have encountered a variety of experiences that have contributed to the creation of cultural and racial hybrids. The immigration status, migratory patterns, and personal struggles of African-Americans give them an authentic (natural) African cultural base, adopted (survivalist) European-American cultural subtype, and adapted (developmentally) African-American culture. Cultural hybrids deriving from ethnicity and racial or biogenetic mixing are many.

3. Framing the Problem

This section addresses some of the issues that are unique to understanding alcoholism in African-Americans and, secondarily, some Native Americans. The patterns of use in these groups have changed over time. Use patterns among African-Americans and Native Americans can be understood in their cultural contexts, which is accounted for by changing social, political, and religious considerations.

Of special significance in studying alcohol use patterns among African-Americans is consideration of the effect of mixing of African-American and Native American cultures at various points in history. These include periods of slavery when runaway slaves were "adopted" by southwestern and southeastern Native American tribes and again during the period of Native American dispersion when Native Americans were placed in urban centers by programs that were meant to promote their acculturation into mainstream society.

3.1. African-Americans

African-Americans are a culturally distinct population bound together by connective factors and forces that give them unity while preserving their heterogeneity. African-Americans encompass descendants of people who originated in Africa and were involuntarily brought to America, people with ties to Africa who had a similar experience in the Caribbean and who have since voluntarily migrated to America, and Africans who are voluntary immigrants. Thus, African-Americans are a highly complex and diverse people, characterized along two dimensions—one in terms of interactions and responses to interactions with European Americans and the other in terms of their own internal dynamics, both as individual personalities and as a collective group.[2]

3.1.1. Major Themes in a Historical Context. While the heterogeneity among blacks is often noted,[3] a quest for identity is the major theme of African-American existence in the Western world. African-Americans have had to contend with transplantation and adjustments: the effects of social, cultural, and environmental contact and changes have been, in many respects, more devastating and intense for African-Americans because of the uniqueness of their journey to the Americas and their experiences in the American world.[4]

Three major conditions characterize the experience of African-Americans in this country: social injustice, societal inconsistency, and personal impotence. These experiences are superimposed on three significant time periods in the lives of African-Americans as described by Nobles[5]: (1) the African experience (prior to 1600); (2) the slavery experience 1600–1865; and (3) contemporary black America 1865 to the present.

Slavery removed African-Americans from their strong cultural heritage and required them to reestablish a cultural identity, while denying them the essence of their very nature as humans. It is this sharing of a common heritage, a common set of experiences, a common culture, and an emotional bond kindled by an awareness of interrelatedness with the preceding generation that defines the ethos of African Americans.

The historical record for African-Americans in this society has consisted of sociocultural adaptation and survival processes. African-Americans' experiences have been profoundly affected by the institutions and processes of slavery, racism, and oppression. The individual and collective character has developed in an environment antithetical to their character, personality and behavior problems. These cultural disruptions have had a profound effect on African-Americans as a whole and are experienced in different ways by African-Americans across gender.

3.1.2. African-Americans—Social Ecology. Eleven and a half percent of the total US population is African-American, 11.2% of the males and 11.8% of the females.[6] The median age of African-Americans in this country is 24.9 years of age (vs. 36.1 years for whites), and 15% of African-Americans are under 15 years of age. Of the 18.4% African-Americans who live in the south, 13.3% are in urban areas. Migration of blacks from the south not only slowed but slightly reversed during the 1970s. Cities with the largest numbers of African-Americans are New York, Chicago, Detroit, Philadelphia, and Los Angeles. The life expectancy of African-Americans in 1983 was 65 years of age for men and 74 years of age for women compared with 72 and 79 years for white men and women, respectively. The age-adjusted mortality rate per 1000 population for African-Americans is 7.7, for whites it is 5.3.

Total birth rates among all groups have dropped since 1970; however, the overall rate of childbearing is still higher among African-American women than women of nonminority groups (2.3 vs. 1.7 per woman). The percent of African-American households headed by women (37.7%) is more than three times higher than that of nonminority households headed by women (10.9%).

One of every three African-Americans (34%) lived below the poverty level in 1981. This rate is consistent with that of Hispanic and Native Americans, but substantially higher than that of nonminorities (11%).

3.2. Native Americans

Native Americans include American Indians, Aleuts, Alaskan Eskimos, and Native Hawaiians. American Indians are the smallest minority group in the United States.

Tribal identity is a more useful way of defining cultural identity for Native Americans, who use a self-identifier as membership in or affiliation with a specific tribe or tribes. Following that, membership in a clan or society within a tribe is described. Statistically, intermarriage is occurring at a higher rate between American Indian women and white men than it is for unions between Indian men and women from other ethnic/racial groups.[7]

3.2.1. Major Themes in a Historical Context. Before the Europeans arrived in this country, there were 2.5 million American Indians in over 300 tribes. In 1890, there were 250,000 left, which represented a greater than 90% reduction in population. This reduction is directly attributable to disease, malnutrition, war, and murder. These forces were partially supported by the federal policy concerning the "Indian problem." The solution gave rise to active attempts to exterminate Indians or remove them from their traditional lands, which brought about relocation policies, extreme poverty, deployment of young people to boarding schools, and the introduction of alcohol and other drugs to Native American people. These policies of extermination gave way to relocation policies in the mid-1800s and have contributed to the extreme isolation of Native Americans in this country.

3.2.2. Native Americans—Social Ecology. In 1980, Native Americans numbered approximately 1.5 million, less than 1% of the total population but two times that of the 1970 census. These increases are probably due to changes in health care, the high birth rate among American Indians and Alaskan Natives, and an increased reporting of identification in this group.[8] The average American Indian family has 4.6 members. The birth rate among American Indians is nearly twice that of other groups, and the average life expectancy is 6 years less. The median age of American Indians is 22.4 years. Nearly one of every four American Indian households is headed by a woman, and approximately half (48%) of American Indian women are employed outside the home. The overall educational attainment of American Indians is the lowest of all minority groups. The 1980 census revealed that fewer than one of three (33%) have graduated from high school and that only 7% hold college degrees. This compares with 79% of African-Americans who have completed high school and 13% who are college graduates. Twenty-nine percent of American Indian families lived in poverty in 1979. One half of all American

Indians live in the western or southwestern United States, 24% on reservations and 8% on historic trust areas in Oklahoma. Most of these reservations have fewer than 1000 residents; one reservation has a population greater than 100,000. Native Americans, along with African-Americans, have the highest rates of injury and death from nondisease causes.[6,9–11]

3.3. Alcoholism

The impact of alcoholism has touched every family in America, either directly (i.e., through having an alcoholic family member, friend, or associate) or indirectly (i.e., through increased costs of insurance policies, increased taxes, or through absenteeism from the workplace). This impact is significantly multiplied when one examines the African-American family, given its preexisting vulnerabilities.[12,13] Alcoholism has been called by Harper[14,15] the number one health and number one social problem in black America.

3.3.1. Drinking in a Cultural Context. There may be important cultural differences among various African-American communities in their tolerance for alcohol consumption, their use of alcohol in ritualized behavior, and the social dislocation secondary to alcohol abuse, as well as the excess morbidity and mortality associated with alcohol use and abuse. Cultural customs, including alcohol-drinking patterns, tend to endure migration despite pressures toward assimilation.[16] Drinking patterns of many African American subpopulations in the United States may represent influences of the European countries that colonized their countries of origin prior to independence or the drinking patterns of African-American descendants of slaves.[17,18] Similarly, cultures prescribe both drug use patterns and control rituals to protect the society and the individuals from disruptive effects of these drugs. These may vary by gender. When cultures mix, drug use patterns and protective rituals may become disassociated from these behaviors.[19]

3.3.2. Drinking in a Historical Context. The patterns of alcohol use have changed significantly among African-American men and women since the 19th century. Heard[20] showed an impact on migration and cultural transformation during the 19th century on epidemiological trends in liver sclerosis mortality in African-American men and women. Superimposed on this migratory and transformatory experience was the experience of African-American women in the work force being hired proportionally more than their white counterparts. Disparate cultural and historical experiences have continued to contribute to widely different sociodemographic profiles of African-American women from white women.

3.3.3. Gaps in the Incident and Prevalence Data. It is well established that there are limitations to the information sources about alcohol abuse prevalence in African-American communities. Many of the surveys currently in use (e.g., High School Senior Survey, National Household Survey, etc), may not represent the true rates of alcohol use or patterns of alcohol consumption in African-American communities. Some parts of the African-American community (i.e., urban-based African-American individuals where there are high rates of school dropouts) may be underrepresented in the High School Senior Surveys. This could lead to a finding of lower rates of alcohol use among those African-American youths who stay in school. The National Household Survey may underrepresent the number of individuals who are in a household if they are being housed temporarily or are not shown on the lease. This may lower the total count in the household survey, thereby leading to an increase in the incidence of alcohol use and abuse in the African-American community. While these issues are not exhaustive and may seem obvious, few published studies consider them.[21]

3.3.4. Alcoholism and African-Americans. The 1990 National Household Survey[22] told that, irrespective of gender, whites consume alcohol in larger percentages than African-Americans. The finding of higher abstinence rates among blacks than whites has been observed by various investigators in various settings.[20,23–25] Whites tend to have their peak years of heavy alcohol consumption between 18 and 25 years of age. Among African-Americans, the ages of 18 to 29 represent a period of high abstinence rates, with heavy drinking increasing dramatically after 30 years of age.[24,25] Even among age-matched whites and African-Americans, African-Americans reported less daily alcohol consumption than whites.[26]

3.3.5. Alcoholism and African-American Women. Only a few studies have focused on alcoholism among African-American women. Those that have, have shown that African-American women are more likely to abstain than their white counterparts,[27,28] but when they drink they suffer consequences sooner.[29,30] Heavy drinking patterns vary by age between African-American and white women. Heavy drinking among African-American women peaks later than for white women.[28,31] The later-onset drinking may be more hidden in African-American women.

4. Women and Drinking: Biosociocultural Context

There are many factors associated with the incidence of alcoholism for an individual. There are biological and sociocultural factors and pharmacological effects. Epidemiological research in the last decade with information on women's drinking include two groups of studies with special ethnic subpopulations; these are large-scale longitudinal surveys focused specifically on women and include alcohol abuse questions.[32–35] Women's drinking seems to be more complex than one might have predicted: there is a need to look not for general changes in women's use but for specific changes within specific sub-populations of women. These changes seem to be influenced by age, race, and ethnicity.

4.1. Biology

Genetic contributions are probably substantial in alcoholism,[36,37] including the propensity for alcoholism and the potential to experience consequences. While much of the work that has been done on racial and ethnic groups has looked at groups as a homogenous population, there has been a significant mating across ethnic groups within this country among African-Americans, Native Americans, European-Americans, and others. Additionally, this country has seen an increase in the voluntary appearance of individuals of mixed racial heritage in the last 20 years, since there were significant numbers of individuals of mixed racial heritage emerging from the institution of slavery. The biological influences on susceptibility to alcohol at varying times are equal to, less important than, or more important than environmental factors.

4.2. Culture

Those cultural factors that may affect a woman's vulnerability to alcoholism include life crisis, social inferiority of her male partners, cognitive distortions, affective distortions (which are based on relationships to others within and outside the group), life stressors, and socioeconomic status, including social class and stigma associated with her drinking.

Culture, tradition, and rituals set the patterns of use that are normative for a collective and control the rituals to protect the individual from ill effects of the substance and to protect others from an individual who is affected by the mood- or mind-altering chemical. When that control is lifted, cultural control over alcohol use patterns fall apart.

4.2.1. Cultural Disruption. Cultural disruption can occur from traumatic, abrupt, or chronic external irritation and erosion in the culture. Involuntary separation from one's homeland or a program designed to eradicate a people are examples of these types of cultural disruptions. People may be removed from access to their culture of origin with resultant adequate, partially adequate, or inadequate substitution provided (e.g., transracial adoption by culturally competent parents who can prepare a minority child for potential experiences in the real world along a continuum to transracial adoption into a family that believes that race and ethnicity is not an important consideration or determinant of access).

4.2.2. Cultural Disruption: Acculturation. Acculturation, which can be viewed as one form of cultural disruption, refers to the complex process whereby the behaviors and attitudes of an identified immigrant change toward the dominant group as a result of exposure to a cultural system that is significantly different.[38]

Many studies that look at large racial and ethnic populations, when conducted by individuals outside of those racial and ethnic groups, do not attach significance to the degree to which individuals within that group are acculturated. There is a wide body of literature that has looked at postimmigration acculturation.[39–43] One area where the acculturation literature has failed to adequately address the issue of acculturation is among African-Americans who do not have the same patterns of immigration and a movement away from cultural immersion toward acculturation in the same patterns that other voluntary immigrant groups show. These studies also fail to address the notion of reimmersion and the experience that is important to Native American groups.

Acculturation occurs when an individual makes a deliberate decision to move away from her cultural norm to one of a variety of end points. One example is moving to a subculture within that culture and immersing oneself in either a negative or a positive iteration of the original culture. Another is an individual who moves away from the culture toward the dominant culture. This movement can occur through assimilation or a moving toward the dominant culture out of attraction or an assimilation and moving away from the subculture out of self-hate. Obviously the end points are much the same but the motivations are entirely different.

4.2.3. Cultural Disruption: Transcultural Marriage. Cultural disruptions can also come about by mixing cultures. When transcultural marriages occur, there can be a development of a hybrid culture that retains some of the elements of both. There can be a loss of definition of both original cultures with resultant values uncertainty. Some transcultural unions result in retention of one culture and sacrifice or loss of the other. The decision to eliminate remnants of one culture might be made by someone moving away from familial/cultural pain. It must be recognized that the individual who makes a decision to cross ethnic/cultural barriers is making a significant statement about their ability to embrace novel customs/beliefs.

Assortive mating occurs among humans.[44] There are studies that suggest that assortive mating plays a role in the familial clustering of alcoholism.[45] If one chooses to "mate" away from one's culture, she or he may "mate" away from other identifiers of self, including familial alcoholism. For example, a woman from a severely affected alcoholic home might choose to marry outside of her culture and at the same time not select an alcoholic mate. The mating decision is so significantly different that major changes are made in more than just the racial/ethnic domain at that time.

4.3. Socialization

Men and women are socialized in different ways and are taught to value themselves for different reasons. Some of this value to self and society may be gender specific, some may be group bound, some both. For example, men may be socialized to derive their value from their ability to support their families and women for their ability to nurture their families.

4.3.1. Women. If a subgroup of women are then socialized to believe that their value comes from bearing children who will be taken from them and, for example, sold to others, that group of women may distort their gender-based value. If the cultural disruption is complete, that group of women may transmit the intergenerational knowledge that to procreate increases one's value. If the cultural disruption is incomplete, the need to procreate and nurture will be transmitted, even in the face of tremendous emotional pain due to the repeated loss of offspring.

4.3.2. Men. A parallel exists for the male members of this culture. If they experience frustration that hinders their ability to provide for their family due to the presence of overwhelming external forces, they could choose one of several responses to lessen the chronic tension between their culture's expectations and their individual reality. Those responses might include: (1) rejecting that which is valued; (2) adopting methods to lessen the emotional experience of that tension; or (3) evaluating external forces and working harder to provide for one's family. Therefore, a man might leave his family, drink to escape his pain, work himself to death, or attribute his inability to achieve in proportion to his output to a lack of self-worth.

4.3.3. Social Class. Socioeconomic factors have been implicated as important determinants of alcoholism. Alcoholism, drinking behaviors, and norms have been found to vary across social class. Socioeconomic status serves as an important, complex source of diversity in research on different ethnic groups. In the United States, many historical and social events have combined to create a situation in which large proportions of members of minority populations are found in lower social classes or identified with lower social classes and the outcomes of low social classes. This has resulted in a tendency for the behaviors related to those members of lower social classes to be generalized to the entire group. Additionally, the criteria for social class categories in the majority culture may not apply directly to categories within minority cultures.[46] Women may derive their social class from their own resources, those of their male partner, or some variant based on the collective resources of those in her household. Whatever the context, in general African-American women compare unfavorably with their white counterparts, despite similarities in work, childbearing, and family roles.[47]

5. Case Study

5.1. Family Genogram

5.1.1. Betsy. Laurel is a 23-year-old African-American female married to a man of German–English descent. She recently delivered a biracial daughter, Betsy, a product of a full-term gestation. Betsy's racial and ethnic pedigree is typical of several generations of the members of her family in that she is biracial. While several members of her family spanning six generations have been biracial, or triracial, most if not all have been culturally immersed in the African-American experience. Betsy's family pedigree can be traced for six generations. Alcohol use histories are available on four generations. All of the children in Betsy's generation are under 5 years of age; therefore, no information is available on her generation. The most distant relatives about which information is available included many individuals born into slavery; their alcohol use histories if ascertained are unreliable.

5.1.2. Laurel (Betsy's Mother). Laurel reports a direct knowledge of her brother's alcohol abuse, including at least one report of driving while under the influence of alcohol. Other members of her generation range from 2 to 26 years of age. There are ten females in her generation and nine males. Five of those individuals (three males and two females) are preadolescent without drinking experiences. Of the eight women in her generation over 13 years of age, four, including Laurel, are abstinent. Of the six males over age 13, one case of alcohol abuse (Laurel's brother) has been identified. Laurel has two brothers, Betsy's uncles, who were both married briefly to Caucasians, and one has a daughter from his marriage.

5.1.3. Diana (Betsy's Maternal Grandmother). Laurel's mother, Diana, while one half Native American (northeastern United States), had limited involvement with her own mother's tribe. Diana was abstinent to alcohol, citing a true allergy to the substance that resulted in full-blown anaphylaxis following consumption of even the smallest amount. Diana has one brother who is an alcoholic. She has two sisters without alcohol-use disorders. Diana's mother, Brenda, married an African-American Catholic and moved off the reservation into a large northeastern United States urban center. Brenda is abstinent. While Brenda visited the reservation frequently, she adopted Catholicism and immersed herself in the culture of that church and the African-American community. Brenda's husband, Felix, identified himself as an African-American Creole, being of mixed French, Spanish, and African-American ancestry, from the costal regions of Louisiana.

Though the focus within their home was on the African-American experience, Diana, Laurel's mother, and her sisters were exposed regularly to their tribal reservation-based relatives and encouraged exposure to and acknowledgement of their Native American culture. Consequently, when Laurel's mother, Diana, died, she was buried in the tribal burial grounds on the reservation following the ceremony in the local Catholic church. Laurel has participated regularly in annual pow-wows on the reservation. One of Laurel's aunts celebrated her marriage in the traditional way of the tribe, including traditional tribal dress.

5.1.4. Clarence Jr. (Betsy's Maternal Grandfather). Laurel's father, Clarence Jr., is one of six siblings. He reports rare use of alcohol. His alcohol use patterns have never been remarkable. He has two male siblings and three female siblings. One male sibling is an alcohol abuser, potentially an undiagnosed alcoholic. One male sibling is a social drinker. Among his three female siblings, one is abstinent and has been most of her life, never having experienced any negative consequences from alcohol but never having enjoyed the effect. A second sister is an alcoholic in recovery. The third may have had an alcoholic-use disorder in the past, but her use of alcohol decreased significantly when diagnosed with a chronic disorder in her early 20s that required medications with a bad alcohol interaction profile. This change in her drinking pattern paralleled her marriage to an African-American male who is abstinent.

5.1.5. Mary and Clarence (Betsy's Great-Grandparents). Clarence's parents, Mary and Clarence are both African-Americans. Clarence Sr. exhibited signs and symptoms of alcohol abuse following his return from World War II. As Mary and Clarence Sr. began to produce their six children, Clarence Sr. found himself working two jobs to support the family, which interfered with his drinking. Mary reports that Clarence Sr.'s alcohol use did not pose a problem to him or their relationship after 1950. Their first son, Clarence Jr., was born in 1947.

Mary's family can be traced back to slavery and includes a number of biracial marriages between African-Americans and Native Americans. Mary has been abstinent for most of her life, not enjoying the effect of alcohol. She had two sisters, one who died in infancy and one who was a social drinker. Among her sister's offspring of three, one female experienced a cocaine-use disorder in the late 1980s and is in remission.

5.1.6. Mary's Family. Mary's mother, Edith, a Catholic of Creole descent who converted to the Southern Baptist faith upon her marriage, was abstinent for all of married life. Her husband, Brad, was a rare user of alcohol.

Edith's parents, Angela and Edward, were of mixed parentage. Angela was a Creole of mixed French, Spanish, and African-American parentage. Her husband, Edward, had one Native American parent (southwestern United States) and one African-American parent, who was a recently freed slave. Edith had one brother who was a known alcoholic.

Mary's father, Brad, was half Indian, half African-American. His Native

American mother was from the southwestern United States. She died when he was a young child, and records regarding her alcohol use patterns are unavailable. John, Brad's father, was an African-American.

5.1.7. Clarence's Family. Clarence Sr. had two sisters who were both abstinent. Clarence Sr.'s mother, LuLu, was the product of a marriage between an African-American woman born in slavery, Melva, and a biracial man, Clarence I, African-American and Native American (mideastern seaboard). LuLu had six siblings; one female sibling was known to be dependent on paregoric, an opioid drug, which was available over-the-counter at that time.

LuLu died 9 years after her marriage to Dick, a biracial African-American and Caucasian man. She left him with three small children, the oldest being Clarence. Following LuLu's death, Dick would often leave the community for extended periods of time to seek work outside of the immediate area. Dick was able to pass for white outside of his community and found the job opportunities for a white man in the late 1920s to be better than those for a black man. Dick was unable to pose as a white man in the surrounding communities because of his long-term residence in that area. Despite these forays into another cultural and racial context, Dick always returned to his community of origin and readily identified with and chose his African-American cultural orientation and racial identity.

Dick's mother, Helen, was the African-American, his father, John, the Caucasian. This relationship did not end in marriage. John's family and John helped provide for Dick while he was growing up in his African-American family and in the community. His affiliation with John's family was accepted and recognized at that time, and his experience was that there were several other biracial members of the community who were recognized as products of liaisons with an imbalance of power between African-American women and Caucasian men.

5.2. Religiosity/Spirituality

While Diana was raised in the Catholic church, her involvement with organized religion sharply declined after her marriage to Clarence Jr., who had no particular exposure to church or religion during his formative years. Laurel expresses no interest in involvement with organized religion, while she does express a belief in God. Clarence Sr. vehemently rejected the notion of a God following the death of his mother when he was 8. His wife, Mary, had been an active participant in the Southern Baptist church, following in the footsteps of her mother, Edith. Edith converted to the Southern Baptist faith from Catholicism, which had been a long-standing tradition in her family, when she married Brad. Mary found her religious beliefs in conflict with those of Clarence Sr., and resolved the issues by withdrawing from participation in the church. Consequently, Mary and Clarence Sr.'s six children had very little exposure to organized religion during their formative years. Among the six siblings, two are nonattenders in organized religious practice; the other four represent affiliation with four different religious organizations. Of those who participate in active religious pursuits, all have affiliated themselves with at least two different groups at different points in their lives.

6. Case Speculation

6.1. Limitations of Case

There are five apparent flaws that affect the reliability and validity of work done across racial and ethnic groups or within racial and ethnic groups. They are: (1) a tendency to generalize findings on a sample to all members of that group; (2) a tendency to compare across racial and ethnic groups without controlling for similarities across all dimensions; (3) limitations on the ability of samples to predict prevalence within groups; (4) a lack of homogeneity within groups; and (5) a reliance on stereotypes that can influence hypothesis development and hypothesis testing in research studies. Merely because an individual can be identified as being a member of a particular racial or ethnic group does not mean that individual represents all members of that group.

Well-controlled pedigree studies provide information to suggest that specific clusters of signs and symptoms, or clinical syndromes, are transmitted through families[48–51] and represent the first stage in the scientific assessment of genetic/biological vulnerability. Family pedigree studies also provide the statistical basis for determining whether different behavioral disorders are transmitted independently.[52] These family pedigree studies, while useful in elucidating some degree of biological vulnerability, are not as useful as adoption studies in identifying discreet genetic risk factors and separating them from cultural influences.

The foregoing contains a number of flaws that severely limit its ability to be representative, relative to alcohol, for the family it describes. The case study presented is included merely to illustrate the diversity of racial/ethnic backgrounds with which any one African-American can present. The information provided regarding alcohol, and secondarily drug, use patterns of members of the family is based entirely on the anecdotal recall of the presenting subject. This anecdotal recall is subject to the same degree of historical overlay and embellishment that would occur in any family. Secondarily, and potentially more important, is the fact that the information being provided relates to certain individual's drug and alcohol use patterns. This information is potentially subject to more protection and distortion over time within families. Furthermore, family pedigree studies are subject to a number of methodological limitations that either cloud the interpretation of findings or severely limit their usefulness and generalizability, even when these studies are well designed.

6.2. "Family Study" versus "Family History Study"

A study by Remmer and Chambers shows that "family studies" in which family members are interviewed reveal higher rates of alcoholism than do "family history studies" in which only alcoholic probans are interviewed.[53] The lifelong expectancy rate for alcoholism among males appears to range from about 3 to 5%; the rate for females is from 0.1 to 1%.[59] Males and females also show different rates of alcohol problems in terms of age of onset and severity of complications. Since there are some differences in the topology of alcoholism between males and females, it is important to generally analyze the data separately as merging of the data may obscure important findings. Critical numbers need to be represented in each sex in order to identify these findings. Clearly this family does not have the numbers to allow those issues to be fully elucidated. Since there are not adequate numbers by sex, there will not be adequate numbers by generation, nor will there by adequate numbers by sex within each generation.

The data with which we are concerned was collected for over six generations spanning over 100 years; this introduces the question of lack of accuracy of historically collected data. These are data that are generally of a hidden nature within family groups and represent that which may be considered some of the worst secrets within a family. Over many years there have been sex differences in the acceptance of drug and alcohol use. Such information regarding women may, in fact, have been more deeply buried the more generations one goes back.

Just as there have been sex differences over time, there have been differences over time in the acceptability of the use of alcohol. Whereas in the 1950s it might have been viewed as being acceptable to have a cocktail after work, in the 1850s that might not have been an acceptable behavior to engage in on a daily basis.

There is evidence that African-Americans in the immediate postslavery period replicated those drinking patterns, of two types, that were available to them on plantations. One was that slaves had their access to alcohol severely limited, the second was that the slavemaster allowed some limited access to alcohol in a way to promote celebration of a productive workweek. Some have suggested that weekend drinking among African-Americans is a direct result of learned patterns in drinking during slavery, and that these patterns are not consistent with the alcohol use patterns of African-America in Western African prior to being brought to this country.[55]

Finally, because of the hidden nature of the information regarding alcohol use, it would be expected that in some families, at least historically, the information that is passed along from generation to generation would minimize the information that is "bad" about previous generations and amplify the information which is "good," such that some records of alcoholism in past generations would be lost.

6.3. Case Speculation

6.3.1. Generational Incidence. Four of eight women over 13 years of age or past the age at risk in Laurel's generation are abstinent. We know from the literature that African-American women in general and in this age group have a higher proportion of abstinence than their white counterparts.

It has been said that "with the turn of the century, the policies of pluralism and assimilation stirred the hope that the 'Indian problem' would go away when Indians forsook their ways of life and blended in with the dominant culture."[56] (p 156) Some of these positions did not lead to total assimilation for many Indians, nor did the American society embrace, honor, or nurture diversity among its peoples. One reason for this is set forth by Trimble:[57] (p 184)

> . . . to meet the fabric of the Indian ethos was an enduring sense of dignity and reverence for traditional custom, legend and spiritualism. This ethos somehow transcended all efforts to control and regulate it, and it managed to bring the Indian into the 20th Century amidst paternalism, poverty, fear, hatred, and frustration.

Diana and her sisters regularly participated in tribal-based activities, and Diana's sister reconnected with a resurgence of Indian identity and pride.[58] Diana's sisters escaped alcoholism even though they had a brother who was an active alcoholic; therefore there may have been gender-specific protective factors in play.

Clarence's siblings consisted of three females, one abstinent, one alcoholic, and one questionable alcohol abuser who experienced the impact of a protective factor associated with chronic disease and her role as a wife and mother, which served as an intervention on the development of her alcoholism.

Laurel's grandparent's generations on both her mother's and father's sides were remarkably absent of alcoholics. Of note is the maternal grandmother who was a full-blooded Native Indian and who was abstinent. This reinforces the finding, often overlooked in discussion of alcohol use, that studies have shown that not all Native Americans are drinkers. There are both heavy drinkers among individuals and groups and abstainers, with fewer numbers of those who drink in moderation.[59] Some studies[60,61] have suggested that there is a maturing out of drinking among women that occurs most often with the onset of family responsibilities, although in one study only the mild-to-moderate drinkers eventually switched to abstention. This abstention from alcohol parallels what we know about the historical patterns of alcohol use in the African-American community.

The patterns of alcoholism and health and social consequences have changed significantly among African-American women over the last two centuries. Following slavery and up until about 1950, African-Americans had low rates of liver cirrhosis mortality, which was attributable to their strong support of abstinence. During the early 20th century, the politics of prohibition moved away from the American temperance movement, which supported antislavery reform, to the white supremacy sects. This shift occurred at the time of migration of African-Americans from the rural South, where abstinence was reinforced by the Southern Baptist tradition, to the North.[20] This migration paralleled the increased use of alcohol at African-American social gatherings and the urbanization of African-American communities. Concomitantly, there was an increase in the number of hospital admissions for African-Americans with alcoholic psychosis in the 1920s. By the 1950s, the cirrhosis mortality for African-American women and men began to rise, doubling between 1950 and 1973.[20]

Betsy's paternal grandfather experienced problems related to alcohol abuse or alcoholism following his return from World War II, and three of his six children later experienced difficulty with alcohol. Two of those three were his female offspring. While Clarence Sr. was not experiencing alcohol problems after 1950, the legacy of his issues that were at one time relieved by alcohol were expressed in the next generation. The fact that Clarence worked harder to achieve stability for his family spoke to his awareness of his inability to be an adequate provider and sets an example of one man's decision to try to overcome issues of inadequate access by overcompensating. It is also of note that this became a protection for him that interfered with his out-of-control alcohol consumption.

He also had a maternal aunt who was an opioid addict, who acquired the drug legally prior to the passage of the Harrison Narcotic Act. While the history of his aunt's opioid addiction was passed from generation to generation, his history is remarkable for an absence of alcoholism. The opioid-addicted aunt was notable for having never married. Marital status and race interact significantly in their relationship to highest usual number of drinks per occasion and abstinence. African-American married women are the most likely to abstain and white married women the least likely.[28]

7. Conclusion

There is a substantial body of research that looks at the multiple causal factors of alcoholism in isolation and in interaction: biophysical, psychological, and sociocultural variables. There is also a substantial body of literature that looks at alcoholism in men. There is a growing body of literature that is beginning to explore gender differences in alcoholism. Finally, there is growing evidence that different racial and ethnic groups differ in the rates of initiation, consequences of use, maintenance of use patterns, and cessation. What is absent in the literature is those gender differences in different racial and ethnic groups.

Close examination of the existent literature that explores different racial and ethnic groups often leads us to conclude that there are high rates of alcoholism among certain groups. These rates may have more to do with socioeconomic conditions of these groups than they do with race and ethnicity. Biogenetic mixing, which occurs in transracial marriage or offspring, is not accounted for in these schemes. Also, cultural disruption through acculturation or transcultural marriage may be more important than originally calculated.

The family genogram presents several interesting findings. One is a consistent low rate of alcoholism among the women in the family. The other is the finding of a repeated pattern of cross-racial marriage and mixing. An incidental finding is that these cross-racial relationships often occur in a generation where significant alcoholism is present. This finding has implications for those who study intrafamilial clustering of alcoholism and the marital patterns of adult children of alcoholics. The finding is consistent with making a radical change that is consistent with both an external indicator (across racial groups) and internal indicators (away from alcoholism).

This is a family where spirituality/religiosity is of minor import in several generations. Many prevention programs highlight the importance of the black church to the African-American community. It is a family that is typical in many regards, but atypical in many respects and illustrates a significant departure from involvement with the African-American church. When trying to define the types of prevention campaigns that work best with different groups, attention should be paid to the African American family with multicultural roots.

It is clear from the literature that patterns of alcohol use evolve from the meanings, attitudes, beliefs, values, and norms that that society assigns to alcohol. A society can have gender differences that influence alcohol's meaning for men and women in that group. There is substantial literature that shows that acculturation has a dramatic effect on drinking patterns among immigrants in the United States and successive generations. It is clear that acculturation occurs in different ways for African-Americazns. The impact of this "acculturation" needs further study. While there have a number of studies on alcohol problems among women of color, which have produced important finding, they also have produced many new questions.

References

1. Fegin J: *Racial and Ethnic Relations*. Englewood Cliffs, NJ, Prentice Hall, 1978.
2. Butler JP: Of kindred minds: The ties that bind, in Orlando MA, Weston R, Epstein L (eds): *Cultural Competence for Evaluators, A Guide for Alcohol Drug Abuse Prevention Practitioners Working with Ethnic/Racial Communities*. Rockville, MD, US Department of Health and Human Services, 1992, p 25.
3. Bell P, Evans J: *Counseling the Black Client: Alcohol Use and Abuse in Black America*. Minneapolis, MN, Hazelden Foundation, 1981.
4. Mintz SW: Forward, in Whitten NE Jr, Szwed JF (eds): *Afro-American Anthropology: contemporary Perspectives*. New York, Free Press, 1970, pp 1–16.
5. Nobles W: African philosophy: Foundations for black psychology, in Jones RH (ed): *Black Psychology*. New York, Harper & Row, 1972, pp 18–32.

6. Bureau of the Census: General Population Characteristics. United States Summary. 1980 Census of Population. Washington, DC, US Department of Commerce, May 1983.

7. John R: The Native American family, in Mindel CH, Habenstein RW, Wright R Jr (eds): *Ethnic Families in America*. New York, Elsevier, 1988, pp 325–363.

8. U.S. Department of Commerce: *American Indian Era and Alaskan Native Village: 1980*. Washington, DC, US Government Printing Offices, 1984.

9. Bureau of the Census: *America's Black Population, 1970–1982: A Statistical View*. Washington, DC, US Department of Commerce, Bureau of the Census, 1983.

10. Bureau of the Census: American Indian Areas in the Last of Native Villages: 1980 Census of the Population. Supplementary Report. Washington, DC, US Department of Commerce, January 8, 1984.

11. Bureau of the Census: American Indian Eskimo and Aleut Populations. Washington, DC, US Department of Commerce, Bureau of the Census, January 8, 1984.

12. *Seventh Special Report to the US Congress on Alcohol and Health*. US Department of Health and Human Services Publication ADM 281-88-0002. Rockville, MD, National Institute on Alcohol Abuse and Alcoholism, 1990.

13. *Report of the Secretary's Task Force on Black and Minority Health*, vol 1: Executive Summary. Washington, DC, US Government Printing Office, 1985.

14. Harper F (ed): *Alcohol Abuse in Black America*. Alexandria, VA, Douglas Publishers, 1976.

15. Harper F, Dawkins M: Alcohol and blacks: Survey of the periodical literature. *Br J Addict* 71:327–334, 1976.

16. Greeley AM, McCready WC, Theisen G: *Ethnic Drinking Subcultures*. New York, Praeger 1980.

17. Harper FD: Research and treatment with black alcoholics. *Alcohol Health Res World* 1022:10–16, 1980.

18. Dawkins MP: Alcoholism prevention and black youth. *J Drug Issues* 18:15–20, 1988.

19. Wolin SJ, Bennett LA, Noonan DL, Teitelbaum MA: Disruptive family rituals: A factor in the intergenerational transmission of alcoholism. *J Stud Alcohol* 41:199–214, 1980.

20. Heard D: The epidemiology of drinking patterns in alcohol related problems among US blacks, in Spiegler L, Tate DA, Aitken S, Christin M (eds): *Alcohol Use Among U.S. Ethnic Minorities*, NIDA Research Monograph 18 DHHS Publications Number (ADM) 89-1435. Rockville, MD, US Department of Health and Human Services, 1989, pp 3–50.

21. Lex B: Review of alcohol problems in ethnic minority groups. *J Consult Clin Psychol* 55:293–300, 1987.

22. National Institute on Drug Abuse: *National Household Survey on Drug Abuse, Population Estimates 1990*. U.S. Department of Health and Human Services Publication ADM 91-1732. Washington, DC, US Government Printing Office, 1991.

23. Heard D: Black–white differences in drinking problems among US males. Presented at the 35th International Congress of the International Council on Alcohol and Addiction, Oslow, Norway, August 1988.

24. Hubbard RL, Schlenger WE, Rachal JV, *et al:* Patterns of alcohol and drug abuse in drug treatment clients from different ethnic backgrounds. *Ann NY Acad Sci* 472:60–74, 1986.

25. Caetano R: Ethnicity and drinking in Northern California: A comparison among whites, blacks and hispanics. *Alcohol Alcohol* 1026:31–44, 1984.

26. Robyak JE, Byers PH, Prange ME: Patterns of alcohol abuse among black and white alcoholics. *Int J Addict* 24(5904):715–724, 1989.

27. Knupfer G, Laurie E: *Characteristics of Abstainers: A Comparison of Drinkers and Non-drinkers in a Large California city* (Drinking Practices Study Report No. 3). Berkely, CA, State Department of Public Health, 1961.

28. Russell M: Alcohol use and related problems among black and white gynecologic patients, in Spiegler L, Tate DA, Aitken S, Christian M (eds): *Alcohol Use among US Ethnic Minorities*. NIAAA Monograph No. 18, DHHS Publ. No. (ADM) 89-1435. Washington, DC, US Department of Health and Human Services, 1989, pp 75–94.

29. Wechsler H, Demone H, Gottlieb N: Drinking patterns of Greater Boston adults: Subgroup differences on the QFU index. *J Stud Alcohol* 41:672–681, 1980.

30. Johnson P, Armor D, Polich S, Stambul H: *US Drinking Practices: Time Trends, Social Correlates and Sex Roles.* Rockville, MD, National Institute on Alcohol Abuse and Alcoholism, 1977.
31. Lillie-Blanton M, Mackenzie E, Anthony J: Black–white differences in alcohol use by women: Baltimore survey findings. *Public Health Rep* 10:124–133, 1991.
32. Aubick AL, Csemy L, Kozeny J: The socio-demographic micro-social and attitudinal contact of Czech women's drinking. Paper presented at the Symposium on Alcohol, Family and Significant Others. A Social Research Institute of Alcohol Studies and Nordic Council for Alcohol and Drug Research, Polenski, Finland, March 1991.
33. Spak F, Hallstrom T WAG (women and alcohol in: Gothenburg). Nordic Council for Alcohol and Drug Research (NAD) Publication No. 14, 1986, pp 127–132.
34. Spak F, Hallstrom T Validation of a screening instrument for use with female populations. Paper presented at the 18th Annual Symposium of the Kettil Bruun Society for Social and Epidemiological Research on Alcohol, Toronto, Ontario, Canada, June 1992.
35. Wilsnack SC, Klassen AD, Schur BE, Wilsnack RW: Predicting onset and chronicity and women's problem drinking: A five-year longitudinal analysis. *Am J Public Health* 81:305–318, 1991.
36. Hill SY: A vulnerability model for alcoholism in women. Focus on women. *J Addict Health* 2:68–91, 1981.
37. Jonsson E, Nilsson T: Alcoholkonsumtion hos monozygota och dizygota tvillinpar (Alcohol consumption in monozygotic and dizygotic pairs of twins). *Nordsk Hygienisk Tidskrift* 49:21–25, 1968.
38. Rogler LH, Malgady RG, Constantino G, Blumenthal R: What do culturally sensitive mental health services mean? The case of Hispanics. *Am Psychol* 42:565–570, 1987.
39. Parrish KM, Higuchi S, Stinson FS, *et al:* The association of drinking levels and drinking attitudes among Japanese in Japan and Japanese-Americans in Hawaii and California. *J Subst Abuse* 4:165–177, 1992.
40. Atkinson DR, Whitley S, Gin RH: Asian-American acculturation and preferences for health providers. *J Coll Stud Dev* 31:155–161, 1990.
41. Sasaki T: Intercultural research of drinking between Japanese American and mainland Japanese: 1 Drinking patterns in problem drinking. *Jpn J Alcohol Drug Depend* 20(1):28–39, 1985.
42. Attneave C: American Indians and Alaska Native families: Immigrants in their own homeland, in McGoldrick M, Pierce J, Giordano J (eds): *Ethnicity and Family Therapy.* New York, Guilford Press, 1982, pp 55–83.
43. Szapocznik J, Kurtines W: Acculturation, biculturalism, and adjustment among Cuban Americans, in Padilla AM (ed): *Acculturation, Theory, Models and Some New Findings.* Boulder, CO, Westview Press, 1980, pp 139–160.
44. Buss DM: Human mate selection. *Am Sci* 73:4751, 1985.
45. Stabenau JR, Hesselbrock VM: Family pedigree of alcoholic and control patients. *Int J Addict* 18:351–363, 1983.
46. Gordon T: Notes on white and black psychology. *J Soc Issues* 29:87–95, 1973.
47. Liepman Mr, Goldman RE, Monroe AD, *et al:* Substance abuse by special populations of women, in Gomberg ES, Nirenberg TD (eds): *Women and Substance Abuse.* Norwood, NJ, Ablex, 1993, pp 214–257.
48. Merikangas KR, Leckman JF, Prusoff BA, *et al:* Familial transmission of depression in alcoholism. *Arch Gen Psychiatry* 42:367–372, 1985.
49. Cloninger CR, Reicht T: Genetic heterogeneity in alcoholism and sociopathy, in Ketys S, Rowland LP, Sidman R, Matthysse S (eds): *Genetics of Neurological and Psychiatric Disorders.* New York, Raven Press, 1983, pp 145–166.
50. Winoknor G, Reicht T, Rimmer J, Pitts F: Alcoholism III: Diagnosis and familial psychiatric illness in 259 alcoholic probans. *Arch Gen Psychiatry* 23:104–111, 1970.
51. Stabenau J: Implications of family history of alcoholism, antisocial personality, and sex differences in alcohol dependence. *Am J Psychiatry* 141:1178–1182, 1984.
52. Cloninger CR, Lewis C, Rice J, Reicht T: Strategies for resolution of biological and cultural inheritance, in Gershon BS, Matthysse S, Breakefield XO, Ciaranello RD (eds): *Genetic*

Research Strategies for Psychobiology and Psychiatry. Pacific Grove, CA, Boxwood Press, 1981, pp 319–332.

53. Remmer J, Chambers DS: Alcoholism: Methodological considerations in the study of family illness. *Am J Orthopsychiatry* 39:760, 1969.

54. Goodwin DW: Is alcoholism hereditary? A review and critique. *Arch Gen Psychiatry* 25(12):545–579, 1971.

55. Brisbane FL: Personal communication, 1994.

56. Fleming CM: American Indians and Alaska natives: Changing societies past and present. In: Orlandi MA, Weston R, and Leonard L, *Cultural Competence for Evaluators: A Guide for Alcohol and Other Drug Abuse Prevention Practitioners Working with Ethnic/Racial Communities.* DHHS, DHS, ADAMHA, OSAP, Pub # (ADM) 92-1884. Rockville MD, US Department of Health and Human Services, 1992.

57. Trimble JE: Stereotypical images, American Indians and prejudice, in Katz PA, Taylor DA (eds): *Eliminating Racism, Profiles in Controversy.* New York, Plenum Press, 1988, pp 181–202.

58. Oetting ER, Beaubas F: Epidemiology and correlates of alcohol use among Indian adolescents living on reservations, in Spiegler L, Tate DA, Aitken S, Christian M (eds): *Alcohol Use Among US Ethnic Minorities.* NIAAA Research Monograph No. 18. Rockville, MD, US Department of Health and Human Services, 1989, pp 239–267.

59. Keith HEHEH D American Indians and alcohol: Epidemiological and social cultural relevance, in Spiegler L, Tate DA, Aitken S, Christian M (eds): *Alcohol Use among US Ethnic Minorities.* NIAAA Research Monograph No. 18. Rockville, MD, US Department of Health and Human Services, 1989, pp 207–222.

60. Lindberg E: Drinking among American Indians, in Gomberg EL, White HR, Carpenter J (eds): *Alcohol, Science and Society Revisited.* New Brunswick, NJ, Rutgers Center for Alcohol Studies, 1982 pp 80–95.

61. Whitaker JO: Alcohol and the Standing Rock Sioux Tribe, II. *Q J Stud Alcohol* 24:80–90, 1963.

Gender Differences for the Risk of Alcohol-Related Problems in Multiple National Contexts

Kaye Middleton Fillmore, Jacqueline M. Golding, Steven Kniep, E. Victor Leino, Carlisle Shoemaker, Catherine R. Ager, and Heidi P. Ferrer

with

Salme Ahlstrom, Peter Allebeck, Arvid Amundsen, Jules Angst, Gellisse Bagnall, Ann Brunswick, Remi Cadoret, Sally Casswell, Nancy DeCourville, Norman Giesbrecht, Bridget Grant, Thomas Greenfield, Joel Grube, Bernd Geuther, Thomas Harford, Ludek Kubicka, Michael R. Levenson, Mark Morgan, Harold Mulford, Leif Ojesjo, David Peck, Martin Plant, Chris Power, Bruce Ritson, Lee Robins, Anders Romelsjo, David Rosen, Ronald Schlegel, Martin Sieber, Soren Sigvardsson, Rainer Silbereisen, Meir Teichman, Richard Wilsnack, and Sharon Wilsnack

Abstract. The primary research question asked is: After holding alcohol consumption constant, will men and women be at equal risk for a variety of alcohol-related problems? Since women are actually at a higher blood alcohol content at the same consumption levels, a physiological argument would suggest that women are at equal or greater risk for alcohol problems than men. However, variation in societal norms surrounding gender roles and/or societal-level stress may mediate the experience of men and women, regardless of the differences in physiology.

Ten cross-sectional general population studies are used. Analyses control for individual-level variables (age, quantity, and frequency of drinking) and societal-level variables (proportion of women in the work force and female suicide rate) that might confound these relationships; cross-study homogeneity is examined.

Kaye Middleton Fillmore, Jacqueline M. Golding, Steven Kniep, E. Victor Leino, Carlisle Shoemaker, Catherine R. Ager, and Heidi P. Ferrer • Institute of Health and Aging, Department of Social and Behavioral Sciences, University of California, San Francisco, California 94143.

Recent Developments in Alcoholism, Volume 12: Women and Alcoholism, edited by Marc Galanter. Plenum Press, New York, 1995.

Controlling for age and alcohol consumption, men and women are equally at risk for self-reported health problems and treatment for alcohol problems, and these findings are homogeneous across studies; the latter suggests that the barriers preventing women from obtaining treatment are not as great as previously thought. Men are at greater risk for reporting loss of control over alcohol, an alcoholic or problem drinker identity, family/job problems, school/job problems, and financial problems, and these findings are homogeneous across studies. The lower risk for women to perceive themselves with drinking problems or to feel "out of control" may be subjected to multiple interpretations; the lower risk for problems of an "acting-out" nature suggests that cultural expectations mediate the relationships between consumption and these problems, endorsing the value of drunkenness and its accompanying behaviors among men.

While men were significantly more highly at risk for symptomatic drinking, accidents, and belligerence, the cross-study findings were not homogeneous. We controlled for "traditional" and "modern" contexts (proportion of women in the work force) and low and high societal stress (female suicide rate) in addition to age and alcohol consumption. The more notable findings were that the presence of societal-level stress elevated the risk of belligerence among men in "traditional" contexts, whereas the presence of lesser stress was associated with equal risk for the genders in "traditional" contexts; these findings were homogeneous. "Modern" contexts were characterized by equal gender risk for belligerence, suggesting that the "modern" roles of women bring with them the latitude to act out their aggressive behavior when drinking to an equal extent as men.

1. Introduction: Gender Differences for the Risk of Alcohol-Related Problems

Numerous studies show that, on average, men report a higher prevalence of heavier drinking, frequent drinking, and alcohol-related problems than women (e.g., for the United States[1]; for Canada[2]; for four countries[3]; for five countries[4]; for quantity per occasion in 20 studies and frequency per month in 27 studies from 15 countries[5]). On the basis of these studies, many analysts have concluded that norms constituting gender roles are critical in mediating consumption patterns, and therefore men, who typically are heavier consumers, are naturally at greater risk for alcohol-related problems.[6] However, women may be at greater risk for experiencing alcohol-related problems should they drink heavily/frequently because their body weight is typically lower than that of men (resulting in alcohol blood levels roughly 20% greater than those of men).[7]

Together, these findings have suggested an interesting research question; namely, if the consumption of men and women is held constant *and* if women are actually at a higher blood alcohol content at the same consumption level, will they therefore experience the same as or more alcohol-related problems as men? A purely physiological argument would suggest that they would. On the other hand, given these same circumstances (i.e., holding the consumption constant), will variation in societal norms surrounding gender roles and/or societal-level stresses mediate between the experience of men and women with respect to their consumption and alcohol-related problems, regardless of the differences in physiology? A sociocultural argument would suggest this to be the case.

The analyses we present herein in part address these questions. We assess the degree to which gender constitutes significant risk among drinkers for *a priori* groups of alcohol problems in ten cross-sectional general population studies from five national contexts (Canada, Federal Republic of Germany, the United Kingdom, Scotland alone, and the United States). The analyses control for individual-level variables (age, quantity of drinking per occasion, and frequency of drinking per month) and societal-level variables (proportion of women in the work force and female suicide rate) that might confound these relationships. They also examine the extent to which these associations are homogeneous across studies.

A research design that entails a cross-level analytic strategy utilizing multiple studies from a variety of social contexts may, in part, address these questions because it is necessary for the universes sampled to embrace variation in norms and stresses experienced by populations. Our analyses are admittedly crude. In the words of Campbell,[8] we are only at the beginning of the beginning because we are attempting to explain how collectivities affect persons over time.[9] This design integrates aggregate-level and individual-level variables that have been postulated to contribute to the risks of gender to alcohol-related problems. Furthermore, they evaluate the degree to which findings from one social context may be generalized to another and specify some traits of national contexts which may contribute to differences in the associations of gender to alcohol-related problems.

1.1. The Individual-Level Evidence

To date, the evidence relating gender to alcohol-related problems is mixed probably, in part, because of different methodological approaches to the question and the wide range of problem domains examined. There is a growing literature that suggests because women experience higher alcohol blood levels at the same dose, they are at higher risk for alcohol-related health problems.[10] Examining female alcoholics compared with male alcoholics, Hill[11] found death rates for females exceeded those for males. Hanna *et al.*[12] found that heavy-drinking women die at younger ages from cardiovascular disease than heavy-drinking men. While problems of detection may result in an underestimation of alcohol-related health problems among women (e.g., physicians may not uncover alcohol problems in women because these problems are often stereotyped as male problems), these findings would suggest that the genders will equally report or that females will slightly exceed males in self-reported health problems in the current investigation.

We will examine gender differences in reported treatment for alcoholism. While it has been argued that women have lesser access to treatment for their alcohol problems as a result of structural or normative barriers[13,14] and while it has been shown that men are the primary utilizers of alcoholism treatment,[15] a recent US community study of multiple-care systems performed by Weisner and Schmidt[16] found that women with alcohol problems were overrepresented in systems not specializing in alcoholism treatment. While the Weisner and Schmidt study is confined to one US community, their observations would lead us to hypothesize that exposure to treatment (which is broadly defined in the analyses herein) will not significantly differ for men and women, after controlling for consumption level and other individual-level variables.

We will examine a number of alcohol-related problems in this chapter— self-reported loss of control over drinking, self-identification as alcoholic or problem drinker, symptomatic drinking, alcohol-related accidents, negative reasons for drinking, and a variety of problems related to lack of demeanor and nonfulfillment of social roles (e.g., belligerence and problems in the familial and job settings and with finances). Here the evidence in the literature becomes more greatly mixed with respect to gender risk for alcohol-related problems.

While Hilton[17] found no significant differences in aggregated problems between US men and women reporting five or more drinks per occasion once a week, Knupfer;[18] aggregating multiple US samples, found that the risk of various groups of problems for women was greater than for men consuming eight or more drinks once a week or more. Recent US and Canadian research has reported that, when controlling for level of consumption, women were equally or more at risk than men for a number of problems, particularly those of the lack of demeanor and social role genre.[19–22] These latter findings, of course, would fall on the side of physiological explanations where high levels of consumption or high blood alcohol would naturally lead to alcohol-related problems irrespective of gender. However, it is posited here that these results may be confounded because the studies from which they emerged were performed in the same *historical era* and in *countries* that share a great deal with respect to societal-level norms and societal-level stresses. For example, it is possible that in the 1980s, both Canada and the United States were exemplars of the "liberation of women" with respect to "nontraditional" gender roles and/or that the roles of women in these places and times were encumbered with considerable stressful circumstances.

This temporal and contextual explanation is posited because gender roles have been interpreted in past research as powerful explanations for drunkenness and associated behaviors of an "acting-out" nature. While gender roles are conceptualized as fluid across and within contexts, they are most frequently linked to cultural stereotypes in which males are more likely to value drunkenness. For instance, Chassin et al.[23] found that adolescent boys thought drinking enhanced their social image while adolescent girls did not. Qualities stereotyping males (e.g., assertiveness) have been positively associated with alcohol problems.[24] When much broader contexts than the United States and Canada have been studied, cultural expectations about drinking have been found to influence the relationships between consumption and nonphysiological problems.[25] In light of these literatures, we hypothesize that there will be gender differences for some nonphysiological alcohol-related problems across social contexts. However, we expect males to be at higher risk overall for the majority of alcohol-related problems (even with drinking level held constant) because it is thought that the prevailing gender norms in the societies studied here are that it is more acceptable for men to engage in drunkenness and associated alcohol-related problem behaviors than for women.

The shortfall of most studies examining the gender–alcohol problems domain is that the work has been confined to one or another context, thus obstructing the degree to which cultural expectations and gender roles within and across cultures and time may operate to mediate the relationships between consumption and the experience of alcohol-related problems.

1.2. The Contextual Evidence

We argue that the context in which people live may mediate the association between gender and alcohol-related problems for those problems in which there are cross-study differences (i.e., cross-study heterogeneity) in gender risk. In other words, the social norms and stresses of an era may *reconfigure* the society or segments of it such that there will be *transitions* in social roles of groups that may constitute new opportunities/conditions/stresses changing the drinking patterns and problems of individuals. In particular, we argue that periods of "modernity" versus "traditionalty" with respect to women's place in the social structure and periods of "higher" or "lower" societal-level stress may remold the gender risk differences for problems.

We use two indicators of traits of nations to determine if these attributes account for some of the remaining variability in the magnitude of the risks of gender differences with alcohol-related problems. Although they are only crude reflections of contextual effects, they are important to integrate into analyses on gender differences because, instead of focusing exclusively on individual drinking to explain variation across social contexts, we should, as Roizen[26] suggests, regard drinking "as an aspect of culture firmly attached or 'glued' to something else in cultural structure—to some other system symbolic, material, cognitive, or whatever—it follows that the understanding of drinking will oblige us to decipher that attachment" (p 12).

First, we examine the national contexts at the time of measurement in each study on the basis of "traditionality" and "modernity" of women's roles, operationalized by the proportion of women in the work force. The choice of this variable relies on research that has shown that employment among women (with education) is a strong predictor of egalitarian gender role attitudes in the United States,[27] and that employed women use alcohol more regularly than unemployed women.[28] The results of specific individual-level investigations of the impact of women's employment on drinking are mixed, although it appears that employment per se and the nature of the employment are implicated in within- and across-gender differences in drinking.[29] Of importance here are studies in which the *context* of the workplace (e.g., the domination of one or the other gender in the work context) has contributed to explaining individual-level drinking patterns among women.[30,31] Extrapolating from the "meso" contextual level (i.e., the workplace context) of these studies, their results suggest that the dimension of gender role "traditionality" and "modernity" (conceptualized herein as a macrolevel variable on the societal-level) may be related to the differential risk of some alcohol-related behavioral problems because, not only might women drink less "excessively" in more "traditional" contexts, but they may not be allowed the permission to drink at all.[26] Furthermore, problems of demeanor and social roles among women in more "modern" contexts may reflect more those of the men about them because, in the Wilsnacks'[29] words, it may be the culture "that weakens the influence of traditional gender-related values and attitudes, with the result that women's drinking and its consequences are affected more by conditions that are not gender-specific" (p 141).

We propose two hypotheses about the relation of eras of "traditionality" and "modernity" to gender risk for drinking problems. First, when cross-study findings are heterogeneous, we expect the risks of problems concerned with demeanor and nonfulfillment of social roles to be equivalent for men and women in societal contexts characterized by more "modern" gender roles. This suggests that these kinds of behaviors among women will more closely resemble those of men in contexts in which women's and men's roles are more similar. We expect the risk of these problems to be greater among men in more "traditional" contexts.

Second, when cross-study findings are heterogeneous, we expect men to be at higher risk than women for alcohol-related problems of a mental and existential nature (e.g., loss of control, symptomatic drinking) in more "modern" contexts. Although we know of no literature directly addressing this hypothesis, we reason as follows. Men have been found to typically "externalize" their problems while women typically "internalize" them.[32] We expect this to be true in contexts of a "traditional" nature where men, in a sense, "own" the behavioral domain of "acting out" when they drink; in fact, it has been argued that one of the major expressions of the male sex role is drinking which provides a way for men to socialize together, to demonstrate their manliness, and to take risks.[33] Now, if this is the case, one must wonder what occurs to men's drinking behavior when the context is much more gender egalitarian. After all, if our first hypothesis is supported, the almost exclusive male-honored traditions of men are being encroached upon by women. We speculate that in "modern" circumstances the opportunities for men to display their masculinity by "acting out" when drinking in all male groups will diminish through social disapproval and, as a result, men will be at higher risk for displaying the symptoms of alcoholism (e.g., they will drink when they had promised not to, report blackouts, skip meals, and so on). Therefore, we speculate quite tentatively that social contexts of a more "egalitarian nature" (i.e., of greater "modernity") will exacerbate these problems among men just as the same contexts likewise exacerbate demeanor and social role problems among women.

Next, we examine the national contexts at the time of measurement in each study on the basis of societal-level stress. Bales[35] advocated measuring societal stress as a predictor of alcoholism (along with measures of norms surrounding drinking behavior and the degree to which the society provides substitute outlets for people to cope with societal stress). The literature related to societal stress and alcohol-related problems is limited because it is primarily confined to aggregate level units of analysis.[36,37] While this literature is less than conclusive with respect to demonstrating causal relationships, it does suggest that there is merit in evaluating measures indicative of societal-level stress.

We use a measure of the suicide rate on the basis of Durkheim's[38] classic work in which it was suggested that these rates are associated with feelings of alienation, disorientation, and dissatisfaction resulting from stress or tension in societies. In particular, we select the female suicide rate as an indicator because it may reflect "moral" stress in societies (as opposed to "material" stress). Specifically, the male suicide rate is linked to economic market fluctuations while the female suicide rate is not, suggesting that the female suicide rate is probably a measure of extreme societal stress and may itself be a product of multiple social stressors in a society.[39] The female suicide rate (compared with the overall suicide rate, the male suicide rate, the divorce rate, and the unemployment rate) is a relatively sensitive cross-sectional predictor of "heavy" drinking[40] and of period effects of alcohol consumption on groups of alcohol problems.[41]

The use of stress as related to drinking patterns and problems also has its roots in studies on the individual level. Cooper et al.[42] summarize the research on the effects of stress on drinking as mediated by gender, citing evidence that "women may be prone to internalize stress-related effects, whereas men may be more likely to use alcohol and exhibit alcohol-related problems as a result of exposure to stressful circumstances" (p 140). Extrapolating to societal-level effects on gender risk, this would suggest that contexts characterized by greater stress will show men to be at higher risk for alcohol-related problems of a demeanor and social role nature, whereas contexts characterized by lower stress will show men and women to be at equivalent risk for these problems. We also tentatively hypothesize that contexts characterized by higher stress will equalize the sexes with respect to alcohol-related problems of a more mental and existential nature. This is because women, more than men, have been found to report symptoms indicating physical and emotional discomfort,[34] and therefore we expect these to increase among women in stressful contexts.

Bales[35] proposed that societal-level stress and social norms in combination predict different rates of alcoholism. Some analysts[43] contend that when a society is "permissive" with respect to alcohol use, alcohol is sufficiently available to be used as an acceptable means for relieving societal stress. Evidence from Horwitz and White[44] on the individual level has suggested that the norms governing the internalization of stress among women and the externalization among men may be mediated by relative gender identity among both men and women. In the spirit of these findings and postulations, we test two hypotheses that should be regarded as exploratory because the unit of analysis is the social context of which we have only limited studies.

First, we have posited higher societal stress will put men at greater risk for problems of a demeanor and social role nature and also that greater "modernity" will equalize the genders with respect to these problems. Therefore, we expect an additive effect of these variables such that contexts of both high societal stress and "modernity" will equalize the risks for men and women. In this vein, we expect that men, more than women, will be at greater risk for demeanor and social role problems in "traditional" contexts in which stress is high.

Second, we have posited that men and women will be at equal risk for mental and existential problems in high-stress contexts and men will be at higher risk in low-stress contexts. We also projected that men will be at greater risk than women for these problems in "modern" contexts and the genders will be at equal risk in "traditional" contexts. We expect an additive effect of these variables such that when both high societal stress and modernity are present, the risks for men and women will not differ. However, we expect that men will be at higher risk for mental and existential problems in low stress, "modern" contexts.

1.3. The Model

The analyses here use a two-tiered approach. First, for each study, gender, age, and individual-level measures of consumption (quantity per occasion and frequency per month) are entered into logistic regression equations predicting drinking problems. There is considerable variation in prevalence by age across highly differing cultures.[3,5] US studies, for example, consistently show that younger people report higher prevalence of heavy drinking and alcohol-related problems more than do older people.[45] Therefore, we enter age as an individual-level variable into our models. We control for quantity and frequency per occasion as well because both have been shown to constitute significant risk for alcohol-related problems in multiple national contexts.[41] The result of interest in these analyses is the odds ratio for gender.

Second, meta-analysis is utilized to combine odds ratios across studies to determine the degree to which findings are replicated (homogeneous). The meta-analysis is repeated blocking for two aggregate-level variables: the proportion of women in the work force and the female rate of suicide of the nation at the time the study took place. We posit that the aggregate level controls will account for some of the remaining variability in the magnitude of risk of gender for problem domains.

Five *a priori* groups of alcohol-related problems (11 measures) are the dependent variables in this paper. The groups of problems are (1) physiological (health) consequences, (2) casualty (accident) problems, (3) mental and existential problems, (4) lack of demeanor and nonfulfillment of social roles.[46] An additional dimension includes (5) "negative" personal reasons for drinking.

2. Methods

Ten studies are used from the archive of the Collaborative Alcohol-Related Longitudinal Project (studies described in ref 47 and in Table I; development of the archive described in ref 48). Only data from drinkers are analyzed here. Studies are from Canada, Federal Republic of Germany, the United Kingdom, Scotland alone, and the United States; periods of measurement range from 1967 to 1986.

Table I. Brief Description of Samples in the Analyses from the Collaborative Alcohol-Related Longitudinal Project Archive

Country	Collaborator	Date T1[a]	Age	T1 N	Sampling frame
Canada	DeCourville	1978	19–22	1,076	Students in schools in two Ontario school districts
FRG	Guether	1975	24–53	9,000	National sample
Scotland-1	Plant	1979	15	1,036	Students in schools in Lothian region
Scotland-2	Ritson	1978	17–79	676	Citizens in Lothian region
UK	Bagnall	1986	13–15	1,586	Students in nine schools from Highlands area, Scotland; Berkshire area England, and Dyfed area, S. Wales
USA-1	Greenfield	1978	18–48	975	University students in Washington State
USA-2	Mulford	1979	17–93	1,535	Citizens of Iowa
USA-3	Wilsnack	1981	21–84	1,313	National sample stratified by alcohol consumption
USA-4	Harford/Grant	1982	17–25	12,686	National sample of United States with supplements of blacks, Hispanics, economically disadvantaged non-black and Hispanic, and young men in military
USA-5	Public domain	1967	21–70+	1,359	National sample

[a]T1, Time 1 or first measurement point.

2.1. The Variables

Variables from the raw data of individual studies were coded to derive compatible constructs for cross-study comparison.

The individual-level predictor variables are: gender (1 = males; 2 = females) age (coded as 9–19, 20–29, 30–49, and 50+), frequency of drinking per month, and quantity of drinking per typical occasion. Quantity measures the consumption of the respondent on a typical occasion, when drinking occurs, by a count of number of cans or bottles of beer, glasses of wine, or number of drinks containing liquor. Frequency measures the total number of drinking occasions occurring in a month for all three beverages.

Alcohol problems are measured as follows:

1. *Physiological consequences* such as cirrhosis or neoplasm of the larynx are infrequently measured in general population surveys because of their rarity. Proxy variables include respondent's reports of any health problems associated with drinking and/or a physician advised the respondent regarding his/her alcohol consumption.

2. *Mental and existential problems* are operationalized by:
   a. *"loss of control"* over drinking which includes (1) drinking is beyond respondent's control and/or (2) respondent keeps on drinking when he or she promised not to and/or (3) respondent becomes drunk when there is a good reason to stay sober;
   b. *self-identifies as "alcoholic" or worries about drinking*, which includes (1) respondent worries about developing a drinking problem and/or (2) respondent self-labels as a problem drinker or alcoholic;
   c. *"treatment" for alcoholism*, which includes inpatient, outpatient, or self-help group;
   d. *symptomatic drinking*, which includes (1) morning drinking and/or (2) shaking associated with drinking and/or (3) blackouts related to drinking and/or (4) tried to cut down or felt should cut down on drinking and/or (5) skipped meals when drinking and/or (6) drinks before a social event because afraid of not getting enough and/or (7) sneaks drinks and/or (8) "tosses" drinks for a stronger effect of alcohol.

3. *Casualty problems* are operationalized as alcohol-related accidents.

4. *Lack of demeanor and nonfulfillment of social roles* are operationalized as:
   a. *belligerence* associated with drinking (e.g., fights);
   b. *family or relative problems*, which includes (1) any spouse or family consequences as a result of respondent's drinking and/or (2) any other family consequences as a result of respondent's drinking;
   c. *school or job problems*, which includes (1) respondent's drinking interfered with job and/or (2) drinking affected promotion or job opportunity and/or (3) drinking caused respondent to quit or lose a job and/or (4) respondent had trouble at school as a result of drinking;
   d. *financial problems* associated with drinking.

5. *"Negative" personal reasons for drinking,* which, according to Room,[49] have questionable theoretical status given their association with puritanical concepts are also considered. They include (1) drinking to forget and/or (2) drinking because tense or nervous and/or (3) drinking because lonesome and/or (4) drinking to gain self-confidence.

For each of the problem categories, an individual respondent is considered positive for the category if she or he reports at least one problem in that category.

Aggregate-level variables are (1) the proportion of women in the work force at the time the study was performed, dichotomized at the median as "high" (greater than 38.6) and "low" (less than or equal to 38.6), (2) the female suicide rate per 100,000 at the time the study was performed, dichotomized at the median as "high" (more than 6.3) and "low" (less than or equal to 6.3). The range of the proportion of women in the work force for the sites was between 36.7 and 41.6; the range of female suicide for the sites was 2.5 and 14.6.

2.2. The Analyses

Meta-analysis is utilized to examine the consistency and average magnitude of the predictive impact of the gender variable.[50] This approach consists of two steps:

1. Derivation of specific effect estimates from the individual studies: The impact of each variable is evaluated using multiple logistic regression[51] with a constant set of covariates. The logistic regression coefficient for gender is exponentiated to obtain an odds ratio for ease of interpretation. For example, if gender had a coefficient of 0.250 in the model of financial problems in one study, the odds ratio would be 1.28. This would indicate that women's odds of financial problems are 28% higher than men's odds in that study, controlling age, quantity of drinking per occasion, and frequency of drinking.
2. After parallel calculation of effect estimates for each gender within studies, meta-analysis is used to combine unstandardized logistic regression coefficients, or log odds, across studies (unstandardized coefficients are recommended for use in meta-analysis by Greenland[52]). General procedures for combining effect estimates across studies are described in Hedges and Olkin[50] and, specifically with reference to the Collaborative Study, in Johnstone *et al.*[48]

Results of within-study analyses are combined using procedures described in Greenland.[52] Each within-study unstandardized logistic regression coefficient is weighted using the reciprocal of the squared standard error of its regression coefficient, i.e., $w_i = 1/SE^2$. Combining across studies yields a weighted average effect estimate (d) for each predictor defined as $d = \Sigma w_i d_i / \Sigma w_i$ with the standard error (s) of the weighted average effect size derived from s = the square root of the reciprocal of the sum of the weights (i.e., $1\Sigma w_i$). Statistical significance of the weighted average effect is assessed using z = b/s which has a standard normal distribution. A test of homogeneity (Q) is defined as $\Sigma w_i(d_i-d)^2$.

We use four statistics to address different hypotheses. First, the p value of the weighted average unstandardized logistic regression coefficient (b) indicates whether gender is statistically significantly related to the individual problems (controlling for age, quantity of drinking per occasion, and frequency of drinking per month) averaged across studies. Second, the Q statistic assesses whether the findings are homogeneous across the multiple studies. A nonsignificant p value indicates homogeneity. The Q statistic is a conservative test to detect heterogeneity because the effect estimates are based on the original sample sizes. However, the significance level of Q is based on the number of effect sizes (i.e., the number of studies) rather than the actual original sample size. With the resulting lower number of degrees of freedom, there is a lower probability of reaching significance. Third, when results are heterogeneous, we evaluate the extent to which characteristics of studies account for their heterogeneity. In this case, societal-level variables ("high" vs. "low" social stress or proportion of women in the work force) serve as study characteristics. For example, results of studies conducted in "high" social stress contexts are compared with results from studies conducted in "low" social stress contexts. This is accomplished by testing the null hypothesis that the average result in "high" contexts is the same as the average result in "low" contexts. This hypothesis is tested using the Q_B statistic,[50(p 154)] which is analogous to a test of between-groups differences in analysis of variance. Fourth, the Q_w statistic evaluates homogeneity in within-group comparisons (e.g., studies taking place in, respectively, "high" and "low" social stress contexts); a nonsignificant p value indicates homogeneity.

3. The Findings

3.1. The Total Sample of Studies

Table II summarizes the meta-analysis from models of individual studies in which gender, age, quantity per occasion, and frequency per month are entered to predict the 11 drinking problems. We first evaluate the statistical significance of the combined effect sizes (the p value from Z). Gender is not a risk factor for health problems, alcoholism treatment, or negative reasons for drinking. When only individual-level variables are controlled, males are at higher risk than females for all other alcohol-related problems.

Next, we evaluate the cross study homogeneity (the p value from Q). The magnitude of the risks differs across studies (i.e., the cross-study findings are heterogeneous) for symptomatic drinking, accidents, belligerence, and negative reasons for drinking. The magnitude of the risks do not differ across

Table II. Summary Statistics for Meta-Analysis for Gender in Unstandardized Logistic Regression Coefficient Estimates Predicting Multiple Measures of Alcohol Problems[a]

	Weighted average odds ratio	95% Confidence interval	p Value from Q[b]	df
Physiological problems				
Health problems	.97	(.75,1.26)	.913	7
Mental and existential problems				
Loss of control	.64[c]	(.51,.79)	.247	6
Alcoholic identity	.69[c]	(.58,.83)	.705	5
Alcoholism treatment	.56	(.25,1.25)	.116	1
Symp. drinking	.73[c]	(.62,.85)	.004	7
Casualty problems				
Accidents	.51[c]	(.33,.77)	.034	4
Lack of demeanor and nonful- fillment of social roles				
Belligerence	.70[c]	(.59,.83)	.000	7
Family/relative	.63[c]	(.50,.79)	.271	4
School/job	.79[c]	(.68,.92)	.065	8
Financial	.58[c]	(.47,.71)	.444	4
Personal reasons for drinking				
Negative reasons	1.05	(.91,1.20)	.007	7

[a]Age, frequency of drinking per month, and quantity of drinking per occasion were controlled in the original regression models in each individual data set.
[b]The Q statistic combines all studies to assess whether the study findings are homogeneous (a nonsignificant p value indicates homogeneity).
[c]p less than 0.001.

studies (i.e., the cross-study findings are homogeneous) for health problems, alcoholism treatment, loss of control, alcoholic identity, family/relative problems, job/school problems, or financial problems.

Figure 1 illustrates the unweighted odds ratios from individual studies and the weighted average for the four problem domains that displayed cross-study heterogeneity. Three observations are noteworthy. First, all of the five studies contributing to the analysis of alcohol-related accidents show men to be at higher risk than women. While these findings attest to variability across studies, they do suggest that men are at least at slightly higher risk than women for alcohol-related accidents. Second, there seems to be a pattern among some studies that if one gender is at higher risk for belligerence, there is equal or higher risk for the other gender for symptomatic drinking. For instance, the study of the general population in Iowa (US-2) shows women are significantly at higher risk for belligerence, while men are significantly at higher risk for symptomatic drinking. On the other hand, a Scottish study of adolescents and a Canadian study of young people show men are at higher risk for belligerence but there are no gender differences for symptomatic drinking. While the majority of these studies show no gender differences for both problems and while there seems to be no other discernible patterning in

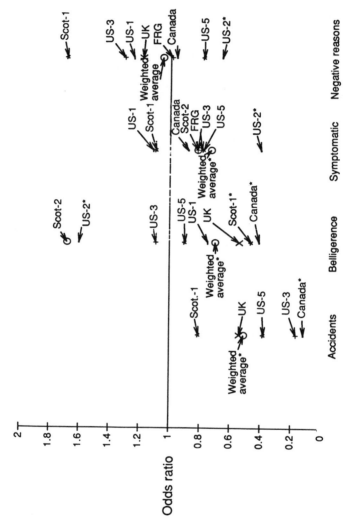

Figure 1. Odds ratios of gender risk to problems in which average risk was heterogeneous across studies. Unweighted odds ratios presented for individual studies.
* = Statistically significant.

the individual results, these outliers will be of interest to us in terms of traits characterizing contexts. Last, although there is considerable variability with respect to gender risk for negative reasons for drinking, only one study (the general population study in Iowa) shows men to be at significantly higher risk. In the next section, we assess whether aggregate-level variables account for some of the remaining variability in risk for these problems.

3.2. Partitioning the Samples by the Proportion of Women in the Work Force

Table III partitions the samples by "low" and "high" female work force participation for the association of gender and problem (controlling for frequency per month, quantity per occasion, and age) for those problems in which the Q_B statistic indicated cross-study heterogeneity.

The Q_B statistic indicates that female work force participation accounts for some of the remaining variability in the magnitude of the risks of gender for symptomatic drinking and belligerence. It does not account for any of the remaining variability in the risks for accidents or negative motivations.

We appraise the strength of the associations when partitioning by female work force participation only for those cases in which it significantly discriminated the two groups. Men have a greater risk of symptomatic drinking in contexts characterized by a higher proportion of women in the work force. There are no gender differences in contexts characterized by a low proportion of women in the work force. Conversely, the average relationship of being male with belligerence is stronger and statistically significant in contexts characterized by a lower proportion of women in the work force; there are no significant gender differences in the risk for belligerence in contexts characterized by a higher proportion of women in the work force.

Last, we appraise the within-group homogeneity (Q_w) for the risks of gender for these two problems. When we block by female work force participation, the association of gender with belligerence is heterogeneous across studies in both "traditional" and "modern" contexts. In contexts characterized by a lower proportion of women in the work force, gender similarity in symptomatic drinking is homogeneous across studies. However, in contexts characterized by a higher proportion of women in the work force, the gender difference is heterogeneous for symptomatic drinking.

3.3. Partitioning the Samples by the Female Suicide Rate

Table IV partitions the samples by "low" and "high" female suicide rates for the association of gender and problems (controlling for frequency per month, quantity per occasion, and age) for those problems in which the Q_B statistic indicated cross-study heterogeneity.

The Q_B statistic indicates that the female suicide rate accounts for some of the remaining variability in the magnitude of the risks of gender for symp-

Table III. Categorical Models for Gender in Unstandardized Regression Coefficient Estimates Predicting Multiple Measures of Alcohol Problems Which Were Heterogeneous When Controlling Only for the Individual-Level Variables: Models Are Partitioned by Low and High Proportions of Women in the Work Force[a]

	Low proportion of women in the work force				High proportion of women in the work force				
	Weighted average odds ratio	95% confidence interval	p value from Q_w[b]	df	Weighted average odds ratio	95% confidence interval	p value from Q_w	df	p from Q_B[c]
Symp. drinking	.86	(.69,1.08)	.854	4	.61[d]	(.49,.77)	.001	2	.031
Accidents	.53[d]	(.35,.82)	.010	2	.45[e]	(.02,1.23)	.301	1	.715
Belligerence	.52[d]	(.42,.65)	.029	3	.99	(.85,1.45)	.022	3	.000
Negative reasons	1.08	(.93,1.29)	.010	3	1.00	(.75,1.21)	.470	3	.560

[a] Age, quantity of drinking per occasion, and frequency of drinking per month were controlled in the original regression models in each individual data set.
[b] The Q_w statistic evaluates homogeneity in within-group comparisons; it accounts for estimates of internal homogeneity within categories (a nonsignificant p value indicates homogeneity).
[c] The Q_B statistic indicates whether groups differ in their mean effect sizes (a significant p value indicates significant differences).
[d] $p < 0.001$.
[e] $p < 0.05$.

Table IV. Categorical Models for Gender in Unstandardized Regression Coefficient Estimates Predicting Multiple Measures of Alcohol Problems Which Were Heterogeneous When Controlling Only for the Individual-Level Variables: Models Are Partitioned by Low and High Female Suicide Rate[a]

| | Low female suicide rate | | | | High female suicide rate | | | | |
	Weighted average odds ratio	95% confidence interval	p value from Q_w[b]	df	Weighted average odds ratio	95% confidence interval	p value from Q_w	df	p from Q_B[c]
Symp. drinking	.64[d]	(.51,.77)	.005	3	.89	(.70,1.14)	.900	3	.027
Accidents	.51[e]	(.23,1.14)	.900	1	.50[f]	(.31,.82)	.010	2	.972
Belligerence	.95	(.74,1.22)	.050	4	.55[d]	(.44,.69)	.005	2	.001
Negative reasons	.87[d]	(.71,1.06)	.100	3	1.22	(1.02,1.46)	.100	3	.013

[a]Age, quantity of drinking per occasion, and frequency of drinking per month were controlled in the original regression models in each individual data set.
[b]The Q_w statistic evaluates homogeneity in within-group comparisons; it accounts for estimates of internal homogeneity within categories (a nonsignificant p value indicates homogeneity).
[c]The Q_B statistic indicates whether groups differ in their mean effect sizes (a significant p value indicates significant differences).
[d]$p < 0.001$.
[e]$p < 0.05$.
[f]$p = 0.005$.

tomatic drinking, belligerence, and negative reasons for drinking. It does not account for the variability in gender differences in risks of accidents.

We appraise the strength of the associations when partitioning by suicide rate context only for those cases in which the female suicide rate significantly discriminated the two groups. The average relationships of gender with symptomatic drinking and negative reasons for drinking are stronger and significant in studies characterized by low female suicide rates with males at higher risk in these contexts; males and females show no significant differences in risk in studies characterized by high female suicide rates. The average relationships of gender with belligerence are stronger and significant in studies characterized by high female suicide rates with males at higher risks in these contexts; males and females show no significant differences in risk in studies characterized by low female suicide rates. Men's risk of negative reasons for drinking is significantly greater than women's in contexts characterized by low female suicide rates but is nonsignificant in contexts characterized by higher female suicide rates.

Last, we appraise the within-group homogeneity (Q_w). While the female suicide rate accounts for variability in the relationships of gender to three of the problems, the findings are heterogeneous for the risk of belligerence in both low and high female suicide rate contexts and for the risk of symptomatic drinking in low female suicide contexts. They are homogeneous for the risk of symptomatic drinking in high female suicide contexts and for the risks of negative reasons for drinking in both low and high female suicide rate contexts.

3.4. Partitioning the Samples by Both the Proportion of Women in the Work Force and the Female Suicide Rate

Table V partitions the samples by "low" and "high" societal stress within contexts of "low" and "high" proportion of women in the work force (controlling for frequency per month, quantity per occasion, and age) for the two problem domains in which both aggregate-level variables accounted for some variability in the risk of gender: symptomatic drinking and belligerence.

We first test for differences in societal stress in "traditional" contexts for belligerence (cells B and D in the table). The Q_B statistic indicates that societal stress in more "traditional" contexts accounts for some of the remaining variability in the magnitude of the risks of gender for belligerence in these contexts. Men are significantly at higher risk than women for belligerence in "traditional" contexts when stress is high; there are no differences in gender risk in "traditional" contexts when stress is low. The findings are homogeneous.

Next, we test for societal stress within "modern" contexts for gender risk for belligerence (cells F and H in the table). The Q_B statistic indicates that stress does not explain variability in "modern" contexts and the cross-study results are heterogeneous.

Table V. Categorical Models for Gender in Unstandardized Regression Coefficient Estimates Predicting Multiple Measures of Alcohol Problems: Models Are Partitioned by Low and High Female Suicide Rate and Low and High Proportion of Women in the Work Force[a]

	Symptomatic drinking	Belligerence
Proportion of women in work force low		
Female suicide rate low	Cell A	Cell B
Weighted average odds ratio	.78	.96
95% Confidence Interval	(.57,1.07)	(.60,1.54)
p value from Q_w[b]	.891	.428
df	1	1
Female suicide high	Cell C	Cell D
Weighted average odds ratio	.94	.44[d]
95% confidence interval	(.70,1.27)	(.34,.56)
p value from Q_w	.719	.680
df	2	1
p from Q_B[c]		.004
Proportion of women in work force high		
Female suicide low	Cell E	Cell F
Weighted average odds ratio	.54[d]	.95
95% Confidence Interval	(.41,.70)	(.71,1.27)
p value from Q_w	.000	.009
df	1	2
Female suicide high	Cell G	Cell H
Weighted average odds ratio	.82	1.08
95% confidence interval	(.55,1.21)	(.71,1.68)
p value from Q_w	—	—
df	0	0
p from Q_B	.081	.598

[a]Age, quantity of drinking per occasion, and frequency of drinking per month were controlled in the original regression models in each individual data set.
[b]The Q_w statistic evaluates homogeneity in within-group comparisons; it accounts for estimates of internal homogeneity within categories (a nonsignificant p value indicates homogeneity).
[c]The Q_B statistic indicates whether groups differ in their mean effect sizes (a significant p value indicates significant differences).
[d]$p < 0.001$.

Figure 2 provides data for the unweighted odds ratios of the individual studies for belligerence, partitioning for societal stress and proportion of women in the work force at time of measurement. The figure illustrates that greater stress in "traditional" contexts elevates the risk of men reporting belligerence for a Scottish and Canadian study; lower stress in "traditional" contexts equates the genders with respect to reported belligerence in a US and Scottish study.

Last we test within "modern" contexts for symptomatic drinking in those contexts charcterized by high and low stress (cells E and G in the table). (We already know that the men are homogeneously at higher risk than women for symptomatic drinking in more "traditional" contexts; therefore, we do not

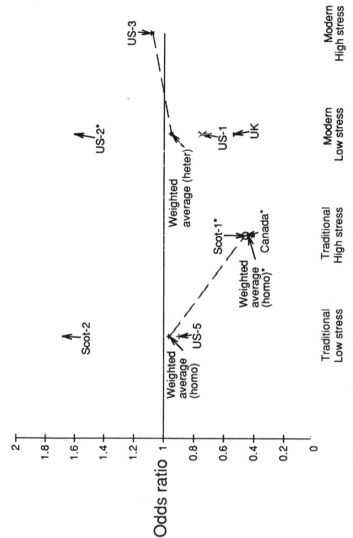

Figure 2. Odds ratios of gender risk for belligerence for individual studies and weighted averages by "traditional/modern" low stress/high stress contexts. * , Statistically significant; homo, cross-study homogeneity; heter, cross-study heterogeneity.

test for societal stress in these contexts.) There are no significant differences in gender risk for symptomatic drinking for high and low societal stress in "modern" contexts (the p value of Q_B is 0.081). There is an indication that men are slightly at higher risk than women for symptomatic drinking when the female suicide rate is low in "modern" contexts. The findings are not homogeneous.

4. Discussion

This study sought to determine whether gender is significantly and homogeneously related to several alcohol-related problems, after controlling for individual-level variables (age, quantity of drinking per occasion, frequency of drinking per month) and, in the cases when the associations of gender and problems were heterogeneous across studies, aggregate-level variables that were hypothesized to confound these relationships. When controlling for age, quantity per occasion, and frequency per month, men and women are equally at risk for self-reported health problems. This finding is homogeneous across studies, supporting our hypothesis that the risk for men and women would be equal or that females would slightly exceed males in reporting these problems. Noteworthy is that the health problems assessed are self-reported from living respondents. Therefore, of course, these methods cannot account for the greater risk from premature death among heavy drinkers due to cirrhosis[53] or other problems related to alcohol.

Although only two studies are considered (one from the United States and the other from Canada), the finding that men and women are equally at risk for treatment supports the hypothesis that if treatment is broadly defined, both men and women will be likely to seek it out. The finding broadens our understanding of previously hypothesized gender differences in the probability of receiving treatment for alcohol-related problems. Some commentators have asserted that women "hide" their drinking[54] and/or women's familial roles prevent them from obtaining treatment.[13] Our results support the findings of Weisner and Schmidt's[16] report of one US community and they also reinforce the summation by Ferrence[55] regarding the notion of the "hidden" female alcoholic:

> . . . we have found little evidence to support the notion that there are a disproportionate number of undetected women problem drinkers. They may be less visible in public because they are less likely to appear intoxicated, to get into fights, or to engage in loud behavior. But these differences reflect general sex differences in socially prescribed norms for behavior rather than those relating solely to drinking. Women problem drinkers are probably no more "hidden" than men from those who are involved in their private lives, their family, friends, physicians and employers. . . . Even for those who are "found," there is no evidence that women are underrepresented compared to men, when those factors that bring people into contact with treatment and social control agents are taken into account. (pp 108–109)

Noteworthy as well is that self-reported data on consumption and alcohol-related problems have been found to be highly reliable,[56,57] suggesting that the allegation that half of the population, namely women, "hide" their drinking is something of an American cultural fantasy.[58]

There are also no gender differences in reporting negative reasons for drinking, but these findings are heterogeneous across studies. Room[49] has questioned the theoretical status of these variables because their prevalence is associated with more puritanical contexts, a hypothesis we are not testing here.

Males are at greater risk than females for reporting loss of control over alcohol, an alcoholic or problem drinker identity, family/job problems, school/job problems, and financial problems. These associations are homogeneous across studies and support the notion from the sociocultural literature that the drinking experiences of men and women are influenced by their gender roles. That is, men are expected to experience these problems whereas women are not, even possibly overcoming women's physiological tendency to have a higher blood alcohol content than men at the same levels of drinking. We were actually quite surprised at the degree of cross-study similarity in these findings; while we expected men to be at higher risk than women, we did not expect the strong homogeneous findings in some problem domains.

Of particular interest is that women are less likely to be at risk to perceive their drinking as "out of control" or to regard themselves as a problem drinker or alcoholic and/or to worry about their drinking. If our interpretation uses the norms of men as the "standard," then the lower risk of these self-labeling processes among women may be due to the reluctance of significant others in the social milieu to bring women's drinking patterns to their attention because alcohol problems are normatively regarded as the property of men. Alternatively, it could mean that the women are less likely to self-identify with "men's problems." Last, it may mean that women feel themselves to be in control and, in fact, are. Remembering that these findings are cross-sectional, we cannot assume that these problems or the drinking practices necessarily represent "chronic states." In addition, some research has shown that men are more likely than women to show longer periods of chronic heavy/frequent drinking and/or alcohol-related problems.[59] Therefore, it is quite possible that women are in control of their drinking for the most part with little reason to self-identify as having a problem. But if our interpretation uses the norms of women as the "standard," then it may be that men are more prone to get into trouble at lower consumption levels because both physiological and normative factors (i.e., it is "manly" to experience and report alcohol-related problems) increase the risk of problems for men, whereas primarily physiological influences are present for women.

The homogeneous findings that men are more at risk for three of the four lack of demeanor and nonfulfillment of social role problems are not surprising. The value of drunkenness among men, the acceptability of it, and its accompanying behaviors (sometimes causing distress, discomfort, and even sacrifice on the part of others) endorse the view that cultural expectations about drinking with respect to gender roles mediate the relationships between consumption and some nonphysiological problems.[25] Therefore, we conclude that in the context of the family, the school, and the job, and also with regard to financial matters, ladies, even when drinking, are more likely to continue to act like ladies, whereas gentlemen are less likely to continue to act like gentlemen.

In three domains of problems, men are significantly more highly at risk, but these findings are heterogeneous across studies: symptomatic drinking, accidents, and belligerence. These problem domains are central to our exploration of societal-level contextual effects.

4.1. Gender as a Risk Factor for Drinking Problems in "Traditional" and "Modern" Social Contexts

It is important to remember that the variation on the "traditionality" versus "modernity" dimension is limited in this comparative study with respect to the proportion of women in the work force. Inclusion of societies with greater range on this dimension into such comparative research would be encouraged in future work of this nature. But despite this limitation, this dimension accounts for variability in the risks of gender for symptomatic drinking and belligerence.

As expected, men are at higher risk for problems of belligerence in "traditional" contexts, while men and women are at equal risk in "modern" contexts. While the cross-study findings are not homogeneous in either context, the average relationships suggest that men are more at liberty than women to "act out" in a negative fashion when drinking when both are in more "traditional" roles; as well, the findings suggest that women are equally at risk to adopt the aggressiveness of men when "modernity" prevails.

Findings of variation in contexts regarding belligerence have been noted elsewhere. Room's[60] discussion of the literature pertaining to differences in the prevalence of belligerence in "dry" versus "wet" contexts (low vs. high per capita consumption of alcohol) describes dry cultures to be characterized by higher rates of violence and social disruption than wet cultures. These observations were validated in our own study's samples (21 studies from 11 countries) in which the risk of quantity per occasion for belligerence was highest in dry contexts.[41] However, per capita consumption of alcohol does not account for variability of gender risk for belligerence (unpublished findings available upon request), whereas the measure of gender norms used herein does. Thus, these findings possibly expand our understanding of the contexts in which the risks among men and women for alcohol-related belligerence, often resulting in social disruption, may arise.

As expected, in studies characterized by more "traditional" contexts, men and women are at equal risk for reporting symptomatic drinking (homogeneous across studies), and in studies characterized by more "modern" contexts, men are at higher risk for these problems (heterogeneous across studies). This was a tentative hypothesis on our part. The findings suggest that there is merit in future work on gender role and contextual effects in studying change among *both* men and women when the roles of one gender change. Although these findings are not homogeneous across studies in "modern" contexts, we interpret them to mean that because the risk of "typical" male behavior associated with drinking (i.e., belligerence) tends to be shared with females in these contexts, the risk of alcoholism-type symptoms (e.g., sneaking drinks) is exacerbated among men. We view this as something of a behavioral trade-off (i.e., when aggressive behavior is equalized between the sexes, the cultural formula may be that men rely on "alcoholismlike" behaviors as an expression of their drinking style to a greater degree than women).

4.2. Gender as a Risk Factor for Drinking Problems in Low- and High-Stress Social Contexts

Societal-level stress (operationalized by the female suicide rate) accounts for variability in the risks of gender for symptomatic drinking, negative reasons for drinking, and belligerence. As expected, in studies characterized by greater societal-level stress, men and women are at equal risk for reporting symptomatic drinking (and also negative reasons for drinking), and in studies characterized by less stress, men are at higher risk for these problems. These findings suggest that higher environmental stress equalizes the sexes with respect to displaying the symptoms of alcoholism and drinking for "negative reasons," because drinking to reduce tension may be regarded as a culturally acceptable means by which to adapt to a stressful environment.

On the other hand, men are at higher risk than women for belligerence in higher stress contexts. We had speculated this to be the case because some research on the individual level has suggested that men are most likely to externalize their reaction to stress in their immediate environment. Our findings here potentially broaden this observation on the individual level to the aggregate level but must be taken cautiously as the findings are heterogeneous within both low- or high-stress contexts.

Noteworthy is that neither societal stress nor the "traditionality/modernity" dimension accounts for the cross-study heterogeneity in the risk of gender for alcohol-related accidents. Other analyses blocking for country of study origin (not presented here) shows the risk of gender for accidents to differ by country of study origin. This suggests to us that other structural factors in these societies, not measured here, are operating to account for these national differences. In particular, we suspect that automobile ownership and driving habits are implicated.

4.3. The Combined Effects of Societal-Level Stress and Societal-Level "Traditionality/Modernity"

Following in the tradition of Bales,[35] we crudely tested for the combination of the two societal-level factors for symptomatic drinking and belligerence when there was heterogeneity within either "traditional" or "modern" contexts. These are extremely exploratory analyses due to the limited sample sizes within each cell.

We learned that men and women were at equal risk for symptomatic drinking in "traditional" contexts and these findings were homogeneous; therefore, we did not partition for stress in those contexts. We also learned that men were at higher risk than women in "modern" contexts, but these findings were heterogeneous. We thus partitioned those studies characterized by "modernity" for high and low stress to test our hypothesis that the presence of stress equalizes the genders with respect to symptomatic drinking. We found that there was a slight tendency for our hypothesis to be supported, namely that the presence of higher stress in "modern" contexts equalized the risk for symptomatic drinking among men and women and that men were at higher risk for symptomatic drinking than women in "modern" contexts characterized by lower societal stress. These are, of course, only very tentative findings with such a small sample size; however, should they be replicated in future research, we speculate that it isn't the "modernity" or the gender roles per se that might equalize the risk of these problems for women, but rather it is external unspecified societal stress.

We learned that men were at higher risk for belligerence than women in "traditional" contexts and that the gender risk did not differ in "modern" contexts. Since within-group heterogeneity was present in both contexts, we tested for the presence of stress, further partitioning these cells. The presence of higher societal-level stress elevated the risk of belligerence among men in "traditional" contexts, whereas the presence of lesser stress was associated with equal risk for the genders in "traditional" contexts. These findings were homogeneous. The findings are of interest (due to the toll taken on societies by alcohol-related belligerence) because when men exceed the risk for belligerence compared with women to allegedly cope with stress, it is in contexts in which women typically have less power than men and are frequently in subservient positions to men. An intriguing research question for the future would be to determine the extent to which alcohol-related belligerent behavior is directed toward women under these circumstances.

As expected, the presence of societal stress in "modern" contexts did not account for variability in the risk of gender for belligerence. Although these findings were heterogeneous, they tentatively suggest that the "modern" roles of women bring with them the latitude to act out their aggressive behavior when drinking to an equal extent as men.

5. Conclusions

This chapter commenced with a discussion of the differences in physiology of the genders versus gender roles as explanatory variables for gender risk. Certainly physiology appears to play a role in health problems, equalizing the sexes, and it possibly plays a role in seeking treatment regardless of gender, once some drinking levels have allegedly become chronic and ill-adapted to the environment. But, for the most part, men continue to win the race, hands down, for the risk of problematic behavior when drinking and even visualizing themselves as problematic compared with women. We interpret this to mean that in the countries studied cultural norms regarding gender roles when drinking put women at lesser risk for most alcohol-related problems.

The few problems that were not homogeneous across studies were of interest with respect to their very contrast—one being "acting like an alcoholic," the other being "'acting out when drinking." The small case study of just two problem domains is only suggestive, but presents the possibility that we might find more variation in the risks of men and women were societies with greater ranges of "traditional/modern" gender roles and societal stressors included in our study. However suggestive, the findings seem, on face value, to hold promise. After all, we know from our history books that there have been convergences of large period effects that have reconfigured the drinking of women (and men). Certainly the Roaring Twenties in the United States massively reshaped drinking for women. Appel,[61] describing the prototypical young woman of that day, states:

> She became a drinking buddy, the flapper was a new model, new although in the sense that the American girl made her appearance on stage [sic]. As "girls" young women did not concern themselves with temperance crusades, they joined the men of their generation as drinking buddies. (p 12)

But while the findings of this study may seem somewhat intriguing, the reader must be counseled with caution to consider their limitations. First, the analyses are cross-sectional. This means that the timing and persistence of some problems to consumption are not accounted for. Our conclusions regarding societal-level factors are limited because both "traditionality/modernity" and societal-level stress are in reality in flux. It also must be recognized that there is ample evidence that both heavy/frequent consumption and the problems of women in the general population have been found to be typically short-lived, not to mention uncommon, compared to those of men. By virtue of men's more chronic heavy or frequent drinking, they are, of course, at a higher risk for experiencing problems. Furthermore, statistical "controls" for consumption may be regarded as inadequate if women's drinking patterns are clustered at the low end of the scale and men's drinking are clustered at the high end. Second, the gender/problem associations that were differentiated by either the proportion of women in the work force or the female suicide rate were sometimes heterogeneous within contexts, meaning that other contextual variables most likely play significant roles in molding these relationships. It is also critically important to note that we have used "macrolevel" contextual variables to partition for individual-level behavior. Models utilizing "mesolevel" contextual variables are needed to understand these relationships, particularly cross-group differences of drinking contexts or the context of the workplace.[31] Third, the study's samples are heavily biased by an overrepresentation from Northern Europe and North America, with measurements taken between 1967 and 1986. The limitations of period of history and geography underscore the chances of finding more variability at the societal level.

Last, there are critiques in the literature regarding the use of meta-analysis. For instance, Wachter[62] has noted that the retrospective application of formal mathematical procedures to combine the results of studies, in the absence of controlled conditions, measurement scales designed to be homogeneous, or rigorously established statistical independence, may limit the validity of conclusions in research syntheses. Additionally, there is a danger that the assessment of prior studies may be reduced to a routinized task in which details of interpretation and the contributions of original investigators are lost in an indiscriminate effort to pool results and determine "overall" effects. However, there are clear advantages in using meta-analysis as an approach to synthesize and interpret the results of multiple studies on a common research question.[63] First, meta-analysis makes use of formal procedures to weight results of varying precision across studies, quantify the consistency of combined effects, and judge the appropriateness of that combination. Second, categorical and continuous modeling approaches available in meta-analysis can identify and evaluate hypothesized explanations for systematic variation in results across studies. This makes it possible to use a single analytic framework to assess the effects of very different types of factors, e.g., design effects and cultural or historical variation, on study differences. Third, the analyses herein use the raw data from individual studies and enlist the collaboration of many of those conducting those studies. These make the coding more accurate and ensure interpretation that takes into account the unique contributions of individual studies.

In a broader context, we must ask ourselves, as does Heath,[64] why does it matter whether the genders are at equal risk for alcohol problems? In our view, this is an important question. Heath reminds us of the symbolic role of alocohol in the social structure, particularly with respect to gender roles, of the extraordinary variation in gender drinking patterns across highly divergent cultures, and of the easy access that women have to alcohol in many cultures, primarily because they are often the producers and sellers of it. Almost 10 years ago, one of the authors of the present analysis was asked to examine the recent alarm over the so-called epidemic of alcohol problems among women in contemporary America.[58] Studying the society's and the scientific community's reactions to drinking patterns and problems of men and women over time in that nation suggested to her that large-scale political and symbolic forces were implicated in the behavioral drinking "rights" of men and women. It is important to keep these observations in mind because if we do not, we run the risk of oversimplifying as well as either overstating or understating our case. Why does it matter? It matters because, according to Heath, our study of gender differences provides "an interface between biology and culture."[64(p181)]

The emphasis on "context" in this chapter derives in part from these broader considerations. Even with the limitations of these analyses and the caveats surrounding them, we believe analyses that address multiple social contexts in cross-level designs will began to fill in the gaps of better understanding human drinking behavior. They will also move us, albeit crudely, toward describing, in Roizen's[26] terms, the "glue" in the social structure to which drinking practices and problems are attached, therefore permitting us to better understand similarities and differences of men and women with respect to the alcohol problems they experience.

ACKNOWLEDGMENTS. This work was supported by a National Institute on Alcohol Abuse and Alcoholism (NIAAA) grant (#RO1 AA07034) and by a NIAAA Research Scientist Development Award (#KO1 AA00073) to Kaye Middleton Fillmore. The Collaborative Project is included in the plan of work of NIAAA as a World Health Organization (WHO) Collaborating Center on Research and Training in Alcohol-Related Problems, and is also affiliated with the WHO Global Program on Prevention and Control of Alcohol and Drug Abuse. Order of authorship in the Collaborative Alcohol-Related Longitudinal Project is designated by the following criteria: (1) the first author has taken principal responsibility for organizing and writing the research paper, (2) persons making substantial contributions follow the first author in alphabetical order, (3) collaborators, having reviewed the paper and its findings in accordance with accuracy and representation of their data and project goals, are listed under "with" on p. 409.

References

1. Hilton ME: The demographic distribution of drinking patterns in 1984, in Clark W, Hilton M (eds): *Alcohol in America*. Albany, NY, State University of New York Press, 1991, pp 73–86.
2. Health and Welfare Canada: *National Alcohol and Other Drugs Survey (1989): Highlights Report*. (Catalogue No. H39-175/1990E). Ottawa, Health and Welfare Canada, 1990.
3. Roizen R: The World Health Organization study of community responses to alcohol-related problems: A review of cross-cultural findings. Annex 41, in Rootman I, Moser J (eds): *Community Response to Alcohol-Related Problems, Phase I* (MNH/83,17). Geneva, Switzerland, WHO, 1981.
4. Helzer JE, Canino GJ, Yeh E-K, *et al*: Alcoholism—North America and Asia. *Arch Gen Psychiatry* 47:313–319, 1990.
5. Fillmore KM, Hartka E, Johnstone DM *et al*: The collaborative alcohol-related longitudinal project: A meta-analysis of life course variation in drinking. *Br J Addict* 86:1221–1268, 1991.
6. Gomberg ES: Historical and political perspective: Women and drug use. *J Soc Issues* 38:9–23, 1982.
7. Ray O, Ksir C: *Drugs, Society and Human Behavior*, 4th ed. St. Louis, MO, Mosby, 1987.
8. Campbell R: Status attainment research: End of the beginning or beginning of the end? *Sociol Educ* 56:47–62, 1983.
9. Huber J (ed): *Macro-Micro Linkages in Sociology*. London, Sage, 1991.
10. McCready BS: Alcoholism, in Blechman EA, Brownell KO (eds): *Handbook of Behavioral Medicine for Women*. New York, Pergamon, 1988, pp 356–388.

11. Hill SY: Physiological effects of alcohol in women. In *Women and Alcohol: Health-Related Issues*. National Institute on Alcohol Abuse and Alcoholism. Research Monograph No. 16 DHHS Publication No. (ADM) 86-1139, U.S. Government Printing Office, 1986, pp 199–215.

12. Hanna E, Dufour MC, Elliott S, *et al:* Dying to be equal: Women, alcohol and cardiovascular disease. *Br J Addict* 87:1593–1597, 1992.

13. Beckman LJ, Amaro H: Personal and social differences faced by women and men entering alcoholism treatment. *J Stud Alcohol* 47:135–146, 1986.

14. Blume SB: Women and alcohol: A review. *J Am Med Assoc*, 256:1467–1470, 1986.

15. Institute of Medicine: *Broadening the Base of Alcohol Treatment*. Washington, DC, National Academy of Sciences Press, 1990.

16. Weisner C, Schmidt L: Gender disparities in treatment for alcohol problems. *J Am Med Assoc* 268(14):1872–1876, 1992.

17. Hilton M: Demographic characteristics and the frequency of heavy drinking as predictors of self-reported drinking problems. *Br J Addict* 82:913–925, 1987.

18. Knupfer G: The risks of drunkenness (*or Ebrietas Resurrecta*): A comparison of frequent intoxication indices and of population sub-groups as to problem risks. *Br J Addict* 79:185–196, 1984.

19. Knupfer G: Problems associated with drunkenness in women: Some research issues, in National Institute on Alcohol Abuse and Alcoholism (ed): *Special Population Issues* (Alcohol and Health Monograph No. 4; Department of Health and Human Services Publication No. ADM 82-1193). Washington, DC, US Government Printing Office, 1982, pp 3–39.

20. Clark WB, Midanik L: Alcohol use and alcohol problems among US adults: Results of the 1979 national survey, in National Institute on Alcohol Abuse and Alcoholism (eds): *Alcohol Consumption and Alcohol Problems* (Alcohol and Health Monograph No. 1. Department of Health and Human Services Publication No. ADM 82-1190). Washington, DC, US Government Printing Office, 1982, pp 3–52.

21. Wilsnack SC, Wilsnack RW, Klassen AD: Epidemiological research on women's drinking, 1978–1984, in National Institute on Alcohol Abuse and Alcoholism (ed): *Women and Alcohol: Health-Related Issues* (Research Monograph No. 16; Department of Health and Human Services Publication No. ADM 86-1139). Washington, DC, US Government Printing Office, 1986, pp 1–68.

22. Robbins C: Sex differences in psychosocial consequences of alcohol and drug abuse. *J Health Soc Behav* 30:117–130, 1989.

23. Chassin L, Tetzloff C, Hershy M: Self-image and social image factors in adolescent alcohol use. *J Stud Alcohol* 48:194–201, 1985.

24. Mosher DL, Sirkin M: Measuring a macho personality constellation. *J Res Personal* 18:150–163, 1984.

25. MacAndrew D, Edgerton R: *Drunken Comportment*. Chicago, Aldine, 1969.

26. Roizen R: Explaining cross-cultural variation in drinking: Some reflections on the WHO community response study. Paper prepared for the International Symposium on Patterns of Alcohol Use and Misuse among Different Populations. Sponsored by the US National Institute on Alcohol Abuse and Alcoholism, Pan American Health Organization, Washington, DC, August 11–15, 1986.

27. Mason KO, Czajka JL, Arber S: Change in US women's sex-role attitudes, 1964–1974. *Am Sociol Rev* 41:573–596, 1976.

28. Parker DA, Harford TC: Gender-role attitudes, job competition and alcohol consumption among women and men. *Alcohol Clin Exp Res* 16(5):159–165, 1992.

29. Wilsnack R, Wilsnack SC: Women, work, and alcohol: Failures of simple theories. *Alcohol Clin Exp Res* 16:172–179, 1992.

30. Haavio-Mannila E: Alkohol, arbete och familj—en jamforelse mellan man och kvinnor (Alcohol, work and family—a comparison between men and women) (Publication No. 15). Helsinki, Nordic Council for Alcohol and Drug Research. [Cited in Haavio-Mannia E (1991) Impact of colleagues and family member on female alcohol use. Paper presented at the Symposium on Alcohol, Family and Significant Others, Social Research Institute of Alcohol Studies and Nordic Council for Alcohol and Drug Research, Helsinki, Finland and ref 29].

31. Kubicka L, Csemy L, Kozeny J: The sociodemographic, microsocial, and attitudinal context of Czech women's drinking. Paper presented at the Symposium on Alcohol, Family and Significant Others, Social Research Institute of Alcohol Studies and Nordic Council for Alcohol and Drug Research, Helsinki, Finland, 1991.

32. Dohrenwend BP, Dohrenwend BS, Gould MS, Link B: *Mental Illness in the United States: Epidemiological Estimates.* New York, Praeger, 1980.

33. Lemle R: Alcohol and masculinity: A review and reformulation of sex role, dependency, and power theories of alcoholism. Paper presented at the American Psychological Association, Toronto, 1984.

34. Biener L: Gender differences in the use of substances for copying, in Barnett RC, Biener L (eds): *Gender and Stress.* New York, Free Press, 1987, pp 330–349.

35. Bales RF: Cultural differences in rates of alcoholism. *Q J Stud Alcohol* 6:480–499, 1946.

36. Brenner MH, Mooney A: Unemployment and health in the context of economic change. *Soc Sci Med* 17:1125–1138, 1983.

37. Wagenaar AC, Streff FM: Macroeconomic conditions and alcohol-impaired driving. *J Stud Alcohol* 50:217–225, 1989.

38. Durkheim E: *Suicide: A Study in Sociology* [Spaulding J, Simpson G (eds)]. Glencoe, IL, Free Press of Glencoe, 1951.

39. La Plante M: Mortality and the business cycle. Unpublished doctoral dissertation. Stanford University, 1985.

40. Ager CR, Ferrer HP, Fillmore KM, *et al:* Aggregate-level predictors of the prevalence of selected drinking patterns in multiple studies: A research synthesis from the collaborative alcohol-related longitudinal study. Paper presented at the 17th Annual Alcohol Epidemiology Symposium, Toronto, Ontario, Canada, June 1–5, 1992.

41. Fillmore KM, Golding JM, Leino EV, *et al:* Relationships of measures of alcohol consumption with alcohol-related problems in multiple studies: A research synthesis from the collaborative alcohol-related longitudinal project. *Addictions,* 84:1994, pp 1143–1156.

42. Cooper ML, Russell M, Skinner JB, *et al:* Stress and alcohol use: Moderating effects of gender, coping and alcohol expectancies. *J Abnorm Psychol* 101(1):139–152, 1992.

43. Linsky AS, Colby JP, Straus MA: Drinking norms and alcohol-related problems in the United States. *J Stud Alcohol* 47:384–393, 1986.

44. Horwitz AV, White HR: Gender role orientations and styles of pathology among adolescents. *J Health Soc Behav* 28:158–170, 1987.

45. Wilsnack RW, Wilsnack SC, Klassen AD: Women's drinking and drinking problems: Patterns from a 1981 national survey. *Am J Public Health* 74:1231–38, 1984.

46. Room R: Alcohol as a cause: Empirical links and social definitions, in von Wartburg JP, Magnenat P, Muller R, Wyss S (eds): *Currents in Alcohol Research and the Prevention of Alcohol Problems.* Toronto, Hans Huber Publishers, 1985, pp 11–19.

47. Fillmore KM, Hartka E, Johnstone BM, *et al:* The collaborative alcohol-related longitudinal project: Preliminary results from a meta-analysis of drinking behavior in multiple longitudinal studies. *Br J Addict* 86:1203–1210, 1991.

48. Johnstone BM, Leino EV, Motoyoshi M, *et al:* The collaborative alcohol-related longitudinal project: An integrated approach to meta-analysis in alcohol studies. *Br J Addict* 86:1211–1220, 1991.

49. Room R: Measurement and distribution of drinking patterns and problems in general populations, in Edwards G, Gross MM, Keller M, Moser J, Room R (eds): *Alcohol-Related Disabilities.* Geneva, World Health Organization, 1977, pp 61–87.

50. Hedges LV, Olkin I: *Statistical Methods for Meta-Analysis.* New York, Academic Press, 1985.

51. Fleiss JL, Williams JBW, Dubro AF: The logistic regression analysis of psychiatric data. *J Psychiatr Res* 20:195–209, 1986.

52. Greenland S: Quantitative methods in the review of epidemiologic literature. *Epidemiol Rev* 9:1–30, 1987.

53. Nicholls P, Dedwards G, Kyle E: Alcoholics admitted to four hospitals in England: General and cause-specific mortality. *Q J Stud Alcohol* 35(3):841–855, 1974.

54. Curlee J: Alcoholism and the "empty nest." *Bull Menninger Clin.* 33:165–171, 1969.

55. Ferrence RG: Sex differences in the prevalence of problem drinking, in Kalant O (ed): *Alcohol and Drug Problems in Women: Research Advances in Alcohol and Drug Problems*. New York, Plenum Press 1980, vol 5, pp 69–124.
56. Midanik L: The validity of self-reported alcohol consumption and alcohol problems: A literature review. *Br J Addict* 77:357–382, 1982.
57. Smith PR, Remington PL, Williamson DF, and Anda RF: A comparison of alcohol sales data with survey data on self-reported alcohol use in 21 states. *Am J Public Health* 80:309–312, 1990.
58. Fillmore KM: "When angels fall": Women's drinking as cultural preoccupation and as reality, in Wilsnack SC, Beckman LJ (eds): *Alcohol Problems in Women: Antecedents, Consequences, and Intervention*. New York, Guilford Press, 1984, pp 7–36.
59. Fillmore KM: Women's drinking across the life course as compared to men's. *Br J Addict* 82:801–811, 1987.
60. Room R: Response to alcohol-related problems in an international perspective: Characterizing and explaining cultural wetness and dryness. Paper presented at "La ricerca Italiana sulle bevande alcoliche nel confronto internazionale," Santo Stefano Belbo (CN), Italy, September 22–23, 1989.
61. Appel C: From temperance to co-dependency or: The discovery of the invisible alcoholic researched in regard to the ideas about women and alcohol in the history of the USA since the 1870s. Presentation prepared for Alcohol Research Group, Berkeley, CA, Morgensternstr.38, D-6000, Franfurt-70, FRG, 1988.
62. Wachter KW: Disturbed by meta-analysis? *Science* 241:1407–1408, 1988.
63. Hedges LV: Meta-analysis. Presented at the First Meeting of the Collaborative Alcohol-Related Longitudinal Project, Berkeley, CA, July 28, 1987.
64. Heath DB: Women and alcohol: Cross-cultural perspectives. *J Subst Abuse* 3:175–185, 1991.

Contents of Previous Volumes

Volume 8

Index

ISBN 0-306-44921-8

90000

9 780306 449215